AF249035

Transfusion-Transmitted Infections

Contributors

Jay E. Menitove, MD
Deputy Director of Medical Affairs
Professor of Medicine
Hoxworth Blood Center
University of Cincinati Medical Center
Cincinati, Ohio

Harold V. Lamberson, MD, PhD
Director, American Red Cross Blood
  Services, Greater Upstate New York
  Region
Professor of Pathology
SUNY Health Science Center
Syracuse, New York

Irvin S.Y. Chen, PhD
UCLA School of Medicine
Jonsson Comprehensive Cancer Center
Los Angeles, California

Jerome A. Zack, PhD
UCLA School of Medicine
Jonsson Comprehensive Cancer Center
Los Angeles, California

Marian T. Sullivan, MS, MPH
American Red Cross
Jerome H. Holland Laboratory
Rockville, Maryland

Alan E. Williams, PhD
American Red Cross
Jerome H. Holland Laboratory
Rockville, Maryland

Paul V. Holland, MD
Center for Blood Research
Sacramento Medical Foundation Blood
  Center
Sacramento, California

Robert L. Randell, MD
Los Robles Regional Medical Center
Thousand Oaks, California

Nancy L. Dock, PhD
Scientific Director, Research and
  Development
American Red Cross Blood Services, Greater
  Upstate New York Region
Department of Pathology
SUNY Health Science Center
Syracuse, New York

Robert G. Westphal, MD
Medical Director
American Red Cross Blood Services
Clinical Professor of Medicine
University of Vermont College of Medicine
Burlington, Vermont

Asa Barnes, MD
Director, Blood Bank of Long Beach
  Memorial Medical Center
Clinical Professor of Pathology
College of Medicine
University of California
Irvine, California

Charles H. Wallas, MD
Director, Blood Bank
Vanderbilt University Medical Center
Nashville, Tennessee

Steve Kleinman, MD
Medical Director
American Red Cross Blood Services, Los
  Angeles
Los Angeles, California

Bruce L. Evatt, MD
Division of Host Factors
Center for Infectious Diseases
Centers for Disease Control
Public Health Service
Atlanta, Georgia

Dale N. Lawrence, MD
Division of Host Factors
Center for Infectious Diseases
Centers for Disease Control
Public Health Service
Atlanta, Georgia

Jeanette K. Stehr-Green, MD
Division of Host Factors
Center for Infectious Diseases
Centers for Disease Control
Public Health Service
Atlanta, Georgia

Edward L. Snyder, MD
Professor, Laboratory Medicine
Director, Pheresis/Transfusion Service
Yale University School of Medicine
New Haven, Connecticut

Gary Stack, MD
Instructor, Laboratory Medicine
Yale University School of Medicine
New Haven, Connecticut

Transfusion-Transmitted Infections

Edited By

Dennis M. Smith, Jr, MD
Director of Laboratories
Chairman, Department of Pathology
Memorial Medical Center
Jacksonville, Florida

Roger Y. Dodd, PhD
Head, Transmissible Diseases Laboratory
American Red Cross
Jerome H. Holland Laboratory
Rockville, Maryland

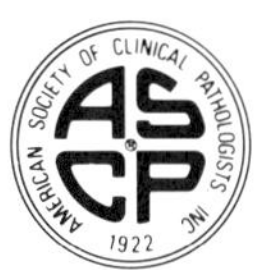

ASCP Press
American Society of Clinical Pathologists
Chicago

Acquisition & Development: Joshua Weikersheimer
Editors: Stephen Borysewicz
       James Losby
Production Manager: Lisa Pollak

Notice

Trade names and equipment and supplies described herein are included as suggestions only. In no way does their inclusion constitute an endorsement or preference by the American Society of Clinical Pathologists. The ASCP did not test the equipment, supplies, or procedures and, therefore, urges all readers to read and follow all manufacturers' instructions and package insert warnings concerning the proper and safe use of products.

Library of Congress Cataloging-in-Publication Data

Transfusion-transmitted infections / edited by Dennis M. Smith, Jr., Roger Y. Dodd.
    Includes bibliographical references.
    Includes index.
    ISBN 0-89189-289-3
    1. Blood—Transfusion—Complication and sequelae.   2. Infection.
3. Communicable diseases—Transmission.   I. Smith, Dennis M.
II. Dodd, Roger Y.
    [DNLM: 1. Blood Transfusion—adverse effects.   2. Communicable
Diseases—transmission.   WB 356 T7747]
RM171.T733   1991
615'.39—dc20
DNLM/DLC
for Library of Congress   91-4561
                                              CIP

Printed in the United States of America.

95 94 93 92 91 5 4 3 2 1

Contents

12

Transfusion of Blood Components Contaminated With Bacteria 195

Section III: Prevention of Transfusion-Transmitted Infections

13

Donor Screening Procedures and Their Role in Enhancing Transfusion Safety 207

14

Donor Testing and its Impact on Transfusion-Transmitted Infection 243

Preface

The emergence of the acquired immune deficiency syndrome (AIDS) in the early 1980s, and the eventual recognition that the agent responsible for this disorder could be spread by blood transfusion, put blood banking and transfusion medicine squarely under public scrutiny. These events ultimately resulted in a new awareness of the risks associated with blood transfusion. There is no issue that concerns both the public and healthcare professionals more than transfusion-transmitted infections.

This book owes its genesis to the lack of a current, comprehensive text on transfusion-transmitted infections. Written by leading scientists, practitioners, and educators in transfusion medicine, this monograph provides needed information for the full gamut of healthcare providers, including physicians who prescribe transfusion, nurses who transfuse blood, medical technologists who frequently interface with nurses and doctors, and medical students and house staff who must learn about the frequency and significance of transfusion-transmitted infections. The information contained in this book is a particularly important resource for individuals participating in discussions concerning informed consent for blood transfusion.

This book contains four distinct sections, encompassing the general safety of blood transfusion, viruses transmitted by blood products, other infectious agents transmitted by transfusion, and prevention of transfusion-transmitted infections. This design allows the reader to locate rapidly the specific information desired and permits minimal redundancy. Specifically, there has been a deliberate attempt to avoid duplication of information among chapters. For example, tests used for screening donated blood for antibodies to the human immunodeficiency virus (HIV) are discussed only in Chapter 14 "Donor Testing and Its Impact on Transfusion-Transmitted Infection" and not in Chapter 4 "Transfusion-Transmitted Human Immunodeficiency Virus Infection." Without such an effort, many chapters would easily have become individual monographs with great duplication of material.

This book addresses not only the major organisms transmitted by transfusion, eg, HIV and the hepatitis viruses, but also many other infectious agents. While these organisms may be seen more rarely or not at all in our country, recent global events, such as expanded international travel and the growing immigration from third-world countries to the industrial world, increase the likelihood of transfusion-transmitted infections. The recent documentation of transfusion-transmitted trypanosomiasis infection in the United States illustrates this point. Thus, once seemingly exotic organisms must be included in any comprehensive text on transfusion-transmitted infection. The final section of this book provides extremely important information on preventing posttransfusion infections, which is, after all, our ultimate goal.

In spite of dramatic recent gains in improving the safety of blood transfusion, a "zero risk" blood supply does not appear imminent because of the many remaining technical and scientific obstacles. Nevertheless, we must remember that currently fewer than 5,000 cases of clinically appreciated transfusion-transmitted disease, and many fewer deaths, occur annually in the United States. This fact must be balanced with the risks faced in everyday life: 1 in 20,000 Americans will die after being struck by an automobile; 1 in 12,500 Americans will die from leukemia; and, over 1,000 Americans die each day from smoking cigarettes. Such comparisons are necessary to provide practitioners and patients with a reasonable perspective from which to consider transfusion-transmitted infections in modern transfusion medicine. We believe that blood transfusion is safer today than ever and hope that this book provides the necessary background for healthcare professionals to understand the frequency, significance, and prevention of these infections.

Transfusion-Transmitted Infections

1
How Safe Is Blood Transfusion?

Jay E. Menitove, MD

Blood is a biologically active substance. At present, viable blood and blood component transfusions cannot be accomplished with "zero risk."[1] The relative safety of blood transfusion, then, requires a comparison of the potential risks and the existing clinical situation. Following is an overview of blood donation and transfusion practices in the United States, a description of adverse consequences associated with transfusion, and a discussion of pharmacologic agents that may prove effective in reducing the need for blood and blood components.

Blood Donation Patterns

Homologous Donations

The number of whole blood collections in the United States increased from 8.5 million units in 1971 to approximately 11.7 million units in 1982, and to approximately 13.2 million units in 1988.[2-5] During the early 1980s, red blood cell use increased approximately 5% annually.[3] This trend halted abruptly, however, in 1983 (Figure 1–1).[6-8] Several factors effecting this change are postulated. They include the introduction of the prospective payment system for hospital reimbursement, heightened fear of transfusion-transmitted diseases following the initial reports of transfusion-associated acquired immunodeficiency syndrome (AIDS) cases, and the loss of health insurance benefits related to unemployment caused by the economic recession that occurred during the early 1980s. As a result, the annual growth rate in blood collections reverted to a net decline in collections from that of the previous year in 1984, and minimal to no growth subsequently.[6-9] Blood usage may have decreased despite an increase in collections since 3% to 5% of units

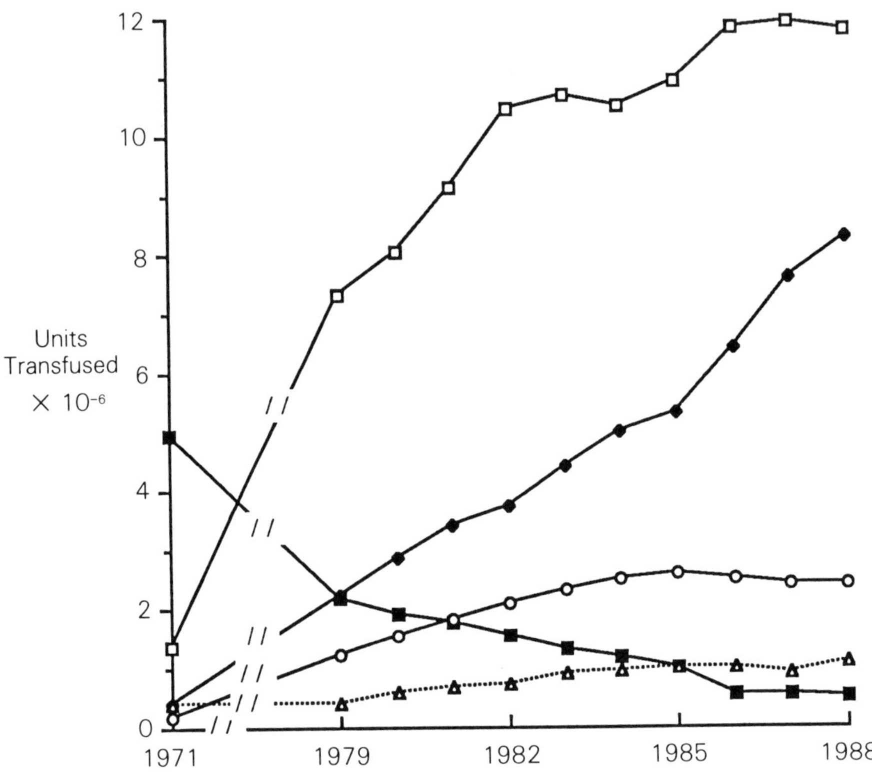

Figure 1–1   Estimated transfusion usage of blood and blood components in the United States from 1971 to 1988. Solid squares indicate whole blood; open squares, red blood cells; closed diamonds, platelet concentrates; open circles, fresh-frozen plasma; and triangles, cryoprecipitate.

collected presently are rejected because of abnormal results of laboratory tests for human immunodeficiency virus antibody (anti-HIV), alanine amino transferase (ALT) and hepatitis B core antibody (anti-HB_c) that were introduced from 1985 to 1987.[5]

Approximately 14.8 million donors present themselves at collection sites each year in the United States. Among these persons, collection from 1.3 million (9%) is deferred, and phlebotomy is unsuccessful in 0.3 million (2%). Of the 13.2 million units collected, 11.9 million (90%) are collected by regional or community blood centers, and approximately 1.3 million (10%) are collected by hospital blood banks.[5]

Overall, 8.8 million individuals make approximately 1.5 per capita donations annually. The median age of these donors is the early 30s, and the median education level includes some college or technical training. The median household income of blood donors is $30,000. Approximately 60% of donors are male and approximately 85% are white. 8500 donations are made per 100,000 age-eligible individuals.[5]

In addition to collections made in the United States, approximately 300,000 units of red blood cells are imported from Western European countries. In general, these red blood cells are a "by-product" of voluntarily donated whole blood obtained for plasma fractionation for derivative production in those countries.

Autologous Donations and Intraoperative Cell Salvage

In 1980, approximately 0.14% of transfused red blood cells were obtained from autologous donors.[8] Autologous units accounted for 0.9% of red blood cell transfusions reported by the American Association of Blood Banks (AABB) institutional members in 1985, 1.5% in 1986, and 3.6% in 1987.[8]

The number of persons depositing autologous units increased 91% between 1985 and 1986 and 125% between 1986 and 1987, according to the AABB.[8] The number of autologous collections is projected to expand and may eventually approximate 10% of all red blood cells transfused at tertiary care hospitals in the United States.[10] A report from the United Kingdom estimated that autologous blood may account for 4% of blood transfusions.[11]

Recently, collection systems that more efficiently salvage blood shed during surgery have been developed. The salvaged blood, washed free of surgical debris, is available for reinfusion within minutes of collection.[12,13] It may be stored for up to 6 hours after the start of collection. AABB member institutions reported a 15.6% increase in the number of patients for whom intraoperative cell salvage was used between 1985 and 1986, and an additional 33% increase between 1986 and 1987.[8] Since many intraoperative cell salvage programs are administered by operating room personnel rather than transfusion service staff, the AABB data probably underreport intraoperative cell salvage activity. As many as 200,000 intraoperative cell salvage procedures were performed in 1987, and it is anticipated that utilization will increase significantly within the next few years.[14]

Directed Donations

Directed or designated units are those donated for a specific patient. In 1986, they accounted for approximately 0.9% of transfused red blood cells, and 2.2% in 1987.[8] The use of directed donations is not expected to expand in the future as rapidly as are autologous collections.

Single-Donor Platelet Donations

Platelet transfusions are prepared by pooling platelet concentrates obtained from donated whole blood. The usual dose is 1 unit of platelet concentrates per 10 kg of body weight. Platelet transfusions may also be prepared by removing platelets from a single donor by apheresis techniques. The equivalent of approximately 6 to 8 units of platelet concentrates is obtained by

Table 1–1   Blood Component Usage in the United States[5]

Whole Blood	No. of Patients Receiving Transfusions/Year	Average No. of Units/Transfusion
Red blood cells	3,100,000	3.5
Platelets (random donors)	125,000	6.0
Platelets (apheresis)	120,000	1.0
Fresh-frozen plasma	480,000	3.3
Cryoprecipitate	4,700	8.0

platelet pheresis of a single donor. Using this calculation, single-donor platelet collections may account for as many as 35% of the platelet concentrates obtained in the United States annually.[5] The use of single-donor platelets has been increasing.

Component Production and Transfusion

Whole Blood and Red Blood Cells

Approximately 12.2 million units of whole blood and red blood cells are transfused annually in the United States (Table 1–1).[5,7,15] In 1988, 3.0% of total red cell components were transfused as whole blood and 87.5% as red blood cells. In addition, 3.9% of the red blood cell components were washed, 2.0% were made into leukocyte-depleted components, and an additional 2.8% of red blood cells were prepared as pediatric units.[8]

The use of whole blood has continued to decrease, from 67.4% of total red blood cell component transfusions in 1971 to 13.0% in 1980 and 3.0% in 1988.[2,8] Frozen-thawed red blood cell usage declined from 2.6% of red blood cell transfusions in 1980 to 1.0% in 1988.[8]

Approximately 8% to 10% of collected units are not transfused because of outdating, breakage, contamination, or abnormal laboratory test results. While the percentage of units that are not transfused has remained relatively unchanged during the past decade, the reasons have. Approximately 7% of units became outdated in 1980, compared with less than 2% in 1987. Currently, 5% to 6% of units collected are not used as a result of abnormal results for tests introduced since 1985. Only 0.2% of donated blood was discarded previously as a result of reactive tests for hepatitis B surface antigen and serologic tests for syphilis.

Platelet Concentrates

Platelet concentrates currently are the only component experiencing increases in usage. Platelet concentrates are prepared from approximately 50% of whole blood units. Production increased from 3.4 million units in 1980 to 5.3 million units in 1985, 7.6 million units in 1987, and 8.2 million units in

1988.[5,7] Approximately 25% of platelet concentrate units are prepared by apheresis. Overall, the platelet concentrate growth rate was approximately 6% to 7% annually through 1986. Random donor platelet concentrates prepared from whole blood collections account for 2% to 3% of the increase. The remainder is attributed to single-donor platelets prepared by apheresis. Approximately 10% of platelet concentrates become outdated.

Fresh-Frozen Plasma

Fresh-frozen plasma (FFP) production underwent expansive growth between 1971 and the early 1980s. FFP preparation increased from 0.18 million units in 1971 to 1.5 million units in 1980, and 2.4 million units in 1987.[2,5] The AABB reported a 4.8% decrease in FFP transfusions between 1985 and 1986, and a further 1.6% decline between 1986 and 1987.[8] Current estimates indicate this trend will continue.

Cryoprecipitated Antihemophilic Factor

In 1980 approximately 582,000 units of cryoprecipitate were prepared. Utilization increased in 1983 and 1984 to approximately 900,000 and 960,000 units annually after the publication of reports linking commercially prepared factor VIII concentrates to AIDS and AIDS-related abnormalities.[2,4,8] Subsequently, heat-treated factor VIII concentrates were introduced and cryoprecipitate utilization stabilized or declined. However, production and utilization increased in 1988 as a result of worldwide shortages of pasteurized or monoclonal antibody purified and viral-inactivated factor VIII concentrates.

Blood Transfusion Patterns

Reports of blood transfusion patterns during the 1970s have been published.[16,19] However, similar data covering transfusion practice in the 1980s are not available. Nevertheless, information presented at three National Institutes of Health Consensus Conferences are available for analysis. In addition, the conferences stimulated further investigation about component transfusion practice and mechanisms for optimizing their use. The first of these conferences was held in September 1984, and addressed FFP usage.[20] The second concerned platelet transfusion therapy and was conducted in October 1986.[21] The third, held in June 1988, dealt with perioperative red blood cell transfusion.[22] The anticipated effect of these conferences is the promotion of appropriate use of blood and blood components and avoidance of transfusion in situations where the benefit is doubtful.

The National Institutes of Health (NIH) Consensus Conference approach assumes that uniform transfusion practice is possible. In fact, transfusion rates for red blood cells and whole blood vary significantly within the United States. For example, red blood cell transfusions were given to 14.9 patients per 1,000 population in the eastern south central part of the United States, compared with only 11.5 patients per 1,000 population in the Pacific region in 1979. Hospitalized patients in the eastern south central region were infused with 60.5 units of red blood cells per 1,000, compared with only 43.4 units per thousand in the mountain states. Certainly, blood utilization patterns are influenced by local medical care delivery practices.[23] Widespread distribution of the NIH Consensus Conference recommendations and increasing requirements for transfusion auditing may lessen these differences.[24] However, use of transfusion therapy requires the application of clinical judgment and some variation in the administration of transfusion therapy is likely to continue.

Whole Blood and Red Blood Cells

Comprehensive evaluations of blood usage patterns were conducted in US hospitals in 1974, 1977, 1979, and 1982–88.[2-9,16-19] Although changes have occurred in surgical procedures and other clinical situations in which blood is used, an increase in the number of elderly persons, who use more blood than younger patients, has kept utilization levels relatively constant. Forty-five thousand hip arthoplasty procedures were performed in 1972 (46% in patients 65 years of age or older), compared with 153,000 in 1981 (72% were performed in patients 65 years of age or older).[25] Two thirds of patients who undergo hip replacement surgery receive transfusions, and each of these patients receives 2½ to 3 units of blood.[16-19]

Surgical patients receive transfusions more often than nonsurgical patients, and older patients receive more blood than younger patients. Patients undergoing operations account for approximately 62% of all transfusion recipients and they use almost 64% of the blood. The average patient undergoing surgery receives 3.5 units of blood, compared with 3.2 units for the average nonsurgical patient. Among patients undergoing surgery, 9.1% received blood transfusions, while only 2.8% of nonsurgical patients received red blood cells or whole blood.[19]

During the 1970s, 44.3% of patients who received transfusions were 65 years of age or older. They received 43.7% percent of all units transfused, despite constituting only 22% of hospitalized patients.[16-19]

Major disease categories of patients receiving transfusions. In 1979, patients treated for malignant neoplasms received 18.7% of red blood cell transfusions. Patients with cardiovascular disease, including cerebrovascular disease, received 16.1% of units transfused. Men undergoing coronary artery bypass graft surgery used 8.4% of transfused blood, and female patients undergoing the same procedure used an additional 4.1%.[16-19] It is estimated that approximately 100,000 coronary artery bypass procedures were performed in 1980, 200,000 in 1985, and 230,000 in 1987.[26] In one study[27] the average age of patients undergoing open-heart surgery was 60 years; 28% were over 65.[27] The percentage of patients undergoing bypass procedures who received transfusions has decreased from almost 100% in the 1970s to approximately 50% to 76% at present.[28-32] The average number of units given to each patient has decreased from 9 to 10 units to 3 to 5 units.

In 1979, patients with nonmalignant diseases of the gastrointestinal tract received 15.7% of all red blood cell units transfused; approximately 60% of these units were given to patients treated medically.[19]

Patients with fractures and traumatic injury, including soft tissue injury, received 12.0% of transfused red blood cell units. Those with anemia, hemophilia, and other diseases of the hematopoietic system utilized 5.2% of transfused blood. Patients undergoing obstetrical procedures and treatment for related complications received 4.3%. Those with bone and joint disease, excluding fractures, utilized 3.5% of red blood cell transfusions, and patients with disease of the respiratory tract and lungs were given 2.8% of the transfusions. Patients treated for liver disease and patients with disease of the kidney and genitourinary tract each received 2.7% of units transfused to all patients. Patients undergoing treatment of gynecologic disease for nonmalignant conditions, including uterine leiomyomas and breast disease, received 2.6% of transfusions.[19]

Special procedures.   Transfusion requirements for patients undergoing specialized procedures such as bone marrow transplantation or liver transplantation have a substantial impact on blood centers serving hospitals with these programs. The overall effect on the nation's blood supply is considerably less. For example, patients undergoing liver transplantation used approximately 5% to 6% of all red blood cells collected by the Central Blood Bank of Pittsburgh between 1981 and 1985.[33] More than 18,600 units of packed cells were transfused during 636 liver transplantation procedures performed on 485 patients. However, only 3,364 liver transplants were performed in the United States between 1981 and 1987; 1,182 in the latter year.[34]

Transfusion trigger.   The "transfusion trigger," in general, has been a hemoglobin level of 6.2 mmol/L or a hematocrit of 0.3.[17,18,35,36] Recently, this concept has been challenged by an expert panel during the NIH Consensus Development Conference on Perioperative Red Cell Transfusion.[22] The panel concluded that healthy patients with hemoglobin values of 6.2 mmol/L or more rarely require perioperative transfusion, and those with acute anemia with hemoglobin values of less than 4.3 mmol/L frequently require transfusion. No evidence was found to support the previously accepted trigger levels. The decision to transfuse red blood cells requires a clinical assessment of the patient's condition aided by appropriate laboratory data (Table 1–2).

The setting in which patients receive care also has an important impact on transfusion practice. Patients with terminal cancer treated in a conventional hospital setting are five to ten times more likely to receive red blood cell transfusions than those receiving care in a hospice or home-care hospice situation.[37]

Platelet Concentrates

Recipients of platelet concentrates can be divided into three broad categories: oncology patients, open-heart surgery patients, and "other" patients. In-

Red Blood Cells
    For volume expansion
    In place of a hematinic
    To enhance wound healing
    To improve general "well-being"

Platelets
    To patients with immune thrombocytopenic purpura (unless there is life-threatening bleeding)
    Prophylactically with massive blood transfusion
    Prophylactically following cardiopulmonary bypass

Fresh-Frozen Plasma
    For volume expansion
    As a nutritional supplement
    Prophylactically with massive blood transfusion
    Prophylactically following cardiopulmonary bypass

---

cluded in the latter category are patients receiving platelet concentrates who are uremic, receive massive transfusions, or have disseminated intravascular coagulation, infection, or other unspecified conditions.

Despite no clear indication for their use, patients undergoing coronary artery bypass graft surgery are reported to receive 33% to 41% of platelet concentrates prepared by regional blood centers.[38,39] However, reports from tertiary care hospitals indicate that less than 20% of platelet transfusions are given to these patients.[28,29,31,40,41]

Approximately 35% to 38% of platelet concentrates are used by patients treated for malignant disorders, and approximately two thirds of that fraction are given to patients with leukemia. The remainder of platelet transfusions are prescribed for patients with "other" disorders.[38,39] Studies of platelet utilization in tertiary care settings suggest that a higher percentage of platelet concentrates are given to patients with hematologic or oncologic disorders. 86% of platelet units were given to these patients and 68% were given prophylactically at one tertiary care center.[40]

Fresh-Frozen Plasma

FFP transfusions have been used for volume replacement, for treatment of coagulopathies associated with massive transfusion, for the treatment of disseminated intravascular coagulation, to replace coagulation factors in patients with liver disease, to reverse the effect of warfarin in patients who are bleeding and face imminent surgery, and for treatment of thrombotic thrombocytopenic purpura. In addition, FFP is occasionally given according to a standard formula; eg, 1 unit of FFP for every 4 units of red blood cells transfused.[42-45]

Many of these uses for FFP have been questioned.[20] A review of the transfusion practice at a tertiary care hospital indicates that as many as 77% of FFP units can be withheld without adversely affecting patient outcome.[46]

A study conducted at a regional blood center indicated that 42% of FFP units are used by patients undergoing open-heart surgery, 23% by patients having other surgical procedures, 26% by patients on the medical service, and 8% by pediatric patients. The trigger for prescribing FFP included bleeding in 43% of transfusion episodes, abnormal results of coagulation studies in 26%, signs and symptoms of hypovolemia in 16%, and "other" explanations in 15%.[42]

Cryoprecipitate

Cryoprecipitate contains fibrinogen, factor VIII, von Willebrand's factor, factor XIII, and fibronectin.

The majority of cryoprecipitate is used to treat patients with hemophilia A, von Willebrand's disease, and hypofibrinogenemia. Cryoprecipitate is also used in the preparation of "fibrin sealants" and as an adhesive in otologic surgery.[47-49] The latter applications involve the addition of thrombin and calcium chloride to cryoprecipitate to promote fibrin clot formation. The preparation is applied to the external surface of vascular anastomosis to prevent leakage, and in the reconstruction of middle ear tissue.

Adverse Reactions Associated With Transfusion Therapy

Blood transfusion has immediate or delayed adverse consequences in as many as 10% to 15% of recipients. Significant acute complications, such as febrile and allergic reactions, occur with a frequency of approximately 1% per unit transfused. Delayed events such as transfusion-transmitted diseases (eg, hepatitis and retroviral infection) occur with a frequency of approximately 0.5% per unit transfused (Table 1–3).

Many of these reactions are not preventable. This underscores the importance of prescribing transfusions only when the benefits clearly outweigh the risks.

Acute Transfusion Reactions

Acute reactions include hemolytic and nonhemolytic transfusion reactions, allergic reactions, hypervolemia, noncardiogenic pulmonary edema, nonimmune hemolysis, and bacterial sepsis.

Acute hemolytic reactions.   Hemolytic transfusion reactions are divided into two categories: acute intravascular hemolysis and acute extravascular hemolysis. Intravascular hemolysis is usually due to ABO incompatibility.

Table 1–3 — Adverse Effects Associated with Blood and Blood Component Transfusion

	Approximate Frequency*	
	Ratio	Percentage
Acute		
Acute hemolytic transfusion reaction	1/25,000	0.004
Febrile, nonhemolytic transfusion reaction	1/200	0.500
Allergic reactions	1/100 to 300	0.200
Hypervolemia	Variable	
Noncardiogenic pulmonary edema	1/5,000	0.020
Bacterial sepsis	Rare	
Anaphylactic hypotensive reactions	1/150,000	0.0007
Complications of massive transfusions (hemostatic defect, hypothermia and metabolic abnormalities)	Unknown	
Delayed		
Delayed hemolytic transfusion reaction	1/1500 to 9000	0.020
Red blood cell alloimmunization	1/100	1.000
Leukocyte/platelet alloimmunization	1/10	10.000
Hemosideosis	Unknown	
Graft-v-host disease	Rare	
Posttransfusion purpura	Rare	
Viral hepatitis	1/1500	0.006
Transfusion-associated AIDS	1/36,000 to 300,000	0.0007
Transfusion-associated malaria	Rare	

*Frequency is presented as risk per unit transfused.

Extravascular hemolysis is usually caused by incompatibility involving other red blood cell antigens and antibodies such as Rh.

The majority of acute hemolytic transfusion reactions are caused by clerical error, choosing a unit of blood intended for another patient in an emergency situation, or laboratory error.[50-52] Acute hemolytic reactions usually occur after infusion of incompatible red blood cells, but may also occur following infusion of incompatible plasma.

Complement and the coagulation pathway may be activated and vasoactive amines may be released. The pathophysiologic consequences include vasomotor instability, cardiorespiratory collapse, disseminated intravascular coagulation, and renal failure. Acute extravascular hemolysis is usually not accompanied by complement activation. Therefore, these reactions generally are less serious than those involving intravascular hemolysis.[53,54]

Febrile nonhemolytic transfusion reactions. Febrile nonhemolytic transfusion reactions are defined by an elevation of temperature of 1 °C or more above the pretransfusion temperature. They occur after approximately 0.5% of transfusions. Since fever is the first sign of a serious hemolytic reaction, it is not possible to determine whether the patient is suffering a hemolytic or nonhemolytic reaction when this sign is observed. Hence, it is advisable to stop the infusion of blood when patients complain of chills or fever.

Febrile nonhemolytic reactions are usually attributed to leukocytes contained in the donor unit and antibodies (eg, leukoagglutinins and HLA-antibodies) directed against these cells.[55,56] Febrile nonhemolytic transfusion reactions are prevented by the transfusion of leukocyte-depleted blood components. Most patients who have an initial febrile reaction do not have a recurrence despite continuation of transfusions of non–leukocyte-depleted components.[57] Red blood cell survival is normal. The reactions, in general, consist of fever and rigors. Occasionally more serious complications such as pulmonary infiltrates occur.[58]

Allergic reactions. Allergic reactions related to blood transfusion include urticaria and, rarely, hypotension or anaphylaxis. They are probably caused by antibodies against plasma proteins. Most urticarial reactions are mild and respond to antihistamine therapy. Patients who develop a few hives during a transfusion are usually treated by temporarily stopping the infusion and administering antihistamines, and then continuing the transfusion if symptoms subside. Red blood cell survival is not compromised.

Approximately 1 in 600 persons are IgA-deficient. Some of these individuals may experience laryngeal edema and anaphylactic reactions as a result of IgG, anti-IgA antibodies directed against IgA in the infused plasma. Patients with a history of anaphylactic transfusion reactions should be evaluated for the presence of anti-IgA antibody. If such antibodies are found, the patients should receive extensively washed red blood cells or plasma from IgA-deficient donors.[59]

Hypervolemia. Patients with chronic anemia are usually normovolemic. They are at risk for developing hypervolemia when the volume of the transfusion surpasses their ability to adjust physiologically. This situation may also occur in patients with hemorrhage if the patient's clinical status is not monitored appropriately. Patients may complain of dyspnea or develop hypertension, pulmonary edema, and cardia arrhythmias. Administration of whole blood should be restricted to patients with active hemorrhage or acute hypervolemia. In general, blood products should be infused slowly over a period of 2 to 4 hours.

Noncardiogenic pulmonary edema. In the plasma of the transfusion, antibodies directed against leukocytes have been implicated as a cause of transfusion-related acute lung injury. These episodes present clinically in a manner similar to that of pulmonary edema. However, ventricular filling pressures are normal or low. Capillary permeability in the lungs is increased and the injury is related, presumably, to fluid leakage into the pulmonary tissue.[60,61]

Nonimmune hemolysis.   Nonimmune hemolysis is caused by exposure of red blood cells to hypotonic solutions (eg, 5% dextrose and water), mechanical stress on erythrocytes during cardiopulmonary bypass, administration of red blood cells under pressure, improper storage, or improper administration through overheated blood-warming devices. Hemoglobinemia and hemoglobinuria may be present. Nonimmune hemolysis, per se, is not associated with adverse consequences. However, the presence of hemoglobinemia or hemoglobinuria requires evaluation by clinicians and may divert attention away from more important aspects of the patient's care.

Bacterial sepsis.   Contamination of blood or blood components with small amounts of bacteria at the time of collection may result in seriously adverse consequences at the time of transfusion since these organisms may proliferate during storage. Psychrophilic organisms survive in red blood cell components that have been stored at 4 °C. Often, they produce endotoxin that causes significant vasomotor instability in transfusion recipients. Other organisms survive and grow in platelet concentrates stored at room temperature. Patients experiencing chills, fever and hypotension shortly after transfusion require evaluation for the possibility of transfusion-associated sepsis.[50-52,62-68]

Delayed Transfusion Reactions

Adverse consequences of blood transfusion may occur several days after transfusion or may not be apparent until several years later. For example, delayed hemolytic transfusion reactions occur 3 to 10 days after transfusion, posttransfusion purpura occurs approximately 7 to 10 days after transfusion, and graft-*v*-host disease may occur several weeks following transfusion. Iron accumulation leading to symptomatic endocrine or cardiac disease and some transfusion-transmitted diseases may not be apparent for many years.

Delayed hemolytic transfusion reaction.   Delayed hemolytic transfusion reactions are caused by the appearance of red blood cell antibodies 3 to 10 days after transfusion. These antibodies may be the result of an anamnestic response or may represent antibody production to newly encountered alloantigens. Delayed hemolytic transfusion reactions are associated with a fall in the hematocrit and hemoglobin levels and jaundice. However, most of these reactions are not associated with serious adverse consequences.[69]

Alloimmunization.   Approximately 1% of recipients of red blood cell transfusions develop alloantibody. Approximately 10% develop anti-HLA antibody.[54] The consequence of development of such antibodies depends on the requirement for further transfusion. In the case of red blood cell recipients, pretransfusion compatibility testing alerts transfusion service personnel to the presence of these antibodies so that red blood cells devoid of the corresponding alloantigens can be selected. Patients with anti-HLA antibody who require multiple platelet transfusions may become refractory to random-donor platelet transfusions and require platelet concentrates to be prepared from HLA-matched donors.[70]

Iron overload.   Each unit of a red blood cell transfusion contains approximately 250 mg of iron. Patients become symptomatic as the result of iron overload when iron stores are in excess of 20 to 30 g. This may occur after the infusion of 80 to 120 units of blood.[71]

Graft-*v*-host disease.   Graft-*v*-host disease may develop in immunocompromised patients such as those with severe combined immunodeficiency disease, bone marrow transplant recipients, and patients whose immune system is compromised by chemotherapy or radiotherapy. The syndrome is considered to be caused by engraftment and proliferation of donor lymphocytes that attack host antigens. Skin, liver, gastrointestinal tract, bronchial mucosa, and lymphoid tissue are most often involved. The problem is avoided by treating blood and cell-containing blood components intended for susceptible patients with 15 to 25 Gy of gamma radiation before transfusion.[72-74]

Posttransfusion purpura.   Posttransfusion purpura is an extremely rare complication of blood transfusion. It usually occurs in patients who have been pregnant or received prior blood transfusions. Most patients affected by this disorder develop profound purpura approximately 7 to 10 days after transfusion. Laboratory evaluation of these patients often reveals the presence of anti-P1[A1] antibody or an HLA antibody. Other antibodies with platelet-specific antigen specificity have also been identified.[75]

Immunomodulatory effects of blood transfusion.   Recently, immunosuppressive effects related to blood transfusion have been reported. Although the interpretation of these reports remain controversial, some investigators have indicated that there is a higher incidence of cancer recurrence in patients undergoing tumor surgery who receive transfusions than in those who do not receive transfusions. Other investigators have reported a higher incidence of postoperative infectious complications among patients who have received transfusions compared with those who have not.[76]

Transfusion-transmitted diseases.   In addition to the above-mentioned delayed adverse consequences associated with transfusion, patients are at risk of contracting transfusion-transmitted diseases. These illnesses are reviewed in detail in subsequent chapters of this book.

Pharmacologic Agents for Reducing
Transfusion Requirements

Avoidance of transfusion should reduce concomitant risk. One method for accomplishing this goal is the use of pharmacologic agents that enhance oxygen-carrying capacity or promote hemostasis. Unfortunately, satisfactory acellular oxygen-carrying compounds have not been developed to date.[77] Bone marrow growth hormones prepared with recombinant DNA, such as erythropoietin, have the potential for stimulating bone marrow stem cells to produce superphysiologic amounts of red blood cells or myeloid elements.[78-81] In the future, the combination of infusion of acellular oxygen-carrying compounds with a brief half-life and stimulation of the bone marrow to produce red blood cells by recombinant human erythropoietin may obviate the need for transfusion therapy for some patients.

An alternative aspect of the use of pharmacologic agents to reduce transfusion requirements involves agents that promote hemostasis, such as 1-deamino-8D-arginine vasopressin (DDAVP) and aprotinin.[82] These agents have been shown to reduce post-operative blood loss after cardiopulmonary bypass surgery and orthopedic surgical procedures.[83-88]

Acellular Oxygen-Carrying Compounds

A perfluorochemical emulsion capable of transporting oxygen composed of perfluorodecalin and perfluorotriperopylamine was used in an investigational study of acutely anemic patients who refused blood transfusion for religious reasons.[77] Patients receiving the compound had no adverse reactions. However, no appreciable benefits were demonstrated. The increase in arterial oxygen content was slight and the half-life of the drug was brief. Currently, other compounds, including chemically modified hemoglobin solutions, are under investigation. It is possible that more effective acellular oxygen-carrying compounds will be developed.

Human Recombinant Growth Factors

Clinical studies with recombinant human erythropoietin in anemic patients undergoing long-term hemodialysis indicate that this agent is capable of raising the hematocrit and the hemoglobin level sufficiently to preclude further transfusion.[80,81] These patients use approximately 200,000 to 400,000 units of red blood cells per year in the United States. Hence, the impact of recombinant human erythropoietin treatment in this patient population may be substantial.

Granulocyte and granulocyte-macrophage colony–stimulating factors and multilineage colony–stimulating factor (interleukin-3) are also available as recombinant DNA–prepared pharmacologic agents.[89-94]. They have been shown to prevent chemotherapy-induced neutropenia and to accelerate recovery from this complication. The long-term benefits and consequences of these factors are speculative. However, it is estimated that shortened periods of marrow aplasia will have a beneficial effect on patients treated for malignant conditions and will reduce these patients' requirement for transfusion support.

Hemostatically Effective Agents

DDAVP has been shown to reduce the need for platelet transfusions in patients undergoing surgery involving cardiopulmonary bypass.[83,84] It has also been shown to correct the bleeding time and promote surgical hemostasis in patients with von Willebrand's disease, uremia, liver cirrhosis, and primary or acquired platelet function defects. It has also been shown to reduce blood loss in patients undergoing orthopedic surgery and in a few patients with acute bleeding and moderate thrombocytopenia.[88,95-100]

Another pharmacologic agent, aprotinin, has also been shown to reduce postoperative blood loss in patients undergoing cardiopulmonary bypass.[86,87] This agent may be effective because it preserves platelet adhesive capacity.[87]

Conclusion

In summary, the rapid growth in red blood cell use that occurred during the 1970s and early 1980s has ceased and currently is in a plateau phase. The use of single donor platelet concentrates is expanding. Fresh-frozen plasma and cryoprecipitate usage is likely to decline as a result of heightened awareness of appropriate indications for the administration of these components. Pressures to assure appropriate use of transfusion therapy are increasing.[20-22,24,38-39,42-46,101-111]

The use of autologous transfusions and intraoperative cell salvage techniques is likely to increase. This is probably related to the perception of risk of transfusion-transmitted diseases.

The introduction of human recombinant-DNA growth factors, such as erythropoietin and G-CSF and GM-CSF, may have a modulating effect on transfusion requirements. Clinical trials using these agents are underway currently.

The median age of the United States population continues to increase and the outlook for expenditures for medical care are anticipated to increase from 10% to 15% of the gross national product within the next decade.[112] These factors are likely to be associated with increased use of blood transfusion. However, emphasis on the appropriate use of blood and blood components, fear of transfusion-transmitted disease, and technological and pharmacological advances are anticipated to have a dampening effect. Ultimately, the use of blood and blood components will be determined by physicians prescribing these resources in the most beneficial manner.

References

1. Zuck TF: Greetings:—A final look back with comments about a policy of a zero-risk blood supply (editorial). *Transfusion* 27:447–448, 1987.

2. *Blood policy and Technology*. Washington, DC, Congressional Office of Technology Assessment, OTA-H-260, January 1985.

3. Polesky HF: Blood banking in the United States: 1981. *Transfusion* 25:304–307, 1985.

4. Menitove JE: Blood utilization, in Wallas CH, McCarthy LJ (eds): *New Frontiers in Blood Banking*. Arlington, VA, American Association of Blood Banks, 1986, pp 1–20.

5. Cumming PD, Schorr JB, Wallace EL: Annual blood facts, United States totals—1986/87, American Red Cross, Washington, DC, 1987 (Document No. B3287-82).

6. Surgenor DM, Wallace EL, Hale WSG, Gilpatrick MW: Changing patterns of blood transfusion in four sets of United States hospitals, 1980 to 1985. *Transfusion* 28:513–518, 1988.

7. Surgenor D, Mac M, Wallace EC, Hao SHS, Chapman RH: Collection and transfusion of blood in the United States, 1982–1988. *N Engl J Med* 322:1646-1651, 1990.

8. American Association of Blood Banks Annual Reports 1983–89, American Association of Blood Banks, Arlington, VA.

9. Marwick C: Six-year slowing noted in previously growing rate of U.S. blood collection and transfusions. *JAMA* 261:968–969, 1989.

10. Toy PT, Stehling LC, Strauss RG, et al: Underutilization of autologous blood donation among eligible elective surgical patients. *Am J Surg* 152:483–486, 1986.

11. Lee D: Annotation. Autologous blood transfusion. *Br J Haematol* 70:135–136, 1988.

12. Popovsky MA, Devine PA, Taswell HF: Intraoperative autologous transfusion. *Mayo Clin Proc* 60:125–134, 1985.

13. Kruskall MS: Intraoperative autotransfusion, in Rossi EC, Simon TL, Moss GS (eds): *Principles of Transfusion Medicine*. Baltimore, Md, Williams & Wilkens, 1991.

14. Dzik WH: Perioperative blood salvage, In *Proceedings of Perioperative Red Cell Transfusion Consensus Conference, National Institutes of Health*, Bethesda, MD, 1988, pp 71–77.

15. Surgenor DMN: Trends in U.S. transfusion activities: 1980–86, In: *Proceedings of Perioperative Red Cell Transfusion Consensus Conference, National Institutes of Health*, Bethesda, MD, 1988, p 21.

16. Friedman BA, Burns TL, Schork MA: A study of blood utilization by diagnosis, month of transfusion, and geographic region of the United States. *Transfusion* 19:511–525, 1979.

17. Friedman BA, Burns TL, Schork MA: An analysis of blood transfusion of surgical patients by sex: a quest for the transfusion trigger. *Transfusion* 20:179–188, 1980.

18. Friedman BA: Patterns of blood utilization by physicians: transfusion of nonoperated anemic patients. *Transfusion* 18:193–198, 1978.

19. Friedman BA, Burns TL, Schork MA: *A Study of National Trends in Transfusion Practice*. Springfield, VA, National Technical Information Service, publication No. 1381125437, 1980.

20. Office of Medical Applications of Research, National Institutes of Health, Consensus Conference: Fresh frozen plasma: indications and risks. *JAMA* 253:551–553, 1985.

21. Consensus Conference on Platelet Transfusion Therapy: National Institutes of Health. *JAMA* 257:1777–1780, 1987.

22. Consensus Conference on Red Blood Cell Transfusion: perioperative red blood cell transfusion. *JAMA* 260:2700–2703, 1988.

23. Chassin M, Brook RH, Park RE, et al: Variations in the use of medical and surgical services by the Medicare population. *N Engl J Med* 314:285–299, 1986.

24. Van Schoonhoven P, Berkman EM, Lehman R: Medical staff monitoring functions blood usage review. In Fromberg (ed), *Medical Staff Monitoring Functions Series*, Chicago, IL, Joint Commission on Accreditation of Hospitals, 1987, pp 1–35.

25. Valvona J, Sloan F: DataWatch: Rising rates of surgery among the elderly. *Health Aff* Fall:108–119, 1985.

26. Killip T: Twenty years of coronary bypass surgery (editorial). *N Engl J Med* 319:366–368, 1988.

27. Winslow CM, Kosecoff JB, Chassin M, Kanouse DE, et al: The appropriateness of performing coronary artery bypass surgery. *JAMA* 260:505–509, 1988.

28. McCarthy PM, Popovsky MA, Schaff HV, Orszulak TA, et al: Effect of blood conservation efforts in cardiac operations at the Mayo Clinic. *Mayo Clin Proc* 63:225–229, 1988.

29. Cosgrove DM, Loop FD, Lytle BW, Gill CC, et al: Determinants of blood utilization during myocardial revascularization. *Ann Thoracic Surg* 40:380–384, 1985.

30. Cosgrove DM: Red cell transfusion in heart surgery, in *Proceedings of Perioperative Red Cell Transfusion Consensus Conference, National Institutes of Health*, Bethesda, MD, 1988, pp 53–55.

31. Goodnough LT, Kruskall M, Stehling L, et al: A multi-center audit of transfusion practice in coronary artery bypass (CABG) surgery. *Transfusion* 72(suppl 1):277a, 1988 (abstract).

32. Giordano GF, Rivers SL, Chung GKT, Mammana RB, et al: Autologous platelet-rich plasma in cardiac surgery: Effect on intraoperative and postoperative transfusion requirements. *Ann Thorac Surg* 46:416–419, 1988.

33. Lewis JH, Bontempo FA, Cornell F, Kiss JE, et al: Blood use in liver transplantation. *Transfusion* 27:222–225, 1987.

34. American Council on Transplantation U.S. Transplant Statistics. American Council on Transplantation, Alexandria, VA, March 31, 1988.

35. Stehling LC, Ellison N, Faust RJ, et al: A survey of transfusion practices among anesthesiologists. *Vox Sang* 52:60–62, 1987.

36. Zauder HL: How did we get a 'magic number' for preoperative hematocrit/hemoglobin level? In: *Proceedings of Perioperative Red Cell Transfusion Consensus Conference, National Institutes of Health*, Bethesda, MD, 1988, pp 29–31.

37. Wachtel TJ, Mor V: The use of transfusion in terminal cancer patients: Hospice versus conventional care setting. *Transfusion* 25:278–279, 1985.

38. Menitove JE, McElligott MC, Aster RH: Where have all the platelets gone? A strategy for monitoring platelet usage. *Wis Med J* 81:11–13, 1982.

39. Silver SS, Rock G, Décary F, Luke KH, et al: Use of platelet concentrate in eastern Ontario. *CMAJ* 137:128–132, 1987.

40. McCullough J, Steeper TA, Connelly DP, Jackson B, et al: Platelet utilization in University Hospital. *JAMA* 259:2414–2418, 1988.

41. Freedman J, Lim C, Wright J: Changing patterns of transfusion practice in a tertiary care hospital from 1977 to 1984. *Can Anaesth Soc J* 33:458–465, 1986.

42. Snyder AJ, Gottschall JL, Menitove JE: Why is fresh-frozen plasma transfused? *Transfusion* 26:107–112, 1986.

43. Blumberg N, Laczin J, McMican A, Heal J, et al: A critical survey of fresh-frozen plasma use. *Transfusion* 26:511–513, 1986.

44. Shaikh BS, Wagar D, Lau PM, Campbell Jr EW: Transfusion pattern of fresh frozen plasma in a medical school hospital. *Vox Sang* 48:366–369, 1985.

45. Braunstein AH, Oberman HA: Transfusion of plasma components. *Transfusion* 24:281–286, 1984.

46. Shanberge JN: Reduction of fresh-frozen plasma use through a daily survey and education program. *Transfusion* 27:226–227, 1987.

47. Rousou JA, Engelman RM, Breyer RH: Fibrin glue: An effective hemostatic agent for nonsuturable intraoperative bleeding. *Ann Thorac Surg* 38:409–410, 1984.

48. Lupinetti FM, Stoney WS, Alford WC Jr, Burrus GR, et al: Cryoprecipitate— topical thrombin blue: Initial experience in patients undergoing cardiac operations. *J Thorac Cardiovasc Surg* 90:502–505, 1985.

49. Silberstein LE, Williams LJ, Hughlett MA, Magee DA, et al: An autologous fibrinogen-based adhesive for use in otologic surgery. *Transfusion* 28:319–321, 1988.

50. Schmidt PJ: Transfusion mortality; with special reference to surgical and intensive care facilities. *J Fla Med Assoc* 67:151–153, 1980.

51. Honig CL, Bove JR: Transfusion-associated fatalities: Review of Bureau of Biologics Reports 1976–1978. *Transfusion* 20:653–661, 1980.

52. Myhre BA: Fatalities from blood transfusion. *JAMA* 244:1333–1335, 1980.

53. Pineda AA, Brzica SM Jr, Taswell HF: Hemolytic transfusion reaction: Recent experience in a large blood bank. *Mayo Clin Proc* 53:378–390, 1978.

54. Walker RH: Special report: Transfusion risks. *Am J Clin Pathol* 88:374–378, 1987.

55. Brittingham TE, Chaplin H Jr: Febrile transfusion reactions caused by sensitivity to donor leukocytes and platelets. *JAMA* 165:819–825, 1957.

56. Perkins HA, Payne R, Ferguson J, Wood M: Nonhemolytic febrile transfusion reactions: Quantitative effects of blood components with emphasis on isoantigenic incompatibility of leukocytes. *Vox Sang* 11:578–600, 1966.

57. Menitove JE, McElligott MC, Aster RH: Febrile transfusion reaction: What blood component should be given next? *Vox Sang* 42:318–321, 1982.

58. Thompson JS, Severson CD, Parmely MJ, Marmorstein BL, et al: Pulmonary 'hypersensitivity' reactions induced by transfusion of non-HL-A leukoagglutinins. *N Engl J Med* 284:1120–1125, 1971.

59. Moore SB: Anaphylactic transfusion reactions: A concise review. *Irish Med J* 78:54–56, 1985.

60. Popovsky MA, Abel MD, Moore SB: Transfusion-related acute lung injury associated with passive transfer of antileukocyte antibodies. *Am Rev Respir Dis* 128:185–189, 1983.

61. Hammerschmidt DE: Of lungs and leukocytes (editorial). *JAMA* 244:2199–2200, 1980.

62. Heal JM, Jones ME, Forey J, Chaudhry A, et al: Fatal *Salmonella* septicemia after platelet transfusion. *Transfusion* 27:2–5, 1987.

63. Braine HG, Kickler TS, Charache P, Ness PM, et al: Bacterial sepsis secondary to platelet transfusion: An adverse effect of extended storage at room temperature. *Transfusion* 26:391–393, 1986.

64. Khabbaz RF, Arnow PM, Highsmith AK, et al: *Pseudomonas fluorescens* bacteremia from blood transfusion. *Am J Med* 76:62–68, 1984.

65. Tabor E, Gerety RJ: Five cases of *Pseudomonas* sepsis transmitted by blood transfusions. *Lancet* 1:1403, 1984.

66. Murray AE, Bartzokas CA, Shepherd AJN, Roberts FM: Blood transfusion-associated *Pseudomonas fluorescens* septicaemia: Is this an increasing problem? *J Hosp Infect* 9:243–248, 1987.

67. Phillips P, Grayson L, Stockman K, et al: Transfusion-related *Pseudomonas* sepsis. *Lancet* 2:879, 1984.

68. Tipple MA, Bland LA, Murphy JJ, et al: Sepsis associated with transfusion of red cells contaminated with *Yersinia enterocolitica*. *Transfusion* 30:207–213, 1990.

69. Pineda AA, Taswell HF, Brzica SM Jr: Delayed hemolytic transfusion reaction: An immunologic hazard of blood transfusion. *Transfusion* 18:1–7, 1978.

70. Duquesnoy RJ, Filip DJ, Rodey GE, Rimm AA, Aster RH: Successful transfusion of platelets 'mismatched' for HLA antigens to alloimmunized thrombocytopenic patients. *Am J Hematol* 2:219–226, 1977.

71. Schafer AI, Cheron RG, Dluhy R, Cooper B, et al: Clinical consequences of acquired transfusional iron overload in adults. *N Engl J Med* 304:319–324, 1981.

72. Von Fliedner V, Higby DJ, Kim U: Graft-versus-host reaction following blood product transfusion. *Am J Med* 72:951–961, 1982.

73. Brubaker DB: Human posttransfusion graft-versus-host disease. *Vox Sang* 45:401–420, 1983.

74. Leitman SF, Holland PV: Irradiation of blood products: Indications and guidelines. *Transfusion* 25:293–303, 1985.

75. Mueller-Eckhardt C: Annotation: Post-transfusion purpura. *Br J Haematol* 64:419–424, 1986.

76. Perkins HA: Transfusion-induced immunologic unresponsiveness. *Trans Med Rev* 2:196–203, 1988.

77. Gould SA, Rosen AL, Sehgal LR, Sehgal HL, et al: Fluosol-DA as a red-cell substitute in acute anemia. *N Engl J Med* 314:1653–1656, 1986.

78. Clark SC, Kamen R: The human hematopoietic colony-stimulating factors. *Science* 236:1229–1237, 1987.

79. Groopman JE: Colony-stimulating factors: Present status and future applications. *Semin Hematol* 25:30–37, 1988.

80. Winearls CG, Oliver DO, Pippard MJ, Reid C, et al: Effect of human erythropoietin derived from recombinant DNA on the anaemia of patients maintained by chronic haemodialysis. *Lancet* 2:1175–1177, 1986.

81. Eschbach JW, Egrie JC, Downing MR, Browne JK, et al: Correction of the anemia of end-stage renal disease with recombinant human erythropoietin: results of a combined Phase I and II clinical trial. *N Engl J Med* 316:73–78, 1987.

82. Editorial: Can drugs reduce surgical blood loss? *Lancet* 1:155–156, 1988.

83. Salzman EW, Weinstein MJ, Weintraub RM, Ware JA, et al: Treatment with desmopressin acetate to reduce blood loss after cardiac surgery: a double-blind randomized trial. *N Engl J Med* 314:1402–1406, 1986.

84. Czer LSC, Bateman TM, Gray RJ, Raymond M, et al: Treatment of severe platelet dysfunction and hemorrhage after cardiopulmonary bypass: reduction in blood product usage with desmopressin. *J Am Coll Cardiol* 9:1139–1147, 1987.

85. Weinstein M, Ware JA, Troll J, Salzman E: Changes in von Willebrand factor during cardiac surgery: effect of desmopressin acetate. *Blood* 71:1648–1655, 1988.

86. Royston D, Bidstrup BP, Taylor KM, Sapsford RN: Effect of aprotinin on need for blood transfusion after repeat open-heart surgery. *Lancet* 2:1289–1291, 1987.

87. Van Oeveren W, Eijsman L, Roozendaal KJ, Wildevuur ChRH: Platelet preservation by aprotinin during cardiopulmonary bypass (letter). *Lancet* 1:644, 1988.

88. Kobrinsky NL, Letts RM, Patel LR, Israels ED, et al: 1-Desamino-8-D-arginine vasopressin (desmopressin) decreases operative blood loss in patients having Harrington rod spinal fusion surgery: A randomized, double-blinded, controlled trial. *Ann Intern Med* 107:446–450, 1987.

89. Morstyn G, Souza LM, Keech J, Sheridan W, et al: Effect of granulocyte colony stimulating factor on neutropenia induced by cytotoxic chemotherapy. *Lancet* 1:667–672, 1988.

90. Socinski MA, Elias A, Schnipper L, Cannistra SA, et al: Granulocyte-macrophage colony stimulating factor expands the circulating haemopoietic progenitor cell compartment in man. *Lancet* 1:1194–1198, 1988.

91. Gabrilove JL, Jakubowski A, Scher H, et al: Effect of granulocyte colony–stimulating factor on neutropenia and associated morbidity due to chemotherapy for transitional-cell carcinoma of the urothelium. *N Engl J Med* 318:1414–1422, 1988.

92. Vadhan-Raj S, Buescher S, LeMaistre A, et al: Stimulation of hematopoiesis in patients with bone marrow failure and in patients with malignancy by recombinant human granulocyte–macrophage colony–stimulating factor. *Blood* 72:134–141, 1988.

93. Nemunaitis J, Singer JW, Buckner CD, et al: Use of recombinant human granulocyte–macrophage colony–stimulating factor in autologous marrow transplantation for lymphoid malignancies. *Blood* 72:834–836, 1988.

94. Donahue RE, Seehra J, Metzger M, et al: Human IL-3 and GM-CSF act synergistically in stimulating hematopoiesis in primates. *Science* 241:1820–1823, 1988.

95. Mannucci PM, Remuzzi G, Pusineri F, Lombardi R, et al: Deamino-8-D-arginine vasopressin shortens the bleeding time in uremia. *N Engl J Med* 308:8–12, 1983.

96. Mannucci PM, Vicente V, Vianello L, et al: Controlled trial of desmopressin in liver cirrhosis and other conditions associated with a prolonged bleeding time. *Blood* 67:1148–1153, 1986.

97. De la Fuente B, Kasper CK, Rickles FR, et al: Response of patients with mild and moderate hemophilia A and von Willebrand's disease to treatment with desmopressin. *Ann Intern Med* 103:6–14, 1985.

98. Pfueller SL, Howard MA, White JG, Menon C, et al: Shortening of bleeding time by 1-Deamino-8-arginine vasopressin (DDAVP) in the absence of platelet von Willebrand factor in Gray platelet syndrome. *Thromb Haemost* 58:1060–1063, 1987.

99. Kobrinsky NL, Tulloch H: Treatment of refractory thrombocytopenic bleeding with 1-desamino-8-D-arginine vasopressin (desmopressin). *J Pediatr* 112:993–996, 1988.

100. Kim HC, Salva K, Fallot PL, et al: Patients with prolonged bleeding time of undefined etiology, and their response to desmopressin. *Thromb Haemost* 59:221–224, 1988.

101. Tomasulo PA, Lenes BA, Noto TA, et al: Automatic special case consultations in transfusion medicine. *Transfusion* 26:186–193, 1986.

102. Coffin CM: Current issues in transfusion therapy: II. Indications for use of blood components. *Postgrad Med* 81:343–350, 1987.

103. Platelet transfusion therapy (editorial). *Lancet* 2:490–491, 1987.

104. Simpson MB: Prospective-concurrent audits and medical consultation for platelet transfusions. *Transfusion* 27:192–195, 1987.

105. Renner SW, Howanitz JH, Fishkin BG: Toward meaningful blood usage review: Comprehensive monitoring of physician practice. *QRB* March:76–80, 1987.

106. Lichtiger B, Fischer HE, Huh YO: Screening of transfusion service requests by the blood bank pathologist: Impact on cost containment. *Lab Med* 19:228–230, 1988.

107. Council on Transfusion Medicine of the ASCP Commission on Continuing Education: The expanded role of the pathologist in transfusion medicine. *Lab Med* 19:672–673, 1988.

108. Murphy S: Guidelines for platelet transfusion (editorial). *JAMA* 259:2453–2454, 1988.

109. Crowley JP, Guadagnoli E, Pezzullo J, et al: Changes in hospital component therapy in response to reduced availability of whole blood. *Transfusion* 28:4–7, 1988.

110. Giovanetti AM, Parravicini A, Baroni L, et al: Quality assessment of transfusion practice in elective surgery. *Transfusion* 28:166–169, 1988.

111. Campbell JA: Appropriateness of blood product ordering: Quality assurance techniques. *Lab Med* January:15–18, 1989.

112. Altman SH, Rodwin MA: Halfway competitive markets and ineffective regulation: The American health care system. *J Health Polit Policy Law* 13:323–339, 1988.

2
Basic Virology

Harold V. Lamberson, Jr., MD, PhD

Some of the most complex and puzzling diseases of humans are caused by viruses. Some viral infections, including hepatitis, AIDS, smallpox, and poliomyelitis, result in significant morbidity and mortality. Other viral illnesses such as influenza, measles, mumps, infectious mononucleosis, and herpes can cause substantial discomfort but are rarely life-threatening. Some viruses, such as cytomegalovirus (CMV), are capable of causing morbidity and mortality in certain clinical settings (congenital infection and infection in an immunocompromised host), while the same virus produces no clinical symptoms in most otherwise-healthy hosts. Other viruses have been linked to leukemia and cancer. Clearly, an understanding of general virology as well as detailed knowledge of certain specific viruses is relevant to blood banking. It is my aim to provide a very brief overview of virology that will provide a useful background for the reader of subsequent chapters of this book.

Definition

Viruses are obligate intracellular parasites that contain either DNA or RNA. They are dependent on host cellular biochemical systems for replication. In other words, viruses are nucleic acid molecules and associated proteins that can invade cells. The virus then uses the host cell as a source of energy and biochemical pathways to direct the replication of viral nucleic acid and the production of proteins encoded in the viral nucleic acid.

The following characteristics of viruses help distinguish them from other infectious agents: (1) viruses may be as small as 20 to 30 nm and are below the level of resolution of light microscopy; (2) viruses possess either DNA or RNA, but not both, and thus RNA can function as the genetic material of viruses; (3) viruses lack ribosomes and complex enzyme systems, although they may contain specialized enzymes such as reverse transcriptase, which catalyzes the synthesis of DNA complementary to the RNA in retroviruses; (4) viral replication is intracellular, directed by the viral genome, and can result in large numbers of virions per infected cell; and (5) viruses exhibit considerable host specificity both at the host species and cellular levels.

Structural Characteristics

Viral nucleic acid is encased in a capsid assembled from identical protein subunits. Capsids either can be helical, resulting in a rodlike virus, or icosahedral, resulting in a spherical virus. Functionally, the viral capsid serves to protect the viral nucleic acid from degradative host enzymes. Depending on the virus, the capsid may be surrounded by an envelope. When present, viral envelopes generally consist of a polypeptide backbone coded by the viral genome together with lipids acquired from host cell membranes and carbohydrates of host cell origin.

The presence of an envelope is an important characteristic that is frequently used to characterize viruses. In addition to characteristic morphology disclosed by electron microscopy, enveloped viruses are inactivated by freezing and thawing, and by chemical agents such as lipid solvents and detergents. Glycoproteins associated with the viral envelope are important in the adsorption of viruses to cell surfaces, in infectivity, and in the host immune response. Structural aspects of viruses are summarized in Figure 2–1.

Classification

Many viruses were first recognized in conjunction with the clinical diseases they produce. Consequently, early classification schemes reflected clinical syndromes, hence, the names measles virus, mumps virus, smallpox virus, hepatitis virus, etc. While such a classification scheme may be clinically useful, it does not lead to any logical taxonomic order. There is currently no comprehensive binomial taxonomic classification system equivalent to that for bacteria. The most widely used system uses virion characteristics, such as nucleic acid type, replication cycle, capsid symmetry, and the presence or absence of an envelope, to classify viruses at the level of family, genus and species. The classification system is under purview of the International Committee on Taxonomy of Viruses (ICTV).[1,2] This classification scheme includes seven families of DNA viruses and 14 families of RNA viruses. Detailed reviews of the classification of viruses can be found in the major general virology texts that served as the basis for this review.[3-6] By convention, names of the major families end in *viridae*. Table 2–1 summarizes some of the characteristics of each family of viruses.

DNA Viruses

The seven families of DNA-containing viruses are *poxviridae, iridoviridae, herpesviridae, adenoviridae, papovaviridae, parvoviridae,* and *hepadnavir-*

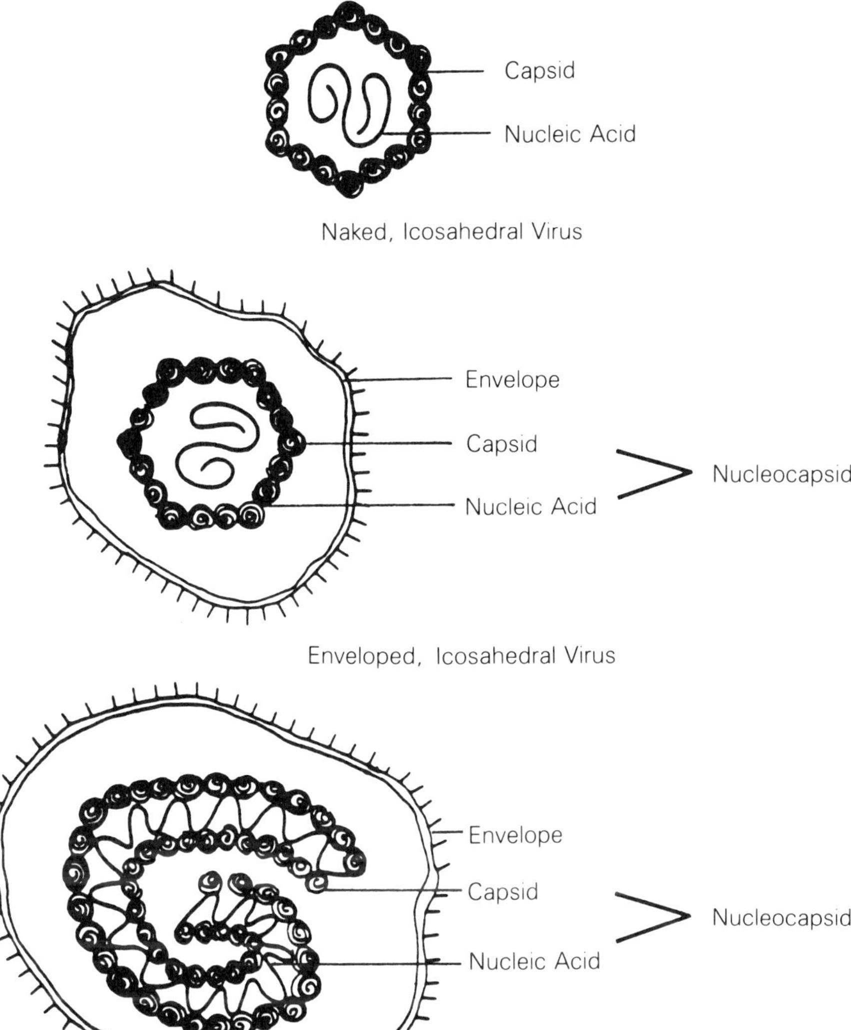

Figure 2–1   Basic structure of human viruses. Viruses consist of a nucleic acid core surrounded by a capsid made up of repetitive protein subunits. The nucleid acid together with the capsid is referred to as a nucleocapsid, which may be either naked or surrounded by an envelope. There are two basic morphologies: icosahedral and helical. (Adapted, with permission, from Davis BD, et al: *Microbiology*. New York, Hoeber Medical Division, Harper & Row, 1967.)

Table 2–1   Classification of Human Viruses

Family	Size, nm	Symmetry	Representative Viruses	Disease Association/Clinical Syndromes
DNA-Containing Viruses: Naked				
Adenoviridae	70-90	Icosahedral	Adenovirus	Respiratory tract infection; gastrointestinal disorders; hemorrhagic cystitis; keratoconjunctivitis
Papovaviridae	55 (papilloma-viruses)	Icosahedral	Papillomavirus	Plantar warts; condylomata accumulata; cervical cancer
	45 (polyoma-viruses)		Polyomaviruses: BK virus JC virus	? Progressive multifocal leukoencephalopathy
Parvoviridae	18-26	Icosahedral	Parvovirus	Usually asymptomatic
DNA-Containing Viruses: Enveloped				
Poxviridae	230 × 300	Complex	Variola Vaccinia Cowpox Molluscum contagiosum Orf	Smallpox Localized skin lesion Localized skin lesion Localized skin lesion Contagious pustular dermatitis
Herpesviridae	100	Icosahedral	Herpes simplex I & II Varicella-zoster Epstein-Barr Cytomegalovirus B-cell lymphotrophic virus	Oral & genital herpes Chickenpox/shingles Infectious mononucleosis/Burkitt's lymphoma Heterophile-negative mononucleosis ?
Hepadnaviridae	42	Complex	Hepatitis B virus	Hepatitis B

Table 2–1 Continued.

Family	Size, nm	Symmetry	Representative Viruses	Disease Association/Clinical Syndromes
RNA-Containing Viruses: Naked				
Picornaviridae	24-30	Icosahedral	Poliovirus	Polio
			Coxsackie A & B	Aseptic meningitis
			Rhinovirus	Common colds
			Echovirus	Diarrhea & respiratory tract infections
			Hepatitis A virus	Hepatitis A
Caliciviridae	35-40	Icosahedral	Calicivirus	Pediatric gastroenteritis
Reoviridae	70-75	Icosahedral	Rotavirus	Pediatric gastroenteritis
			Colorado tick fever virus	Encephalitis
RNA-Containing Viruses: Enveloped				
Togaviridae	60-70	Icosahedral	Alphaviruses: "group A arboviruses"	Equine encephalitis: Eastern, Venezuelan, Western
			Sindbis; Ross River virus; chikungunya; o'nyong-ngong	Viral syndrome, including fever, rash, arthritis, arthralgia
			Rubivirus: rubella virus	German measles
Flaviviridae	45-55	Icosahedral	"Group B arboviruses"	
			Yellow fever virus	Yellow fever
			Dengue virus	Fever, rash, arthralgia
			St Louis encephalitis virus	Encephalitis
			Japanese encephalitis virus	Encephalitis
Arenaviridae	50-300	Helical	Lymphocytic choriomeningitis	Encephalitis (often fatal)
			Tacaribe viruses	Hemorrhagic fever (frequently fatal)
			Lassa virus	

Continued.

Table 2–1 Continued.

Family	Size, nm	Symmetry	Representative Viruses	Disease Association/Clinical Syndromes
Bunyaviridae	80-110	Helical	"Group C arboviruses" Rift Valley fever virus Hantann virus California encephalitis virus group	Retinitis, fever, arthralgia Korean hemorrhagic fever Fever, rash, encephalitis
Coronaviridae	80-130	Helical	Human coronavirus strain HCV-229E	? Upper respiratory tract infections
Filoviridae	80 (diameter) variable length	Helical	Marburg virus; Ebola virus	Acute hemorrhagic fever (frequently fatal)
Orthomyxoviridae	80-120	Helical	Influenza A, B, C	Epidemic Influenza
Paramyxoviridae	150-300	Helical	Paramyxovirus Parainfluenza Mumps Virus Morbillivirus: measles virus (rubeola) Pneumovirus: respiratory syncytial virus	Croup/Common Cold Parotitis, Orchitis, Meningoencephalitis Measles/Subacute Sclerosing Panencephalitis Pneumonia & bronchiolitis in children
Rhabdoviridae	180 × 75	Bullet-shaped helical	Lyssavirus: rabies virus	Encephalitis (almost always fatal)

Table 2–1　Continued.

Family	Size, nm	Symmetry	Representative Viruses	Disease Association/Clinical Syndromes
Retroviridae	100	Icosahedral	Oncovirinae 　HTLV-I 　HTLV-II	Adult T-cell leukemia/Tropical Spastic Paresis Hairy cell leukemia
			Lentivirinae: (Visna group) 　HIV-1 　HIV-2	AIDS
Incompletely Characterized				
Non-A, non-B hepatitis agent	27	Naked icosahedral	Non-A, non-B hepatitis virus(es)	Hepatitis: 90% of posttransfusion cases
Delta hepatitis virus	36	Circular RNA envelope of HBsAg protein	Delta agent	Hepatitis: always associated with hepatitis B infection
Chronic infectious neuropathic agents	Unknown	Unknown	Kuru agent Creutzfeldt-Jakob agent	Acute spongiform encephalopathies Kuru Creutzfeldt-Jakob disease

idae. Following is a brief review of each of these families with emphasis on the human pathogens in the group. More detailed descriptions of each of the families will be found in references 1 through 6.

Poxviridae are relatively large, 230 × 300-nm, brick-shaped, double-stranded DNA viruses that are pathogenic in several animal species, including humans. Human pathogens in this family include variola (smallpox), vaccinia, cowpox, orf (contagious pustular dermatitis), and molluscum contagiosum. Of the poxviruses, only variola major, the smallpox agent, appears to be capable of causing significant morbidity and mortality in man. Fortunately, previous vaccination programs appear to have eliminated smallpox, with the last two cases occurring in 1978 as a result of laboratory exposure. Currently, the only known reservoirs for the virus are the laboratories of the Centers for Disease Control (CDC), Atlanta, and the Research Institute for Viral Preparations, Moscow. Vaccinia has been used in the past to stimulate protective immunity to variola but is no longer administered for this purpose. Vaccination by this technique was not without complications since vaccinia itself is capable of causing systemic infection, especially in immunocompromised hosts. Recent advances in recombinant DNA techniques have made it possible to insert foreign gene sequences into vaccinia, with the virus then serving as a vector for the foreign gene. This approach to vaccine development would seem to be justified only when the potential benefit outweighs the risks of vaccinia infection. Of note are complications in patients with AIDS that is undiagnosed at the time of exposure to vaccine.[4]

Iridoviridae are enveloped DNA viruses that infect swine, frogs, fish, insects, and mollusks. Only one iridovirus is known to infect mammals (the African swine fever virus). None are known to infect man.

Herpesviridae are enveloped, double-stranded DNA viruses that replicate in the nucleus and acquire an envelope by budding from the nucleus into the cytoplasm. There are five generally recognized human herpes viruses (properly named human herpesvirus 1 through 5) and commonly referred to as herpes simplex virus type 1 (HSV-1; HHV-1), herpes simplex virus type 2 (HSV-2; HHV-2), varicella-zoster virus (VZV; HHV-3) Epstein-Barr virus (EBV; HHV-4), and human cytomegalovirus (HCMV; HHV-5). A proposed addition to the herpes family is human B-cell lymphotropic virus (HBLV; HHV-6) as described by Gallo's group.[7] Human herpes viruses share important biologic properties including cell association, and the ability to produce life-long latent infection, with reactivation often in conjunction with immunosuppression of the infected host.

Herpes simplex 1 and 2 most commonly cause vesicular lesions of the oropharynx, eye, skin and genitalia. It is often said that HSV-1 causes infection above the waist and HSV-2 below the waist. This is an empirical observation and does not represent viral specificity. Varicella-zoster virus (HHV-3) causes chickenpox as a primary infection, usually in children. Reactivation of varicella-zoster virus infection in adults causes shingles, a painful vesicular rash following dermotomal pattern. EBV (HHV-4) is frequently asymptomatic in children but in adolescents and young adults causes infectious mononucleosis. EBV is associated epidemiologically with Burkitt's lymphoma and nasopharyngeal carcinoma. Additionally, the EBV genome has been detected in these tumors. Human CMV (HHV-5) infection most commonly results in asymptomatic infection in the immunocompetent host, but can cause a heterophil-negative, mononucleosislike syndrome. In general, primary infections with human CMV are clinically more severe in the immunocompromised host. Since human CMV is transmissible by cellular blood components from some donors who are seropositive for antibody to human CMV, and human CMV infection can cause severe disease in certain clinical situations, including the fetus in utero, low birth weight premature infants, and immunocompromised adults, it is of concern to blood bankers.

Adenoviridae are double-stranded DNA viruses that infect many species of animals. There are presently 41 recognized human serotypes. Some are highly prevalent but have no known pathogenicity. The clinical symptoms caused by different serotypes vary, and include respiratory tract infections, gastrointestinal disease, hemorrhagic cystitis, and keratoconjunctivitis. Some adenoviruses are capable of establishing latent or masked infection in lymphoid tissue.

Papovaviridae is a contraction derived from papilloma-polyoma-simian vacuolating agent. These naked, double-stranded DNA viruses can be classified into two groups based on size. The papillomaviruses have 55-nm capsids. Human papillomaviruses cause a variety of warts, including plantar warts, anogenital warts (condylomata acuminata), and condylomas of the uterine cervix. Accumulating evidence links human papillomavirus to malignant neoplasms of the cervix, vagina, and uterus. Polyomaviruses have 45-nm capsids and include simian vacuolating virus (SV 40) and B.K. and J.C. viruses of man. B.K. virus has been isolated from the urinary tract of immunosuppressed renal transplant patients and J.C. virus from a patient with progressive, multifocal leukoencephalopathy and the initials J.C. The latter virus is recognized as the agent causing progressive, multifocal leukoencephalopathy. The nomenclature serves to confuse students of virology, since J.C. virus bears no relationship to Creutzfeldt-Jakob disease, a chronic progressive fatal infection of the central nervous system of man, which is caused by an as yet incompletely characterized transmissible agent.

Parvoviridae are single-stranded DNA viruses that infect several animal species, including man. Human parvoviruslike agent was discovered fortuitously by Cossart and colleagues[8] while screening blood donors by counterimmunoelectrophersis for hepatitis B surface antigen using polyvalent human sera. Parvoviruslike infection is common and asymptomatic in healthy children. Serologic evidence of recent parvovirus infection has been reported in patients with sickle cell disease in aplastic crisis.[4]

Hepadnaviridae consist of a relatively small, partly double-stranded, partly single-stranded DNA molecule together with a DNA polymerase and a lipoprotein (hepatitis B surface antigen: HBsAg) envelope. Hepatitis B is the only virus of this family recognized to infect man. Included in the family are the hepatitis B viruses of woodchucks, ground squirrels, ducks, and tree squirrels. Hepatitis B virus is highly infectious and transmissible by blood and body fluids of viremic hosts. This virus is reviewed in detail in Chapter 6: "Transfusion-Associated Hepatitis."

RNA Viruses

RNA-containing viruses include the picornaviridae, caliciviridae, togaviridae, flaviviridae, arenaviridae, bunyaviridae, coronaviridae, filoviridae, orthomyxoviridae, paramyxoviridae, rhabdoviridae, reoviridae, birnaviridae, and retroviridae.

Picornaviridae are small ("pico"), 24- to 30-nm, single-stranded RNA–containing viruses with no envelope. The picornaviridae contain four genera: enterovirus, cardiovirus, rhinovirus, and apthovirus. The genera enterovirus includes several important human pathogens, among them poliovirus, Coxsackie A and B viruses, echoviruses (*enteric cytopathic human orphan*), and hepatitis A virus (human enterovirus 72). Enteroviruses are acid-stable, a characteristic that enables them to survive the acid conditions of the stomach and reproduce in the intestinal tract.

Enteroviruses cause a wide spectrum of clinical disease including poliomyelitis, hepatitis A, aseptic meningitis, diarrhea, upper respiratory tract infections, herpangina, and pleurodynia. While the coxsackie A viruses are a cause of the common cold, this syndrome is more frequently caused by rhinoviruses. There are more than 100 serotypes of rhinoviruses. Presumably their antigenic variation and serologic diversity contributes to the frequency of the common cold. The subgroups cardiovirus and aphthovirus are not considered to be important human pathogens.

Caliciviridae are relatively small (35- to 40-nm), nonenveloped, single-stranded RNA–containing viruses. Some evidence indicates that calciviruses may be associated with pediatric gastroenteritis.

Togaviruses are enveloped, 60- to 70-nm, RNA–containing viruses. "Toga," Latin for cloak, is descriptive of the envelope with its associated spikes. Important human pathogens in this group include members of the genera alphavirus and rubivirus. Alphaviruses were previously classified as the "group A arboviruses," recognizing their dependence on an insect vector (mosquito or tick). Pathogenic alphaviruses include eastern equine encephalitis, Venezuelan equine encephalitis, and western equine encephalitis. Other alphaviruses include chikungunya, o'nyong-ngong, sindbis, and Ross River viruses, which produce similar clinical symptoms including fever, rash, arthritis, and arthralgias.

The sole member of the subgroup rubivirus is the rubella virus, the etiologic agent of German measles. While rubella infection is generally self-limited and of no major consequence in the postnatal period, it is well known to cause congenital defects, including deafness, heart disease, eye defects, growth retardation, thrombocytopenic purpura, osteitis, hepatitis, pneumonia, encephalitis and cerebral damage, especially when the infection occurs during the first 3 months of pregnancy. Two additional subgroups in the family togaviridae, artervirus and pestivirus, cause disease in animals but not in humans.

Flaviviridae were previously classified as the "group B arboviruses" in the family togaviridae. However, flaviviruses are antigenically distinct and their replicative cycle sufficiently different from the togaviruses to designate a discreet family. The flavivirus family (latin *flavus*, yellow for the prototype yellow fever virus) are 45- to 55-nm enveloped viruses with icosahedral nucleocapsids. Transmission of flaviviruses generally involves an insect vector (mosquitos or ticks). Human pathogens include the yellow fever virus, dengue virus, St Louis encephalitis, Japanese encephalitis and other encephalitic viruses. The hepatitis C virus has some characteristics of the flavivirus family.

Seven families of RNA-containing viruses (arenaviridae, bunyaviridae, coronaviridae, filoviridae, orthomyxoviridae, paramyxoviridae, and rhabdoviridae) share the common characteristic of helical nucleocapsids surrounded by an envelope.

Arenaviridae are characterized morphologically by well-defined envelopes enclosing two helical nucleocapsids. Arenaviridae are natural parasites of rodents, in which they characteristically produce lifelong, asymptomatic infections. The same viruses infect humans and may produce fatal encephalitis (lymphocytic choriomeningitis virus) or hemorrhagic fever, which is frequently fatal (tacaribe viruses and lassa virus).

Bunyaviridae were formerly categorized as the "group C arboviruses." There are currently four subgroups within the family, each containing several serologically related viruses. Several members of the bunyaviridae family are pathogenic in man, causing symptoms such as fever, rash, encephalitis, and hemorrhagic fever.

Coronaviridae derive their name from the characteristic large, petal-shaped spikes attached to the envelope. Several members of the family are pathogenic in animals, but no major human pathogens have been recognized. An association with upper respiratory tract disease is possible.

Filoviridae is proposed as a new family with unique morphology, consisting of filaments of uniform diameter (80 nm), but variable length (up to 14,000 nm). There are two members of this family, the Marburg virus and the Ebola virus, both of which cause an acute hemorrhagic fever that is frequently fatal.

The former family myxoviridae (a term denoting affinity of these viruses for glycoproteins) has been reclassified as two families, orthomyxoviridae and paramyxoviridae. Both families include agents of considerable medical significance. The family orthomyxoviridae includes one subgroup of three species: influenza virus type A, type B, and type C. Influenza viruses possess two types of glycoprotein spikes on the envelope, which function as hemagglutinins or as neuraminidase. Hemagglutinins are responsible for adsorption of the virus to host cell receptors. The ubiquitous orthomyoviridae are the cause of epidemic influenza.

The family paramyxoviridae includes three subgroups: paramyxovirus, morbillivirus, and pneumovirus. Paramyxoviridae that are important in humans include the parainfluenza viruses, which cause respiratory tract infections, and the mumps virus. The morbillivirus of importance to humans is the measles (rubeola) virus, which is also considered to be the agent of subacute sclerosing panencephalitis, a chronic degenerative disease of the central nervous system. The genus *Pneumovirus* includes respiratory syncytical virus, an important human pathogen causing pneumonia and bronchiolitis in infants and children.

Rhabdoviridae have a characteristic bullet or brick shape. There are several members of this family that are pathogenic in animals. However, the only member of direct significance to man is the rabies virus, a lyssavirus.

Reoviridae are double-stranded RNA–containing viruses. They are not enveloped and they characteristically have two distinct capsid shells. There are six subgroups of reoviridae, but only two cause human disease: rotavirus, which commonly causes acute gastroenteritis in humans, and Colorado tick fever virus, which can cause encephalitis.

Birnaviridae are double-stranded RNA–containing viruses, with a diameter of approximately 60-nm of icosahedral symmetry. There are no known human pathogens in this group.

The retroviridae are of major importance to blood banks and are discussed in detail in Chapters 3 through 5. The retroviridae family is characterized by a common morphology, the presence of reverse transcriptase, and the presence of two identical strands of RNA. Virions contain a coiled nucleocapsid surrounded by a core shell and an envelope. The reverse transcriptase is a unique characteristic of retroviruses from which they derive the ability to produce DNA that is complimentary to the viral RNA. This complimentary proviral DNA can be integrated into the host cellular DNA. Thus, through the action of reverse transcriptase, viral RNA serves as a template for the production of complimentary DNA, which is apparently randomly inserted into and copied with the host cellular DNA. This unique attribute of retroviruses provides the fundamental basis for their ability to produce lifelong infections and to transform host cells. There are currently three subfamilies recognized within the family retroviridae: oncovirinae, lentivirinae, and spumavirinae. Oncornavirinae are oncogenic and cause leukemias, lymphomas, mammary tumors and neuronal tumors in animals. The oncornavirinae subfamily includes HTLV-I, which causes adult T-cell leukemia and tropical spastic paraperesis in man, and HTLV-II, which is associated with hairy cell leukemia. Lentivirinae share the above-noted characteristics of oncornavirinae but do not transform cells. Lentiviruses are sometimes referred to as the "visna group" of viruses. Visna is well known to veterinarians as a slow virus disease of sheep. Human immunodeficiency virus type I (HIV-I, formerly HTLV-III or LAV) is a member of the lentivirinae subfamily. The third subfamily, the spumavirinae, are recognized for their ability to cause the formation of multinucleated giant cells with a foamy appearance in cell culture. No members of this subfamily are recognized to be human pathogens.

Finally, there remain some important etiologic transmissible agents that are either incompletely characterized or do not fit into the classification system described. The agent of non-A, non-B hepatitis has not been isolated and cultured as yet. Chapter 6 reviews the current knowledge of non-A, non-B hepatitis. Recent advances in identification of viral gene sequences associated with non-A, non-B hepatitis should permit further characterization of the non-A, non-B agent.

Hepatitis delta virus will be reviewed in Chapter 6. The delta agent is a defective virus that has an obligate requirement of coinfection with hepatitis B virus. The delta agent consists of self-associated RNA, a corresponding delta protein, and an outer coat of HBsAg.

There is a group of chronic, progressive, fatal infections of the central nervous system known as the subacute spongiform encephalopathies. Two such diseases of man are kuru and Creutzfeldt-Jakob disease. Kuru is characterized by cerebellar ataxia, progressing to total incapacitation and death over a period of 3 to 9 months. Fortunately, the incidence of kuru, which is limited to the New Guinea highlands, has been decreasing steadily, presumably as a result of cessation of certain cannibalistic rituals. Creutzfeldt-Jakob disease is a rare disease of the central nervous system characterized by rapidly progressing dementia, with myoclonus and progressive motor dysfunction. The disease is usually fatal. The agents of kuru and Creutzfeldt-Jakob disease, while clearly transmissible, are not recognizable as virions by electron microscopy. The term "prion" (acronym for proteinacious infectious particle) has been coined to represent this class of infectious agents, the nature of which remains undetermined. Transmission of Creutzfeldt-Jakob disease is known to occur by direct tissue-to-tissue contact following transplantation but not by sexual means nor from mother to child across the placenta. Reports of transmission have been reported in recipients of human derived pituitary growth hormone. This observation, along with the theoretical possibility of transmission by blood transfusion requires that potential blood donors who have received human pituitary derived growth hormone be permanently deferred. A review of slow virus infections can be found in references by Gajdusek[9] and Johnson.[10]

Biology of Viral Replication

Intact infectious virions lack energy-producing metabolic pathways and are in fact inert. Only by entering a susceptible host cell and redirecting the intracellular events can a virus replicate and under certain circumstances produce clinically recognizable disease. The molecular biology of the interactions of the virus and host cell is extremely diverse and complex. There are however, certain common themes that provide a useful background for the understanding of the interaction of specific viruses with host cells. Viral infection is often considered as a series of steps that includes attachment, penetration, replication, and release of infectious viral progeny.

The first step in the interaction of virus and host cell is *attachment* or *adsorption* of the virus to the cell surface. This process generally involves specific glycoprotein receptor molecules on the cell surface and complimentary "antireceptors" on the virus. Specificity of the interaction between receptors and antireceptors is a determinant of susceptibility of cells to infection with a particular virus. One example of relevance to blood bankers is the role of the CD4 molecule as a cellular receptor for HIV-1. HIV-1 infects cells that express the CD4 molecule. Included are CD4(+) lymphocytes, peripheral blood monocytes, and certain tissue macrophages. Indeed, much of the pathobiology of HIV-1 is determined by the receptor specificity during the attachment phase of the infection.[11,12]

Attachment is followed by *penetration* and *uncoating* of the viral nucleic acid, allowing viral enzymes and nucleic acid access to cellular biochemical pathways. Nonenveloped viruses enter the host cell by translocation of the entire virus across the plasma membrane or by pinocytosis. Many enveloped viruses (eg, herpesviruses) enter by fusion of specific viral envelope protein with the cellular plasma membrane, releasing viral constituents into the cytoplasm.

Attachment, penetration, and uncoating are collectively referred to as the *eclipse phase* of viral infection. This terminology reflects the in vitro observation of a decrease in the number of detectable infectious virions in conjunction with these events. An increase in the number of infectious particles requires subsequent replication and release of the virus.

Viral multiplication involves the organization and execution of the expression and replication of viral genome. Details of viral multiplication are difficult to summarize in general terms since the sequence of molecular biologic events is a characteristic of the virus and its interaction with the infected host cell. A few generalizations are, however, possible and serve as a useful framework for the understanding of the events in the replicative cycle of specific viruses. One generalization is eukaryotic cells synthesize their own messenger RNA (mRNA) exclusively in the nucleus by transcription of cellular DNA. Eukaryotic cells lack the ability to synthesize viral mRNA from a viral RNA genome, and eukaryotic cells lack the enzymes to transcribe viral DNA in the cytoplasm.

Some further generalizations are possible based on the genetic materials of the virus. The genomic RNA of some single-stranded RNA viruses is capable of serving directly as mRNA. By convention, such viruses are designated (+)-stranded. Picornaviruses are (+)-stranded RNA viruses. Picornavirus RNA binds directly with host cellular ribosomes, resulting in translation to a polyprotein that on cleavage gives rise to viral proteins that include a viral polymerase that synthesizes a complimentary (−)-stranded RNA. The newly synthesized minus strand then serves as the template for additional (+)-strands that can serve as messengers or templates for additional (−)-strands or as the genome of progeny virus. Since the genomic RNA serves directly as mRNA using the host cell's protein-synthesizing capabilities, it is logical that naked (+)-stranded RNA extracted from virions can be infectious.[13]

Other RNA viruses, including the orthomyxoviruses, paramyxoviruses, bunyaviruses, arenaviruses, and rhabdoviruses are (−)-stranded RNA viruses. Since only (+)-stranded RNA can serve as mRNA and eukaryotic cells lack the necessary enzymes to produce mRNA from viral genomic RNA, these viruses require a viral transcriptase for the synthesis of (+)-stranded RNA to serve as mRNA and as template RNA for the synthesis of additional (−)-strands. Consequently, purified naked (−)-stranded viral RNA is not infectious.[12]

As previously noted, the retroviridae share as a common characteristic the presence of a reverse transcriptase that uses the viral genomic RNA as a template to produce viral DNA. The viral RNA is then digested by a viral ribonuclease and a complementary strand of DNA is synthesized. This double-stranded DNA is then apparently inserted randomly into the host cellular DNA.[13,14]

Of the DNA viruses, the papovaviridae, parvoviridae, and herpesviridae genomes are all transcribed and replicated in the nucleus using host cellular transcriptional enzymes. As a consequence, purified DNA from these viruses is infectious.[13]

The poxviridae differ in that initial transcription takes place in the cytoplasm and hence requires viral transcriptional enzymes.[13]

The hepatitis B virus, of the family hepadnaviridae, is unique in that the partially double-stranded genomic viral DNA is converted to supercoiled DNA and then transcribed into mRNA and genomic RNA. A viral reverse transcriptase then synthesizes the viral progeny genomic DNA.[13]

In summary, replication of viral nucleic acids, as well as transcription and translation to the proteins coded in viral gene sequences, is a complex series of events that is generally under the direction of viral gene products that serve as regulators of the various events. On completion of expression of the viral genome, progeny viral nucleic acid is encased in viral structural protein. Intact progeny viruses are then released either by death and lysis of the infected cell or by budding of the virus such that an enveloped virus is released, often without destruction of the infected host cell.

Laboratory Diagnosis of Viral Infections

With the recognition of recently discovered pathogenic human viruses such as HIV and HTLV-I, progress in the elucidation of non-A, non-B hepatitis, detailed knowledge of hepatitis B, and an appreciation of the potential for ubiquitous viruses such as cytomegalovirus (CMV) to cause disease, a working knowledge of the laboratory diagnosis of viral infections is of increasing importance in blood banking and transfusion medicine. General methods of viral diagnosis include viral isolation, direct detection of viral gene products or viral nucleic acid sequences in patient specimens, and detection of host serologic response to viral antigens.

Viral Isolation

Since viruses are obligate intracellular parasites, it follows that laboratory propagation of viruses involves the use of living cells. The previously described events of attachment and the molecular events involved in intracellular viral replication often result in considerable specificity at the virus–host cell level. This specificity can determine both the species and cell type that will support viral propagation. Many viruses with pathogenic potential for man can be isolated from an appropriate clinical specimen with a relatively limited num-

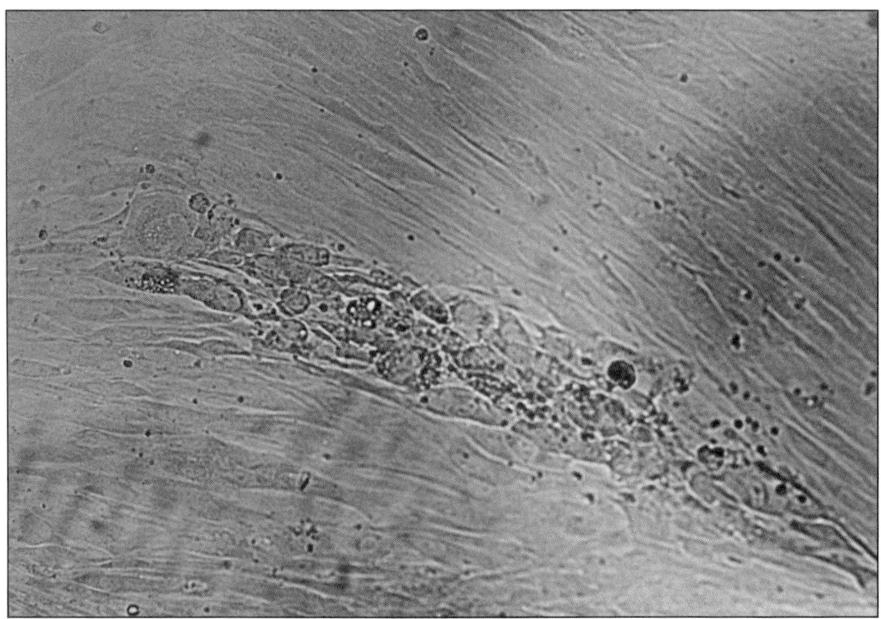

Figure 2–2   This photomicrograph demonstrates the cytopathic effect (CPE) resulting from the infection of human foreskin fibroblasts with CMV. At center are foci of rounded, refractile, degenerating cells that are frequently described as having a ground glass–like appearance. Foci of CPE are surrounded by uninfected fibroblasts. The focal nature of CPE produced by CMV is related to the fact that CMV is cell-associated and spreads from cell to cell in the tissue culture monolayer.

ber of cell lines. Three types of cell cultures are routinely used in clinical diagnostic laboratories: primary cultures, which are prepared by trypsinizing fresh tissue such as monkey kidney or human amnion; semicontinuous cell lines such as human embroyonic lung or human foreskin fibroblasts, which can be subcultured for 30 to 40 passages; and continuous cell lines such as the Hela cell line derived from a human cervical cancer, which can be grown in culture indefinitely. In routine clinical diagnostic work, the presence of a virus in cell cultures can be recognized by the production of a characteristic cytopathic effect, the hemadsorption of reagent erythrocytes added to the culture, or direct or indirect immunofluorescence staining. Additional techniques for the detection of viruses in culture include visualization by electron microscopy, detection of viral antigen by enzyme-linked immunosorbent assay (ELISA), detection of viral enzymes such as reverse transcriptase, or the direct detection of viral nucleic acid sequences. Figure 2–2 illustrates the typical cytopathic effect of a human herpes virus in laboratory culture. Depending on the strain of virus and the inoculum size these cytopathologic characteristics take 2 to 4 weeks to develop. Demonstration of the presence of viral antigens in the culture can expedite the diagnostic process substantially. Figure 2–3 illustrates the utility of immunofluorescence in rapid viral

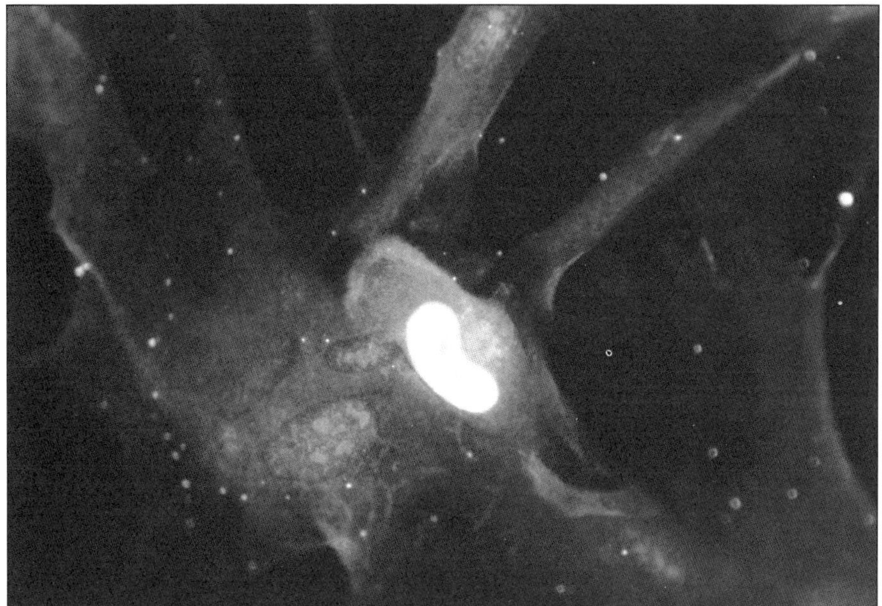

Figure 2–3   Indirect immunofluorescence staining to identify CMV in cell culture. This photomicrograph shows intense, homogeneous fluorescence in the nucleus of a cell infected with CMV. Staining is with mouse monoclonal anti immediate early protein followed by fluorescein conjugated antimouse immunoglobulin (magnification, X 400). Photo courtesy of Ellyn Lentz.

diagnosis. Figure 2–3 shows specific staining of viral "early antigens" 2 days after inoculation of the culture. Staining is with a mouse monoclonal antibody to a CMV "early antigen." Increasing availability of monoclonal antibodies surely will contribute to the availability of rapid viral diagnostic methodologies. Monoclonal antibodies are adaptable to ELISA techniques in addition to immunofluorescence techniques. Hemadsorption is not illustrated but results from the adsorption of reagent erythrocytes to the hemagglutinin proteins present on the envelopes of some viruses such as influenza. Figure 2–4 illustrates the in situ hybridization of a radiolabeled probe for the J fragment of the CMV genome to CMV-encoded nucleic acid in CMV-infected human fibroblasts. In addition to the demonstration of CMV nucleic acids in infected cell cultures, this probe has also been used to detect CMV-coded nucleic acid in peripheral blood mononuclear cells.[15,16]

Many viruses of interest to blood bankers cannot be grown in the cell lines routinely used for diagnostic viral isolation. Some can be cultured using more specialized techniques, while others such as hepatitis B virus and non-A, non-B hepatitis viruses have not been isolated in culture and are propagated only by primate inoculation.

Growth of the retroviruses requires specialized culture conditions. Commonly, blood or body secretions, often containing host cells, are cocultivated

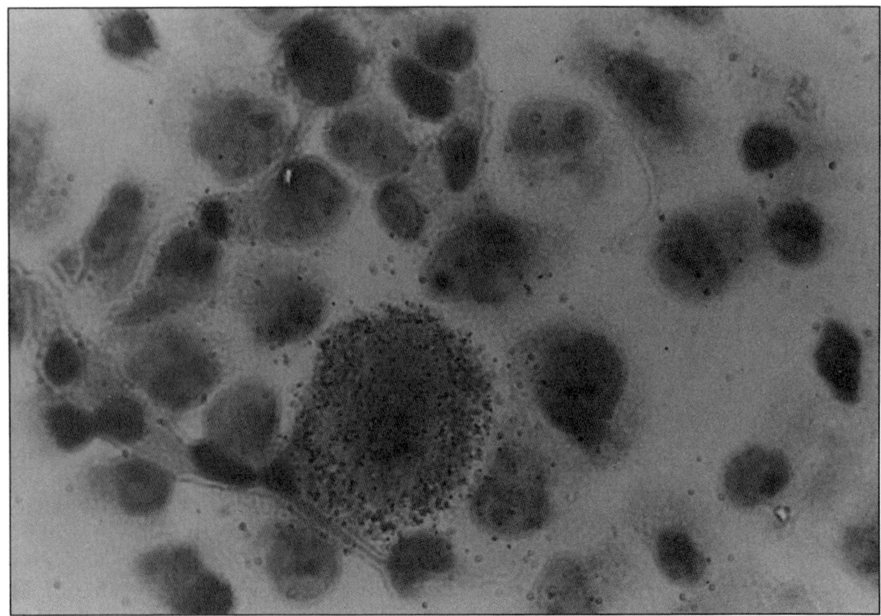

Figure 2–4   In situ hybridization. This photomicrograph shows a human foreskin fibroblast cell infected with CMV (laboratory strain AD169) that has been hybridized with a CMV-specific probe, yielding black grains at the sites of specific nucleic acid hybridization. Other cells in the field are uninfected. The cells have been incubated 48 hours in the presence of cytosine arabinoside to inhibit DNA replication (magnification, × 400). (Photomicrograph provided by B.A. Forbes, State University of New York Health Science Center, Syracuse.)

with a susceptible lymphoid cell line (eg, H-9, CEM) with the addition of growth promoting factors such as T-cell growth factor (interleukin-2). While retroviruses often cause characteristic cytopathologic changes, their presence is often detected by assaying cultures for the presence of reverse transcriptase. Since reverse transcriptase is produced by all retroviridae, it is a nonspecific marker for retroviruses. Detection of specific viral proteins using either polyclonal or monoclonal antibodies in antigen-capture ELISAs is often both a sensitive and specific indicator of virus propagation. Hybridization of specific probes to viral nucleic acid extracted from cultures and the polymerase chain reaction (PCR) are also adaptable for the demonstration of virus in culture. Finally, electron microscopy with direct visualization of virus particles can often provide specific verification of the presence of viruses in culture and clinical specimens.

While many viruses can be propagated in the laboratory and others can be propagated by animal inoculation, interpretation of culture results requires that both the sensitivity and specificity of the culture and detection systems be considered. It is essential that both routine clinical diagnostic and research laboratories appropriately utilize positive and negative controls to establish maintenance of appropriate sensitivity and specificity. Finally, the inherent limitations of a negative viral culture must be appreciated. Specimen quality, inoculum size, state of the viral infection in the patient, and the growth requirements of the virus can all contribute to a negative viral culture. In fact, since hepatitis B and the non-A, non-B viruses have not been isolated in cell cultures, and the isolation of retroviruses requires specialized techniques, these viruses are routinely diagnosed by serologic techniques. Similarly, while CMV is routinely recovered from appropriate clinical specimens of patients with an active CMV infection, viral isolation is of no practical value for the purpose of detecting infectious blood donors. Fortunately, serologic methods for the detection of viral antigens and antibody are adaptable for large-scale, rapid screening of donor specimens. Texts by Lennette,[17] Specter and Lancz,[18] and Grist and colleagues[19] are sources of more detailed information on techniques for viral isolation.

Viral Serology

While a variety of techniques are available for the detection of viral antigen-antibody reactions, ELISA is readily adaptable to the production laboratory setting for the purpose of screening for the presence of viral antigen or antibody. ELISA has all but completely replaced radioimmunoassays since it obviates the need for radioactive material and yields similar sensitivity and specificity. For some purposes, such as the detection of total antibody to CMV, agglutination of antigen-coated latex beads, gelatin particles, or erythrocytes is a suitable alternative. Selection and interpretation of serologic assays requires an understanding of the biology of the virus-host interaction and performance characteristics of the available assays, as a review of the serologic characteristics of HIV-1 infection serves to illustrate.

The "typical" serologic profile of HIV-1 infection is summarized in Figure 2–5. After exposure to the virus there is an initial incubation period during which the host is asymptomatic and viral culture is negative and viral antibody is undetectable. Following this incubation period, infection progresses to an acute phase that may include the symptoms of acute HIV-I infection (fever, flulike illness) and during which viral cultures are likely to be positive. This phase may be clinically asymptomatic, with virus present in the circulation and antibody levels below detectable limits, a situation of concern to blood bankers. This phase is often referred to as a "serologic window" during which a donor can be asymptomatic, seronegative, viremic, and infectious. This phase is followed by antibody production and seroconversion. The sequence of antibody development to specific viral antigens is probably determined both by the biology of the host-virus interaction and the performance characteristics of the assays used to detect antibody. For example, western blot analysis of early seroconversion specimens frequently shows antibody to viral core protein (p24) to be present before formation of antibody specific for viral envelope antigens (gp41, gp120/160). Using other assays, antibody to envelope glycoproteins may be simultaneously present or even proceed the presence of anti-p24. Proper interpretation of results in this seroconversion

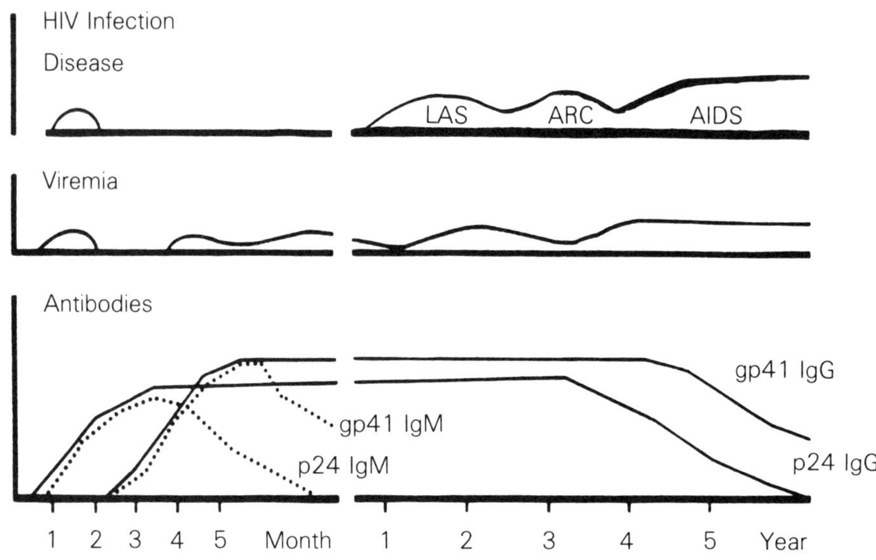

Figure 2–5   Course of infection with human immunodeficiency virus (HIV). LAS indicates lymphadenopathy syndrome; ARC, AIDS-related complex. (Reprinted, by permission, from Deinhardt F: Diagnostic tests for HIV Infection, in: Allain JP, Gallo R, Montagnier L, eds. *Human Retroviruses and Disease They Cause: Symposium Highlights.* Abbott Park, IL, Abbott Laboratories, 1988.)

phase requires a detailed understanding of the performance characteristics of the assays used. Fortunately, this period of seroconversion is usually of brief duration and in most cases antibody to several viral antigens appear and persist throughout the course of the infection. However, the possibility of a prolonged seronegative window period in HIV infection has been described.[20] Reversion to seronegativity in terminal HIV infection due presumably to the combined effect of immunosuppression and overwhelming viremia has also been described.[21] Assays for the direct detection of HIV antigen in the initial seronegative window period and in the late phases of infection were under investigation at this writing.[22]

Interpretation of positive screening tests requires confirmation of the specificity of the reaction since there is potential for serologic cross-reactivity with other retroviruses or reactivity with nonviral antigens contaminating the viral antigen used in preparing screening assays.[23] Figure 2–6 shows a typical seroconversion profile as detected by western blot confirmatory testing. Other useful confirmatory assays include immunofluorescence using HIV-I–infected cells as the source of antigen and assays using recombinant-based viral antigens.

Finally, it must be noted that the typical serologic response described probably represents a significant oversimplification of the serologic events associated with HIV-I and other retroviral infections. Furthermore, the timing

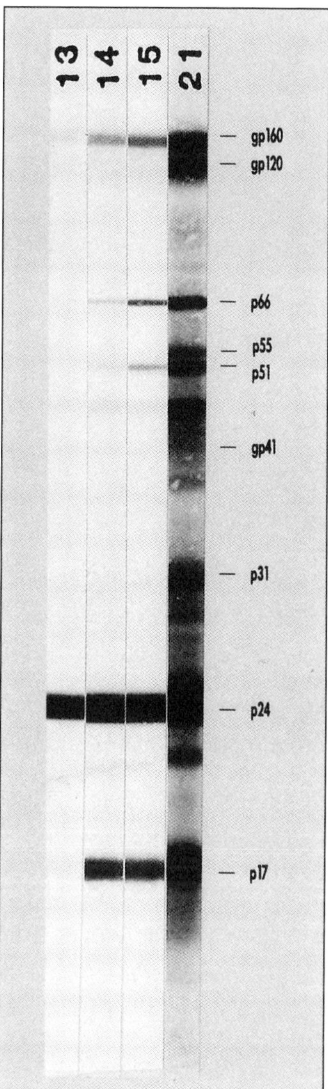

Figure 2–6   Typical seroconversion after human immunodeficiency virus infection as detected by Western blot.

of serologic events associated with exposure to a virus represents a dynamic interaction between the host and the virus. Proper interpretation of results requires a detailed knowledge of the characteristic host response to the virus as well as the natural history of infection with the virus of concern. Knowledge of variations in the response to the virus of concern is also essential. For example, there are several fundamental differences in the serologic response to hepatitis B infection compared with HIV. Antigenemia is readily detected during the acute phase of hepatitis B infection, presumably because hepatitis

Table 2–2   Serologic Response to CMV

Type of Infection	IgM	Anti-EA	IFA	IHA	CF
Congenital*	+ (cord +)	+	+	+(R)	+(R)
Perinatal[†]	+ (cord −)	+(R)[‡]	+(R)	+(R)	+(R)
Acquired	+(R)	+(R)	+(R)	+(R)	+(R)
Carrier (urine, cervix)	±	±	+	+	+
Past (latent)	−	−	+	+	+

*Viral culture positive at birth.

[†]Viral culture negative at birth but positive 2 or more weeks after exposure.

[‡]R indicates rising titer.

B surface antigen is produced in quantities that are in excess of the need for assembly of virions. Antigenemia in acute HIV infection apparently occurs at a much lower level. Antibody to HIV is considered to represent active infection, even if attempts to isolate virus are unsuccessful. Antibody positivity is clearly a marker for infectivity with respect to HIV. By contrast, antibody positivity to HBsAg indicates recovery from the infection with immunity and loss of infectivity since hepatitis B virus does not ordinarily produce a persistent infection. On the other hand, for reasons not completely understood, hepatitis B can in a minority of infections result in a prolonged infection characterized by fluctuating levels of antigen and antibody. With a detailed knowledge of the serologic events associated with a specific virus, assays for IgM antibody or antibody to specific viral antigens may contribute to serologic diagnosis. An example is summarized in Table 2–2, which shows the characteristic serologic profiles of CMV infection.

The fact remains that serologic responses represent a dynamic interaction between the virus and the host and are subject to substantial biologic variability. This is an inherent limitation in serologic approaches to viral diagnosis. Newer techniques to detect viral gene sequences both in clinical specimens and cell cultures offer considerable promise both for elucidating the events associated with infection and for closing the gaps resulting from the inherent limitations of viral culture and serology.

Viral Gene Sequence Detection

As described above, viruses are classified in part on the basis of their nucleic acid composition. Viruses contain either DNA or RNA but not both. Molecular biologic techniques such as dot-blot analysis, restriction endonuclease digestion, and Southern or northern blot analysis are readily adaptable to the study of viruses and infected cells.

The basis for these techniques resides in the basic biochemical structure of nucleic acids. According to the model developed by Watson and Crick, DNA is made up of strands of the nucleotides: adenine (A), thymine (T), guanine (G) and cytosine (C). These purine (A,G) and pyrimidine bases (T,C) are held together by a covalently linked deoxyribose-phosphate backbone. Through hydrogen bonding, adenine and thymine and guanine and cytosine pair, forming a complementary strand of DNA. The strong tendency to form the base pairs A-T and G-C is known as *hybridization* and is the basis of probe technology. RNA is similar to DNA but differs in that the sugar is a ribose sugar, uracil (U) replaces thymidine, and the molecule is usually single-stranded. As noted above, retroviridae have as a characteristic reverse transcriptase that synthesizes a complementary DNA molecule from viral RNA. DNA and RNA are organized such that three adjacent bases form a codon for a specific amino acid. *Probes* are single strands of nucleic acid with a label, usually phosphorus 32 or biotin-avidin, attached to them. Probes are selected to represent a unique DNA/RNA base sequence that is complementary to the viral sequence to be detected. One source of the probes is from the viral nucleic acid of the target virus. For example, viral DNA is extracted from cell cultures, purified, and digested with enzymes called *restriction endonucleases*, which are bacterial enzymes that bind to specific DNA sequences and cleave the DNA at that site. This cleavage at specific sites produces a series of specific fragments that are determined by the specificity of the restriction endonuclease and the base sequence of the nucleic acid being digested. Fragments from the endonuclease digestion can be separated by electrophoresis in gel. Specific sequences of viral DNA can then be recovered and inserted into bacterial plasmids and replicated in quantity in bacteria. Alternatively, base sequences can be synthesized by chemical methods in the laboratory. A discussion of gene isolation and molecular cloning can be found in the report by Macleod.[24]

Labeled nucleic acid probes prepared from subgenomic restriction endonuclease fragments of viral genomes show promise as diagnostic reagents. Nucleic acid probe techniques are potentially of particular value in detecting viruses that are difficult to recover in culture.

A basic requirement and sometimes limitation of this approach is the need for a suitable clinical specimen from which viral nucleic acid can be recovered in sufficient quantity for detection as the target for hybridization with the labeled reagent probes.

Binding of nucleic acid probes can be detected by in situ hybridization, as demonstrated in Figure 2–4. While this technique offers the advantage of localizing the site of target nucleic acid sequences, it is not particularly adaptable as a rapid diagnostic technique since the procedures are technically challenging and interpretation of results can be tedious. Sensitivity is also a consideration since the number of copies of target nucleic acid may be small.

An alternative is to isolate, denature, and bind nucleic acid to a solid support such as nitrocellulose. Labeled probes are allowed to hybridize under appropriate conditions with immobilized nucleic acids. The nitrocellulose filters are then washed, dried, and autoradiographed with X-ray film. This tech-

Specimen DNA is Extracted & Mixed with:

Specific Viral DNA Primer Pairs
DNA Polymerase (*Taq*)
Nucleic Acids
Reaction Buffer
↓
Reaction Mixture Placed in DNA Thermal Cycler

Specimen DNA is Denatured at High Temperature
Primers Anneal to Their Specific Viral DNA Sites at Cool Temperature
Replication of Specific Viral DNA Sequences is catalyzed by DNA Polymerase
(*Taq*)
↓
DNA Thermal Cycler Repeats This Reaction until Reagents are Consumed

Each Cycle Takes Approximately 10 min
The Copy Number of Specific Viral DNA Sequences is Amplified Exponentially by
Repeating this Cycle
25 Standard Cycles can Yield 1 Million–Fold Increase in DNA
For example, <0.1 μg of Specific Viral DNA will be Amplified to 2 μg in 4 h

Figure 2–7   Polymerase chain reaction for DNA amplification.

nique has been used for the rapid diagnosis of CMV in urine[25] and buffy coats[26] of immunosuppressed patients.

A refinement of the dot-blot procedure involves the isolation of DNA followed by restriction endonuclease digestion, gel electrophoresis, and electrophoretic transfer of DNA fragments to nitrocellulose. Probes can then be applied to the nitrocellulose sheet on which DNA fragments have been immobilized. This procedure is known as Southern blotting, since it was developed by E. M. Southern.[27] A variant of the Southern blotting technique is the northern blotting technique in which different conditions are used that permit the binding and detection of RNA fragments. Southern and northern blotting, like dot blotting, require the recovery of sufficient quantities of nucleic acid to be detectable.

A particularly promising technique with greatly enhanced sensitivity for detecting specific DNA sequences is the PCR. With PCR, starting with as little as a single gene copy, DNA sequences can be copied or amplified 1 millionfold or more.[28] Figure 2–7 summarizes the PCR technique. The technique requires short pieces of DNA that are synthesized to be complementary to the purines and pyrimidines flanking the regions of DNA to be amplified.

These synthesized sequences are known as primers and define the ends of the DNA to be duplicated. A thermostable DNA polymerase is added to the mixture of target DNA, primers, and nucleotide triphosphates and the mixture is repeatedly cycled to temperatures that allow the synthesis and dissociation of newly synthesized copies of the target DNA. Typically, 25 to 30 cycles are completed, with each cycle doubling the number of DNA copies synthesized. Thus, 25 cycles results in a 10^6-fold increase in copies. Newly synthesized DNA copies are either detected by DNA fragment analysis or with DNA probes specific to the sequences being sought.[28]

While PCR offers great potential for the diagnosis of infectious diseases and further elucidation of the biology of viral infection, it is at present a research technique. Current limitations include the lack of general availability of primer pairs and the lack of standardization of procedures. Additionally, because of the ability to make millions of copies from a single copy of a target gene sequence, meticulous attention to the possibility of interference from inadvertent contamination should be a major concern.

In summary, complete viral diagnosis requires a coordinated application of techniques for viral culture, serologic study, and detection of gene sequences. Serologic techniques are and will likely remain for the foreseeable future the mainstay in the production blood bank. There appears to be some potential for adaptation of procedures for the detection of viral gene sequences to clinical diagnostic virology. These same procedures also are essential to elucidating the biology of viral infections.

Epidemiology

More than 400 distinct viruses can infect man. Some viruses almost universally produce serious morbidity and mortality when infection occurs (eg, smallpox, rabies). Others produce self-limited illnesses that may result in considerable discomfort and inconvenience (eg, rhinovirus infection). Yet other viruses may cause frequent infection but infrequently cause clinical disease (eg, CMV). The balance between viruses and humans involves several interdependent viral and host factors. Those factors influencing the balance between viruses and humans include the geographic prevalence of the virus, human and nonhuman reservoirs of the virus, mode of transmission of the virus, ability of the virus to mutate, portal of viral entry into the host, site of primary replication of the virus, spread of the virus within the infected host, tropism of the virus (cellular receptors and permissivity of cells), and host responses to viral infection, including humoral immunity, cellular immunity, and interferon production.

For some viruses, geographic variations in prevalence may relate to requirements of the life cycle of the virus. The epidemiology of the arthropod-borne viruses serves to illustrate this point. There are over 400 arthropod-borne viruses, of which about 60 infect man. Some are transmitted by mosquitoes, others by ticks, and others by mites. Most have specific amplifying vertebrate hosts that include birds, monkeys, pigs, horses, wild mammals, and humans. Specificity of the arthropod vector and the amplifying host contributes to the determination of the geographic distribution of the virus.[4,6] For other viruses, such as HIV-1, a complex geographic distribution presumably is explained primarily by the modes of transmission of the virus. Prolonged viremia in infected humans serve as the reservoir, with transmission occurring through sexual or parenteral exposure, primarily to blood. Geographic distribution of viruses can be altered by vaccination practices. In the extreme this can lead to essential elimination of the virus from the population (eg, smallpox).

Modes of transmission of viruses include human (with acute infection or with chronic carrier state) to human, arthropod to human, and other animal to human. Of these modes, the first is the most relevant to transfusion medicine. Human-to-human spread may be by aerosols of the respiratory system, fecal-oral contact, water, breast milk, sexual contact, percutaneous exposure to blood and other infectious fluids, and mucous membrane exposure, including hand-to-mouth and hand-to-conjunctiva. Some viruses are extremely contagious, others, fortunately, are very much less so.

Most viruses that are readily spread person-to-person cause acute, self-limited infection of short duration and usually yield prolonged immunity. This basic characteristic greatly simplifies our task with respect to blood transfusion. This furnishes an explanation for the extremely infrequent transmission of hepatitis A by blood transfusion. Hepatitis A, readily transmitted by the fecal-oral route, has a relatively short incubation period (3 to 4 weeks), with the virus present primarily in the feces for 2 weeks preceding and several weeks after the onset of symptoms. Hepatitis A virus may be present in blood, but only briefly. Furthermore, a substantial proportion of the population has been exposed to hepatitis A virus and has protective immunity. Human-to-human transmission from virus carriers is of more concern to blood bankers. Infections that are inapparent or characterized by recovery from illness with persistence of the virus represent a particular challenge. Persistent or intermittent asymptomatic viremia is the sine qua non for transmission of infection by blood transfusion. Viruses that have this potential include hepatitis B, hepatitis non A–non B, the herpes viruses (particularly CMV), the retroviruses (HIV, HTLV-I), and the slow viruses (Creutzfeldt-Jakob disease). Because primary infections with these agents can be completely asymptomatic and the presence of infectious viruses in blood can be lifelong, current strategies for prevention of transmission rely both on the exclusion of donors who are likely to be infected and on laboratory diagnosis of the infectious carrier state.

Pathogenesis of Viral Infections

Application of molecular biologic techniques to specific viruses and the cells they infect has led to an explosive increase in our knowledge of the pathogenesis of viral infections. Generalizations are somewhat difficult; however, certain basic principles of viral pathogenesis can be summarized. To initiate infection, viruses need to come in contact with cells that they can attach to and penetrate. The example of the CD4 molecule serving as the receptor for HIV has been referenced above. Following penetration, the host cell must be capable of supporting viral replication. To produce clinical symptoms, the virus must be capable of altering cell function or causing cellular injury or death. Host defenses, including humoral immunity, cellular immunity, and other mechanisms such as interferon production, can modulate the viral infection and contribute to the pathogenesis. For the viruses that cause asymptomatic prolonged viremia, it is important to recognize that infection persists, often in the presence of detectable levels of neutralizing antibody and detectable cellular immunity. Furthermore, while some viruses are capable of killing cells directly, the immune response directed against viral antigens and modified host cellular antigens can contribute to the pathogenesis of the infection. The immune complex phase of hepatitis B infection with vasculitis, arthralgia, skin rash, and fever is an example of the direct role of the immune response in the pathogenesis of hepatitis B virus infection.

Prevention and Treatment

Specific chemotherapeutic treatment of viral infections has lagged behind the treatment of bacterial infections. The basis for our lack of antivirals is to be found in the nature of viruses. As described above, viruses by themselves are inert and lacking in the molecular machinery for their own propagation. Many viruses are essentially nucleic acid with a protective protein shell. Hence, the biochemical and molecular events supporting viral replication involve the virus-host cell interaction. Drugs that have been very useful for studying the in vitro molecular biology of viruses (eg, dactinomycin, puromycin, quanidine hydrochloride) have proved either too toxic or ineffective in the treatment of infection. It has, therefore, been difficult to identify drugs that inhibit viral activity without disrupting host cellular metabolism. At present, five drugs are in general use for the treatment of systemic viral infections. These drugs are amantadine, acyclovir, ribavirin, vidarabine, and zidovudine (azidothymidine or AZT).[29]

Amantadine has a very narrow spectrum of activity that is limited to influenza A. Its use is generally reserved for patients who are at high risk because of significant morbidity or mortality during influenza A epidemics. It is given both prophylactically and as specific therapy. Rimantadine is similar to amantadine both in chemical structure as well as in activity. At this writing it was not licensed for clinical use in the United States.[29]

Ribavirin is a synthetic nucleoside that inhibits the enzymes required for viral nucleic acid synthesis. It has a broad spectrum of activity and has been demonstrated to shorten symptoms of influenza A, influenza B, and respiratory syncytial virus infection. Ribavirin is under evaluation in patients with HIV infection.[29] Acyclovir is a synthetic nucleoside that inhibits thymidine kinase, an enzyme coded for by some herpes viruses. Acyclovir is useful in the treatment of herpes simplex infections but it has not been shown to be effective in the treatment of CMV infection. The lack of efficacy in CMV infection is explained by the fact that CMV does not code for thymidine kinase.[29]

Zidovudine is a thymidine analogue that is incorporated by viral reverse transcriptase (HIV) into DNA, leading to interruption of DNA synthesis. While there is no evidence that use of zidovudine results in a virologic cure of HIV infection, it clearly is of therapeutic benefit.[29]

One drug, ganciclovir (DHPG), appears to be inhibitory to CMV in vitro and shows some promise of clinical efficacy. Relapses are, however, apparently common when administration of the drug is discontinued and it cannot, therefore, be considered to be a definitive therapeutic agent.[29] Gancyclovir has been recently approved for the treatment of CMV retinitis in immuno-compromised patients.

Production of interferons has been mentioned above as a host response to viral infections. Host cells infected with certain viruses produce a series of soluble, biologically active substances known as interferons, which are glycoproteins that do not exhibit specificity with respect to the virus that initiated their synthesis. Interferons modulate host cellular events. Modification of host cellular metabolism has a protective effect not only against the virus that stimulated interferon production, but against a wide variety of un-related viruses. Interferons clearly play a protective role during viral infection and there is substantial interest in their efficacy as therapeutic agents. Current classification of interferons recognizes three distinct classes: (1) interferon alpha, which is produced by peripheral blood leukocytes and lymphoid cells (recombinant-based interferon-alpha has also been synthesized); (2) inter-feron beta, which is of fibroblastic origin; and (3) interferon gamma, which is produced by immunologically stimulated lymphocytes. There are many ongoing studies of the interferons as antiviral and antitumor agents.[4,29]

Hyperimmune globulin preparations represent an additional approach to the prevention and moderation of specific viral infections. Hepatitis B immune globulin is of proven efficacy for the prevention of hepatitis B infection fol-lowing exposure to the hepatitis B virus. Varicella-zoster immune globulin is of demonstrated efficacy in the prevention of chickenpox in children who have had close contact with a person with chickenpox. CMV hyperimmune globulin has demonstrated some promise in the treatment of CMV infection in renal and bone marrow transplant recipients.

Since the above-described therapeutic agents are few and of limited ef-ficacy, prevention of exposure is the best strategy for preventing CMV disease in immunocompromised patients. Vaccines may be live attenuated strains of the virus (eg, measles, mumps, rubella, oral polio vaccine), inactivated whole virus (eg, influenza), purified fractions of inactivated viruses (eg, Heptavax™, hepatitis B) and recombinant-based viral protein (eg, Recombivax™, hepatitis B). Hepatitis B vaccine of both types is of demonstrated safety and efficacy and is recommended for prophylaxis of all individuals at increased risk for hepatitis B infection. There is currently no clinically available vaccine for CMV and the prospects for development of a live attenuated vaccine are not good because of the concerns surrounding latency, lifelong infections, and the potential for oncogenicity. Continuing efforts to produce a vaccine for the prevention of HIV infection are referenced in Chapter 13 and in a recent review by Matthews and Bolognesi.[30]

References

1. Andrews CH: Nomenclature of Viruses. *Nature* 173:260–261, 1954.
2. Matthews REF: Classification and nomenclature of viruses. *Intervirology* 17:1–199, 1982.

3. Melnick JL: Structure and classification of viruses, in Belshe RB (ed.): *Human Virology*. Littleton, MA, PSG Publishing Co, 1984, pp 1–28.

4. Joklik WK: *Virology*. East Norwalk, CT, Appleton & Lange, 1988.

5. Matthews REF: Viral taxonomy for the non-virologist. *Ann Rev Microbiol* 39:451, 1985.

6. Murphy FA: Virus taxonomy, in Fields BN (ed): *Virology*. New York, Raven Press, 1985, pp 2–25.

7. Salahuddin SZ, Ablashi DV, Markham PD, et al: Isolation of a new virus, HBLV, in patients with lymphoproliferative disorders. *Science* 234:596–601, 1986.

8. Cossart YE, Field AM, Cant B, Widdows, D: Parvovirus-like particles in human sera. *Lancet* 1:72–73, 1975.

9. Gajdusek CD: Unconventional viruses causing subacute spongiform encephalitis, in Fields BW (ed): *Virology*. New York, Raven Press, 1985, pp 1519–1557.

10. Johnson TC: Persistent-latent slow virus infections and viral oncogenesis, in Paterson PY, Sommers HM (eds): *The Biological Clinical Basis of Infectious Diseases*. Philadelphia, WB Saunders, 1985, pp 45–69.

11. Dalgleish AG, Beverly PC, Clapham PR, et al: The CD4 (T4) antigen is an essential component of the receptor for the AIDS retrovirus. *Nature* 312:763–767, 1984.

12. Maddon PJ, Dalgleish AG, McDougal JS, et al: The T4 gene encodes the AIDS virus receptor and is expressed in the immune system and the brain. *Cell* 47:333–348, 1986.

13. Roizman B: Multiplication of viruses, in Fields BW (ed): *An Overview in Virology*. New York, Raven Press, 1985, pp 69–127.

14. Haseltine WA, Wong-Staal F: The molecular biology of the AIDS virus. *Sci Am* 259:52–62, 1988.

15. Shuster E, Beneke JS, Tegtmeier GE, et al: Monoclonal antibody for rapid laboratory identification of cytomegalovirus infections: Characterization and diagnostic application. *Mayo Clinic Proc* 60:577–585, 1985.

16. Schrier RD, Nelson JA, Oldstone MBA: Detection of human cytomegalovirus in peripheral blood lymphocytes in a natural infection. *Science* 230:1048–1051, 1985.

17. Lennette EH: *Laboratory Diagnosis of Viral Infections*. New York, Marcel Dekker, 1985.

18. Specter S, Lancz GJ: *Clinical Virology Manual*. New York, Elsevier, 1986.

19. Grist NR, Bell EJ, Follett EAC, Urquhart GED: *Diagnostic Methods in Clinical Virology*. Boston, Blackwell Scientific Publications, 1979.

20. Ranki A, Valle SL, Krohn M, et al: Long latency precedes overt seroconversion in sexually transmitted human-immunodeficiency-virus infection. *Lancet* 2:589–593, 1987.

21. Lange J, Goudsmit J: Decline of antibody to HIV core protein secondary to increased production of HIV antigen. *Lancet* 1:448, 1987.

22. Stramer SL, Heller JS, Coombs RW, Ho DD, Allain JP: Transmission of HIV by blood transfusion. *N Engl J Med* 319:513–514, 1988.

23. Dock NL, Lamberson HV, O'Brien TA, et al: Evaluation of atypical human immunodeficiency virus immunoblot reactivity in blood donors. *Transfusion* 28:412–418, 1988.

24. Macleod A: Molecular Cloning, in Macleod A (ed): *Molecular Biology and Human Disease*. Boston, Blackwell Scientific Publications, 1984, 3–20.

25. Chou S, Merigan TC: Rapid detection and quantitation of human cytomegalovirus infection in urine through DNA hybridization. *N Engl J Med* 308:921–925, 1983.

26. Spector S, Rua JA, Spector DH, McMillan R: Detection of human cytomegalovirus in clinical specimens by DNA-DNA hybridization. *J Infect Dis* 150:121–126, 1984.

27. Southern EM: Detection of specific sequences among DNA fragments separated by gel electrophoresis. *J Mol Biol* 98:503–517, 1975.

28. Landegren U, Kaiser R, Caskey CT, Hood L: DNA diagnostics: molecular techniques and automation. *Science* 242:229–237, 1988.

29. Simon HB: Immunizations and chemotherapy for viral infections. *Sci Am Medicine Section XXXIII*, 1988, Ch 7, pp 1–7.

30. Matthews TJ, Bolognesi DP: AIDS vaccine. *Sci Am* 259:120–127, 1988.

3
The Biology of Retroviruses

Jerome A. Zack, PhD
Irvin S.Y. Chen, PhD

Retroviruses have been implicated in a wide variety of diseases in animals and humans. This group of viruses is unique in that it uses a double-stranded DNA intermediate to replicate a single-stranded RNA genome. In man, human T-cell leukemia viruses type I (HTLV-I) and type II (HTLV-II) have been implicated as the causative agents of some forms of leukemia and neurologic disorders; AIDS is caused by HIV. These agents are transmitted sexually, during or shortly after birth, and by administration of contaminated blood and blood products. In this chapter we discuss the basic structure and replication cycle of retroviruses in general, and concentrate specifically on human retroviruses in the areas of gene function and biology.

Taxonomy

Retroviruses are members of the Retroviridae family, based on their RNA genome and reverse transcriptase activity.[1] Members of this family are highly related in their basic genomic structure, chemical composition, and life cycle.[2] The Retroviridae family consists of three subfamilies: the Oncovirinae, which includes transforming retroviruses and their relatives; the Spumavirinae, whose members induce persistent infections and a foamy vacuolization of infected cells; and the Lentivirinae, which include visna virus and HIV, and induce slow, progressive diseases, often with neurologic manifestations.

The Virion

The salient features of all retroviral particles are similar. These include a single-stranded RNA genome consisting of two molecules, usually identical, that resemble eukaryotic messenger RNA (mRNA) packaged in a protein core.[3] This core also contains 20 to 70 copies of the virally encoded proteins necessary for conversion of the single-stranded RNA genome into double-stranded DNA (reverse transcriptase), integration, and proteolysis, as well as cell-derived molecules.[4] The core is surrounded by an envelope consisting of virally encoded glycoproteins and host-derived lipids obtained when the virus is released from the cell by budding. The envelope contains the molecules responsible for binding to virus receptors on target cells. Figure 3–1 shows a schematic representation of a typical retroviral virion.

The Retroviral Life Cycle

The life cycle of retroviruses contains several discrete steps. These viruses must first enter a susceptible host cell. Once the virus has entered, it converts its RNA genome into DNA, which must then integrate into the host genome to form the provirus. The viral genes are expressed and the virion is assembled. After assembly the retrovirus exits the host cell by a process known as budding, at which time it obtains its envelope.

Entry Into a Susceptible Host Cell

The first step in the retroviral life cycle is adsorption of the virion onto the target cell. Retrovirus attachment is believed to be mediated by specific receptors for the retroviral envelope glycoproteins on the cell surface. Binding sites on susceptible cells for purified envelope glycoproteins can be saturated and quantitated.[5] To date, however, only the receptor for HIV has been identified. This is the CD4 molecule, found on a subset of T lymphocytes and on macrophages.[6-8] Although the receptor for HTLV-I/-II has not been identified, it is not CD4, as CD4($-$) cells are susceptible to infection by these viruses. Penetration of the cell by the virion is believed to be mediated by endocytosis of the virion-receptor complex.[9] In addition to endocytosis, a slightly different mechanism of virus entry seems to operate in the infection of some cells by HIV. In this case, fusion of infected cells with uninfected cells, mediated by an envelope glycoprotein–CD4 interaction, can transfer the virus.[10] After penetration, the retroviral envelope is removed in the cytoplasm.[11]

Reverse Transcription

The virion particle contains two copies of the genomic RNA template, reverse transcriptase, and the cell-derived transfer RNA (tRNA) primer. Upon entry into a host cell, synthesis of viral DNA occurs in the cytoplasm, resulting in a linear DNA molecule containing identical repeat segments at each end. Figure 3–1 illustrates these duplicated sequences (see below for a discussion of the retroviral genome).

The reverse transcription process is very complex.[11,12] Briefly, the reaction is primed by the host tRNA contained in the virion, which hybridizes to a

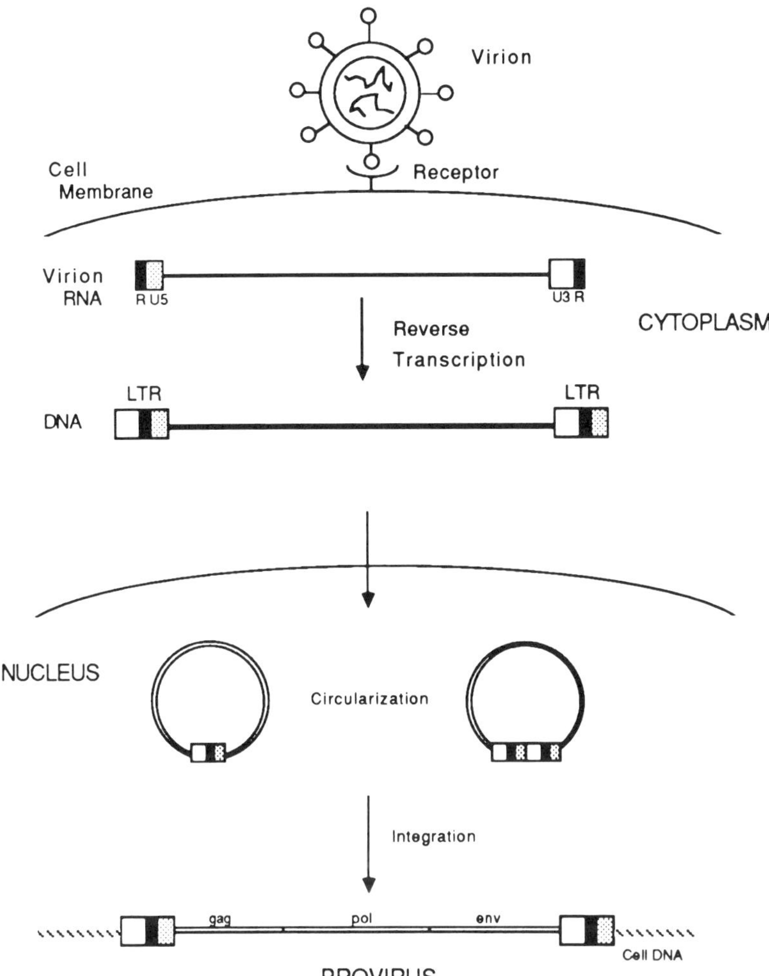

Figure 3–1   The retroviral life cycle. To initiate the replicative cycle, the retrovirus first binds a specific surface receptor and enters the target cell. Virion RNA is illustrated. The unique 5′ (U5) and unique 3′ (U3) sequences, as well as the terminal redundant sequences (R) of the RNA are shown. During reverse transcription of RNA to DNA, the U5 and U3 sequences are duplicated to form the long terminal repeats (LTRs). After reverse transcription, the viral DNA enters the nucleus where some circularizes. It is uncertain if linear or circularized viral DNA with one LTR or two LTRs is the immediate precursor to integration. Both circular forms are shown here. After integration into host cell sequences, the viral DNA is termed a provirus. Once integrated, the viral genes can be expressed, and progeny viruses formed.

site adjacent to the U5 region of the viral RNA molecule. Polymerization of the first (minus) strand proceeds through the 5' repeat (R) region, forming an RNA:DNA hybrid region. An enzyme (RNase H) present in reverse transcriptase then digests away the RNA in the hybrid, forming a single-stranded DNA segment. This remaining sequence is complementary to the R region of the viral RNA molecule. It is thought that this single-stranded segment is available to hybridize to the R region at the 3' end of the genomic RNA. This now can act as a primer, allowing the reverse transcriptase to switch templates and synthesize the remainder of the minus strand. A second similar template-switching event is needed in the synthesis of the complementary (plus) strand of the linear genomic DNA. Recent evidence suggests that the first template-switching event involves translocation of the initial single-stranded DNA stretch to the R region at the 3' end of the *other* virion RNA molecule (an interstrand transfer), while the second switching event appears to be an intrastrand transfer.[13] Thus, both copies of the RNA found in the virion are necessary for efficient reverse transcription.

Integration

Integration of the retroviral DNA genome into the host's DNA is essential for replication. Integration is dependent on virally encoded proteins and sequences in the long terminal repeats (LTRs). Each species of virus always integrates into the cellular DNA using precisely the same nucleotides near the end of the LTRs. However, the cellular DNA sequences involved in this process appear to be random.[14,15] During integration, the putative product of reverse transcription loses two base pairs (bp) at the terminus of each LTR, and a short region of host DNA (4 to 6 bp) is duplicated on either side of the LTRs.[14-16] Before integration, the retroviral DNA migrates from the cytoplasm into the nucleus, where some circular DNA forms can be found. It is not yet known if the immediate precursor for integration is a linear or circular form of retroviral DNA.[17] The process of integration is dependent upon expression of the viral integrase (IN) gene; mutations in this region allow reverse transcription of genomic RNA, entry of the viral DNA into the nucleus, and circularization, but inhibit the formation of the integrated provirus.[18-20] A cell-free in vitro model system for retroviral integration has recently been developed.[17] Proviruses formed in this reaction have the same structure as those formed in vivo. This system should help elucidate further the events required for retroviral integration.

In addition to the need for the viral integrase, certain sequences in the LTRs also appear to be important in provirus formation. The LTRs of retroviruses contain short inverted repeat sequences (2 to 13 bp) at their termini.[21-26] Deletions of sequences at the LTR termini abolish the ability of retroviruses to integrate into the host cell's DNA; however, they do not appear to affect entry into the nucleus or circularization of the viral genome.[27] These integration-defective mutants retained the ability to produce virus, but at a much lower level than integration-competent strains.

Assembly and Release

After expression of the viral genes, cores are assembled in the cytoplasm.[4] Packaging of genomic RNA into these cores is facilitated by specific viral sequences. These cores then associate with envelope glycoproteins located in the cell membrane, and the complete virion is released from the cell by budding.[28] During the process of budding, the virion obtains its envelope, which is derived from the host cell's lipid bilayer and contains virion-encoded glycoproteins and host-derived molecules.

The Retroviral Genome

The retroviral genome consists of two identical molecules of single-stranded RNA, each of which is base-paired with a single host-derived tRNA molecule. This tRNA is used as a primer for DNA synthesis during reverse transcription of the viral genome. The genomic RNA molecule resembles host mRNA molecules in that each contains a methylated cap structure at the 5′ terminus (a 7-methyl guanosine triphosphate (GTP) attached to the terminal residue encoded by the virus that is methylated at the 3′ position of the ribose) and a polyadenylated (poly-A) sequence at the 3′ terminus.[3] A short repeated sequence (R) is found immediately following the cap structure, and once again immediately preceding the poly-A tract. Sequences unique to either the 5′ or 3′ end of the RNA (U5 and U3, respectively) are located adjacent to the R regions (Figure 3–1). The primer binding site is located approximately 100 to 200 nucleotides from the 5′ end of most retroviral genomic RNA molecules.[3] The internal stretches of the genomic RNA molecule include the regions encoding the genes for the structural proteins (Gag), the viral polymerase or reverse transcriptase (Pol), and the envelope glycoproteins (Env). During the complex reverse transcription of genomic RNA into viral DNA, the unique 3′ (U3) and unique 5′ (U5) regions of the viral RNA are duplicated to form the LTR found at each end of the linear viral DNA. Following reverse transcription, some of the linear viral DNA circularizes. One of these DNA forms, most likely the linear, inserts into the host cell's genome to form the integrated provirus (Figure 3–1).

The LTR

The LTRs of retroviral DNA contain regions responsible for controlling virus expression and signals for synthesizing and processing virally encoded mRNAs. During reverse transcription, the unique 5′ and 3′ regions of the RNA genome are duplicated to form the LTRs. This process results in two LTRs, one at the 5′ end of the viral DNA, and the other at the 3′ end, both having the organization U3-R-U5.

U3. The U3 region of most retroviral LTRs does not contain an open reading frame, and is therefore noncoding.[29] This region contains the TATA box, the promoter for RNA synthesis. The U3 regions of the LTRs of human T-cell leukemia viruses types I (HTLV-I) and II (HTLV-II) contain three 21-bp repeat sequences upstream of the promoter that interact with viral *trans*-activating proteins (the *tax* gene products) to increase expression of genes linked to the LTR.[30,31] The U3 regions of these viruses also contain sequences that signal the site of polyadenylation onto mRNA. The HIV-1 LTR contains sequences in the U3 region that bind to cellular factors such as NF_xB, and increase transcription of viral genes following mitogenic stimulation of the host cells.[32-34] There is a second distinct region in the HIV-1 LTR upstream of the NF_xB binding site that appears to down-regulate basal LTR activity and mitogen responsiveness.[35] This region is known as the negative regulatory element.

The R region.   The R ("redundant") region of the LTR is derived from the terminal repeated sequence found at both the 5′ and 3′ ends of the genomic RNA molecule. This sequence enables the reverse transcription process to switch templates from the 5′ to the 3′ end of the genomic RNA, allowing polymerization of a full-length DNA copy. This region also contains the consensus sequences required for ribosomal binding and initiation of translation. Signals for polyadenylation of mRNA are also present in the R region.[3,29] The R region of the HIV-1 LTR contains sequences (TAR) responsive to the *trans*-activating protein (Tat) of the virus, which increases transcription from the LTR.[35,36]

U5.   The function of the U5 region of the retroviral LTR is still uncertain. However, it has been shown that sequences in the R-U5 region of the HTLV-I LTR are required for maximal expression of genes linked to the LTR.[37] These sequences function in an orientation-independent fashion; however, there is a strict requirement for their localization. It is possible that this region affects the translational efficiency of the viral RNA.

The *gag* Gene

The *gag* gene products are virion-associated proteins that form the internal structure or core of the virion. The retroviral core surrounds the genome and its associated reverse transcriptase. The core proteins are not covalently attached to the retroviral genome. These proteins are encoded on a full-length genomic mRNA molecule. Gag proteins are first made as a large precursor polypeptide that is enzymatically cleaved by the viral protease into smaller polypeptides. In the case of HTLV-I, this cleavage results in three Gag gene products: p19, p24, and p15.[38,39] HIV encodes three Gag proteins, all of which arise from a 58-kilodalton (kd) precursor. The major Gag protein (p24) is phosphorylated, while a slightly smaller protein (p17) is myristylated. The remaining protein has a molecular weight of 15 kd.[40,41]

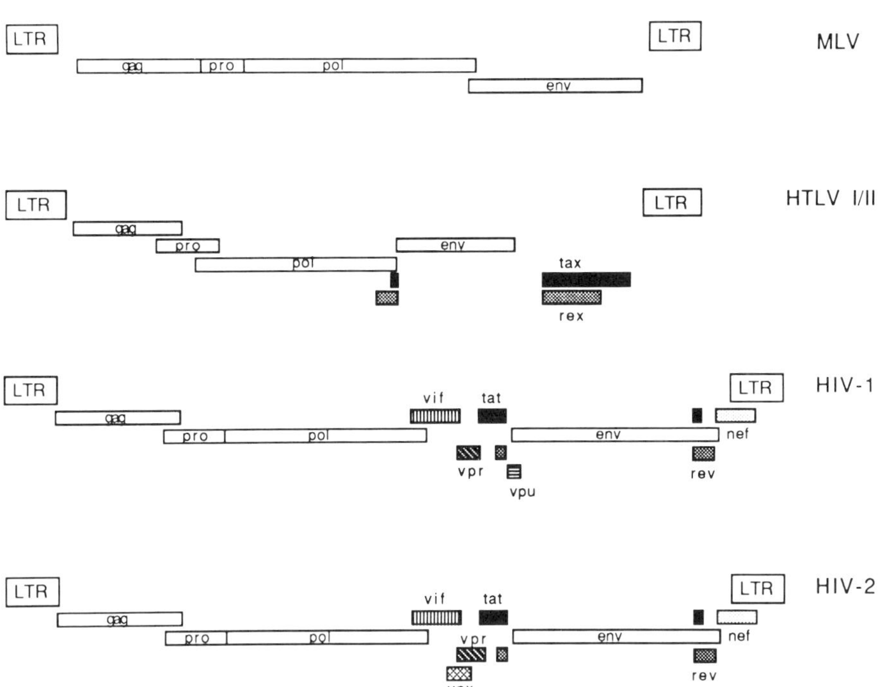

Figure 3–2   Retroviral genome structures. The structures of murine leukemia virus (MLV), HTLV-I and HTLV-II, and HIV-1 and HIV-2 are shown schematically for comparison. Individual genes are indicated as boxes and are labeled. The positions of the genes are representative of their location in the genome. Broken boxes indicate splicing, and overlapping genes represent different reading frames. Individual genes are discussed in the text. "Pro" is the viral protease gene.

The *pol* Gene

The *pol* gene encodes the viral polymerase (reverse transcriptase), along with the viral integrase.[18-20] In murine retroviruses, the viral protease is also encoded in the *pol* gene; however, in avian retroviruses it is localized in *gag*, and in HTLV it is encoded by an alternate reading frame overlapping *gag* and *pol* (Figure 3–2). Reverse transcriptase is responsible for converting the RNA genome into double-stranded DNA. This molecule also has RNase H activity; that is, an RNA-degrading activity specific for RNA/DNA hybrid molecules. The viral protease cleaves the large *gag* precursor into the core proteins, and the integrase assists in the insertion of the viral DNA into the host cell genome. mRNA for the *pol* gene products is transcribed as a full-length genomic message and separated from *gag* sequences during translation. This occurs by various mechanisms in different viruses, such as the presence of stop codons or frame-shifting mechanisms.[28]

The *env* Gene

The *env* (envelope) gene encodes the surface glycoproteins of the virion. This gene is expressed via a spliced subgenomic mRNA. The translated envelope precursor is glycosylated and cleaved to yield two glycoproteins that are both present at the virion surface.[4,42] The envelope proteins are obtained by the virion as it buds out of the infected cell. In the case of HIV-1, the envelope precursor is a 160-kD glycoprotein cleaved into 120-kD and 41-kD proteins.[40,43-46] The smaller HIV Env protein, gp41, is a transmembrane protein[46] that anchors gp120 in the membrane. The exterior glycoprotein, gp120, binds the receptor for HIV, the CD4 molecule, present on target cells,[6,7,47] allowing infection of the cell. The HTLV-I Env proteins include a 46-kD external glycoprotein (gp46) and a 21-kD transmembrane protein (gp21).

Oncogenes

Certain retroviruses contain genes other than *gag, pol,* and *env.* This new genetic information is attained by a process known as transduction. These new sequences are responsible for the transforming potential of these viruses, and are known as viral oncogenes (v-*oncs*).[48,49] Usually these sequences are inserted into the internal stretches of the viral genome at the expense of one or more of the normal viral genes. This generally renders the virus replication-defective, and dictates its requirement for a replication-competent helper virus to allow its reproduction. V-*onc* sequences are derived from normal cellular genes incorporated into the viral genome. However, the cellular sequences usually contain mutations that appear to alter their normal function. It is also thought that placing these cellular sequences under the control of the powerful retroviral promoter found in the LTR allows for aberrant high-level expression, or expression at an inappropriate time in the cell's differentiation or replicative cycle, which could lead to transformation. Currently, close to 30 different v-*onc* sequences have been identified. The cellular homologues to the v-*oncs* are known as proto-oncogenes, and their involvement in malignant neoplasms in humans is the subject of intensive investigations.

The human retroviruses linked to cell transformation (HTLV-I and -II) have not transduced cellular transforming sequences. These viruses are believed to transform cells by other mechanisms that will be discussed below.

Transformation by retroviruses. As discussed above, certain animal retroviruses contain cell-derived information that contributes to their oncogenic potential. The protein products of these v-*onc* sequences have varied mechanisms of action that lead to transformation of the host cell. Some of these products act as growth factors or growth factor receptors; others appear to function as intracellular messengers. Another group of viral oncogenes has the ability to bind to DNA, and may directly influence the expression of cellular genes important in growth regulation.[28,48,49] Retroviruses containing oncogenes form tumors rapidly in animals (usually in a matter of a few weeks), and are known as acutely transforming viruses. Other animal retroviruses appear to transform cells by inducing the expression of cellular genes. Integration of the strong retroviral promoter in the vicinity of genes important in growth regulation (cellular proto-oncogenes such as c-*myc*) appears to alter their expression, and can lead to malignant transformation.[28] This process is known as promoter insertion, and may involve increased overall expression of the cellular gene or an alteration of its temporal expression.[28,48,49] Retroviruses that transform cells by this type of mechanism generally require a long time to form tumors in animals, and are known as chronically transforming viruses. This long latency period may be due to the low frequency of integration events at the appropriate site in the cell genome.

The human transforming retroviruses HTLV-I and HTLV-II transform normal human peripheral blood T-cells in vitro, rendering them proliferative in the absence of exogenous interleukin 2 (IL-2), a growth factor required for proliferation of normal T cells.[50-53] Infection in vitro only occurs when uninfected cells are cocultured with infected cells; cell-free virions are generally noninfectious. Transformation of newly infected cells occurs after approximately 1 month in culture. During the first 4 to 8 weeks after coculture, the transformed cells (which are mostly CD4[+]) exhibit polyclonal integration of HTLV proviruses. After long-term culture, however, a few dominant transformed clones displaying an oligoclonal pattern of HTLV integration are observed. This latter event is probably due to selection pressures occurring during culture.

In contrast to the transforming retroviruses of animals, HTLV-I and HTLV-II do not transform cells because of a transduced oncogene. Promoter insertion is also not operative, as there is not a common integration site for HTLV in adult T-cell leukemia.[54] Alternate models for T-cell transformation by the HTLVs exist. Both of these viruses contain sequences that can *trans*-activate the expression of viral messages,[55-58] as well as certain cellular genes such as those encoding IL-2 and the IL-2 receptor.[59-63] It is thought that the *trans*-activation of cellular genes involved in growth control might be responsible for transformation. When introduced into transgenic mice, the *trans*-activating gene (*tax*) of HTLV-I induces mesenchymal tumors.[64] To date, however, there has been no direct evidence that the *tax* gene product alone can transform T lymphocytes.

In addition to *trans*-activation, the HTLVs may also use other gene products in the transformation process. Purified HTLV virions have been shown to be mitogenic for T lymphocytes, most likely mediated through the envelope glycoproteins.[65-67] This mitogenic activity does not require infection by HTLV, as heat-inactivated virions produce similar effects. Mitogenic stimulation of surface receptors on an infected cell might lead to increased proliferation of that cell, and allow subsequent changes to occur, resulting in transformation. This activity may also be important in establishing infection by the HTLVs, and in the polyclonal proliferation of lymphocytes seen following infection in vitro and in vivo. These two models for T-cell transformation by the HTLVs are not mutually exclusive. The activation state of the T cell is important for retroviral gene expression. Mitogenic stimulation by the virion or its products may allow increased production of the *tax* gene, resulting in transformation of the cell. Alternatively, increased proliferation plus *trans*-activation by *tax* may be required for a secondary mutation in a cellular sequence to occur, leading to the transformed phenotype.

Additional Genes Contained in Human Retroviruses

In addition to the normal retroviral genes, *gag, pol,* and *env,* HTLV-I/-II and HIV-1/-2 contain other sequences important in the viral life cycle. Although some of these genes perform similar functions, those found in the HTLVs are not related in sequence to those found in the HIVs. A schematic representation of the genetic structure of these viruses is shown in Figure 3–2. The functions of many of these genes have not yet been elucidated. Some of these genes have been given numerous names. To avoid confusion, a unifying nomenclature for these genes has been proposed.[68]

Additional Genes Found in the HTLVs

The genomes of HTLV-I/-II contain, in addition to the normal retroviral structural genes, two distinct overlapping regulatory genes that encode three proteins. These genes are discussed individually below.

tax.   The *tax* gene ("*trans*-activator of expression"; previously known as *x, x-lor, tat*-1, and *tat*-2) encodes a protein designated p40[taxI] in HTLV-I and p37[taxII] in HTLV-II.[58,69,70] This gene is located at the 3′ end of the virus, and is encoded by a doubly spliced mRNA molecule.[71,72] The protein product of the *tax* gene is required for replication of the virus,[73] and acts in *trans* to increase the rate of transcription from the viral LTR.[55,56,74,75] The observation that the *tax* gene product may regulate the expression of certain cellular genes[60-63] makes *tax* an attractive candidate for the gene responsible for malignant transformation.

rex.   The remaining two additional proteins produced by the HTLVs are encoded by the *rex* gene. The *rex* gene ("regulator of expression") is encoded on the same subgenomic mRNA as the *tax* gene, but uses an alternate overlapping reading frame.[76-78] HTLV-I encodes a 27-kd and 21-kd species (termed p27[rexI] and p21[rexI], respectively).[76,77,79,80] The larger of the proteins is required for efficient *gag* gene expression, and appears to function through a posttranscriptional modification mechanism.[79,80] The corresponding proteins expressed by the *rex* gene of HTLV-II are 26 and 24 kd.[78] The *rex* gene of HTLV-II modulates the *trans*-activating effect of the *tax* gene product, and may help regulate viral mRNA expression in infected cells.[81]

Additional Genes Found in HIV-1 and HIV-2

The human immunodeficiency viruses have a complex regulatory system not found in other retroviruses. To date, there are seven known open reading frames (ORFs) with protein-encoding potential, in addition to the normal retroviral structural genes. Most of these additional genes are found in both HIV-1 and HIV-2. Figure 3–2 illustrates the genetic structure of the HIVs.

tat.   The *tat* gene ("*trans*-activator of transcription"; previously known as *tat*-III) produces a protein that interacts with specific sequences in the R region of the HIV LTR to stimulate the expression of genes linked to the LTR.[35,36] This gene is required for HIV replication and may cause as much as a 1000-fold increase in viral gene expression. The *tat* product is encoded on a subgenomic spliced mRNA molecule.[82]

rev.   The *rev* gene ("regulator of expression of virion proteins") was initially known as *art* or *trs*. The *rev* gene product is also encoded on a subgenomic spliced mRNA molecule. Deletions in this gene are lethal to the virus. The *rev* gene product augments expression of the Gag and Env proteins[83,84] and may affect processing and transport of incompletely spliced mRNA transcripts.[85] The effect of *rev* is mediated by direct binding to a region in full-length or singly spliced RNA known as the Rev-responsive element.[86-88]

nef.   The *nef* gene ("negative factor," previously known as 3' ORF, *orf*B, and F) is found at the 3' end of the virus, overlapping the LTR. The product of the *nef* gene is a 27-kd protein (p27) that is highly immunogenic.[89] It has been reported that deletion mutations in the *nef* gene do not alter virus replication or cytopathic effects[90]; however, other studies have shown that deletions in this gene actually increase virus production approximately five-fold.[91] This latter result suggests that the *nef* gene down-regulates virus production; hence its name, an acronym for "negative factor." The *nef* gene product contains both a guanine nucleotide (GTP)-binding activity and a GTPase activity.[92] These are qualities reminiscent of the characteristics of G-proteins, molecules thought to be important in intracellular signal transduction. This protein can be phosphorylated and contains a myristic acid residue at the *N*-terminus,[92] suggesting that it may interact with molecules at the cell surface. Indeed, the *nef* gene product does appear to down-regulate the expression of the CD4 molecule on the surface of T-lymphocyte cell lines.[92] Although Nef was previously thought to down-regulate virus expression by negatively interacting with sequences in the LTR,[93,94] recent results suggest that Nef does not decrease virus expression.[95,96] Hence, the function of Nef remains unclear.

vif.   The *vif* gene ("virion infectivity factor," previously known as SOR, *orf*A, Q, and P') overlaps the 3' end of *pol*, and ends before the coding region for *env*. This gene encodes a 23-kd protein.[97-99] This gene does not appear to be required for viral replication or cytopathic effect; however, *vif* deletion mutants are 100 to 1000 times less infectious than wild-type viruses.[100,101] Expression of *vif* appears to allow efficient transmission of cell-free virions, as well as infection by cell-to-cell contact in vitro.

vpr.   The *vpr* gene ("virion protein R"; previously known as "R") is an ORF that overlaps *vif* and terminates before the first coding exon of *tat*. This gene is thought to encode a protein consisting of 78 amino acids, which is immunoreactive with serum derived from HIV-infected persons.[102] As yet, there is no known function for *vpr*. A frame-shift mutation in this region, which would produce a truncated *vpr* protein, had no effect on virus infectivity, replication, or cytopathicity.[103]

vpu.   The *vpu* gene ("virion protein U") is found in some HIV-1 isolates and encodes both a 15-kd and a 16-kd protein. Antibodies against these proteins are found in patients' serum following infection. *vpu* is not present in HIV-2 or the related simian immunodeficiency virus (SIV). All HIV-1 isolates contain *vpu* sequences in their genomes; however, many lack an initiating methionine or contain a stop codon in this reading frame that would truncate the protein.[104,105] The function of the *vpu* gene product is not yet known; however, cells infected with *vpu* mutants accumulate high levels of intracellular viral structural proteins and produce low amounts of progeny virus. This suggests that *vpu* has a role in virus assembly or maturation.[105]

vpx.   The *vpx* gene ("virion protein X") is an open reading frame found only in HIV-2 and SIV, but not HIV-1. This gene is located between the *pol* and *env* genes of these viruses. Antibodies to the purified 14-kd *vpx* gene product of SIV cross-react with a homologous 16-kd protein in HIV-2. The *vpx* gene product is found in substantial amounts in the virion particle. The actual function of the *vpx* gene product is not known, but it appears to be able to bind single-stranded nucleic acids and may function as an RNA-binding protein in vivo.[106]

Recent epidemiologic studies have shown that many individuals have been exposed to both HIV-1 and either HTLV-I or HTLV-II.[107-112] This raises questions regarding possible interactions between these different viruses, and whether co-infection could be a cofactor for AIDS. There is some suggestion that persons dually infected with HTLV-I and HIV-1 have lower indices of immune function and may have an increased risk of progression to AIDS than those infected with HIV-1 alone.[113] Two different mechanisms of interaction between HIV and the HTLVs have been shown. The HTLV *tax* protein can *trans*-activate the LTR of HIV-1, but only following deletion of certain sequences in the HIV-1 LTR.[33] This mechanism may act to increase expression of HIV-1 in some cells containing both viruses, but most likely only if the HIV LTR is altered. The second mechanism involves mitogenic stimulation of HIV-1–infected cells by HTLV particles or viral products. When quiescent peripheral blood T cells harboring inactive HIV are mitogenically stimulated by purified HTLV-I virions in vitro, HIV production is induced. Cells stimulated similarly before infection by HIV also produce HIV, whereas unstimulated cells do not.[67] This model of HTLV-induced stimulation of HIV production does not require coinfection of the same cell, as external stimulation of mitogen receptors on the surface of the HIV-infected cell would give the same result. This stimulation could be provided by free HTLV particles, or by contact with an HTLV-infected cell displaying the mitogenic viral product (see above) on its cell surface. Another interaction between human retroviruses is also conceivable. Although not yet documented, the immunodeficiency caused by the HIVs could lead to an increased severity of HTLV-associated disorders in coinfected individuals. This could result from an inability of the immune response to remove the coinfecting virus or infected cells.

Conclusion

The human retroviruses show a complex biology and regulation not seen in more commonly investigated animal retroviruses. There are as yet many unanswered questions regarding gene function, control of expression, and pathogenesis of these viruses. Further investigation into the basic mechanisms involved in the replication and life cycle of retroviruses is needed before effective therapies can be developed. Targeting research and therapeutic regimens toward aspects of the viral life cycle that differ significantly from cellular processes (such as reverse transcription and *trans*-activation) may eventually lead to reagents that will reduce considerably the morbidity and mortality caused by these agents. As the incidence of infection by the HTLVs is rising, routine screening of blood and blood products for these viruses has been instituted in the United States to reduce transmission of these agents. A greater understanding by the public of the transmission and biology of retroviruses will also lead to a decreased incidence of disease.

References

1. Fenner F: The classification and nomenclature of viruses. *Intervirology* 6:1–12, 1975.
2. Teich N: Taxonomy of retroviruses, in Weiss R, Teich N, Varmus H, Coffin J (eds): *RNA Tumor Viruses.* Cold Spring Harbor, NY, Cold Spring Harbor Laboratory, 1982, pp 25–207.
3. Coffin J: Supplement of genome structure, in Weiss R, Teich N, Varmus H, Coffin J (eds): *RNA Tumor Viruses.* Cold Spring Harbor, NY, Cold Spring Harbor Laboratory, 1982, pp 261–368.
4. Dickson C, Eisenman R, Fan H, Hunter E, Teich N: Protein biosynthesis and assembly, in Weiss R, Teich N, Varmus H, Coffin J (eds): *RNA Tumor Viruses.* Cold Spring Harbor, NY, Cold Spring Harbor Laboratory, 1982, pp 513–648.
5. De Larco J, Todaro GJ: Membrane receptors for murine leukemia viruses: Characterization using the purified viral envelope glycoprotein, gp71. *Cell* 8:365–376, 1976.

6. Dalgleish AG, Beverley PCL, Clapham PR, et al: The CD4 (T4) antigen is an essential component of the receptor for the AIDS retrovirus. *Nature* 312:763–767, 1984.

7. Klatzmann D, Champagne E, Chamaret S, et al: T-lymphocyte T4 molecule behaves as the receptor for human retrovirus LAV. *Nature* 312:767–768, 1984.

8. Maddon PJ, Dalgleish AG, McDougal JS, et al: The T_4 gene encodes the AIDS virus receptor and is expressed in the immune system and the brain. *Cell* 47:333–348, 1986.

9. Mims CA: Virus receptors and cell tropisms. *J Infect Dis* 12:199–204, 1986.

10. Stein BS, Gowda SD, Lifson JD, et al: pH-independent HIV entry into CD4-positive T cells via virus envelope fusion to the plasma membrane. *Cell* 49:659–668, 1987.

11. Varmus H, Swanstrom R: Replication of retroviruses, in Weiss R, Teich N, Varmus H, Coffin J (eds): *RNA Tumor Viruses.* Cold Spring Harbor, NY, Cold Spring Harbor Laboratory, 1982, pp 369–512.

12. Varmus H, Swanstrom R: Supplement replication of retroviruses, in Weiss R, Teich N, Varmus H, Coffin J (eds): *RNA Tumor Viruses.* Cold Spring Harbor, NY, Cold Spring Harbor Laboratory, 1985, pp 75–134.

13. Panganiban AT, Fiore D: Ordered interstrand and intrastrand DNA transfer during reverse transcription. *Science* 241:1064–1069, 1988.

14. Shoemaker C, Goff S, Gilboa E, et al: Structure of a cloned circular Moloney murine leukemia virus molecule containing an inverted segment: Implications for retrovirus integration. *Proc Natl Acad Sci USA* 77:3932–3936, 1980.

15. Shimotohno K, Temin HM: No apparent nucleotide sequence specificity in cellular DNA juxtaposed to retrovirus proviruses. *Proc Natl Acad Sci USA* 77:7357–7361, 1980.

16. Hughes SH, Mutschler A, Bishop JM, Varmus HE: A Rous sarcoma virus provirus is flanked by short direct repeats of a cellular DNA sequence present in only one copy prior to integration. *Proc Natl Acad Sci USA* 78:4299–4303, 1981.

17. Brown PO, Bowerman B, Varmus HE, Bishop JM: Correct integration of retroviral DNA in vitro. *Cell* 49:347–356, 1987.

18. Donehower LA, Varmus HE: A mutant murine leukemia virus with a single missense codon in *pol* is defective in a function affecting integration. *Proc Natl Acad Sci USA* 81:6461–6465, 1984.

19. Panganiban AT, Temin HM: The retrovirus *pol* gene encodes a product required for DNA integration: Identification of a retrovirus *int* locus. *Proc Natl Acad Sci USA* 81:7885–7889, 1984.

20. Schwartzberg P, Colicelli J, Goff SP: Construction and analysis of deletion mutants in the *pol* gene of Moloney murine leukemia virus: A new viral function required for establishment of the integrated provirus. *Cell* 37:1043–1052, 1984.

21. Ju G, Skalka AM: Nucleotide sequence analysis of the long terminal repeat (LTR) of avian retroviruses: Structural similarities with transposable elements. *Cell* 22:379–386, 1980.

22. Shimotohno K, Mizutani S, Temin HM: Sequence of retrovirus provirus resembles that of bacterial transposable elements. *Nature* 285:550–554, 1980.

23. Sutcliffe JG, Shinnick TM, Verma IM, Lerner RA: Nucleotide sequence of Moloney leukemia virus: 3' end reveals details of replication, analogy to bacterial

transposons and an unexpected gene. *Proc Natl Acad Sci USA* 77:3302–3306, 1980.

24. Scott ML, McKereghan K, Kaplan HS, Fry KE: Molecular cloning and partial characterization of unintegrated linear DNA from gibbon ape leukemia virus. *Proc Natl Acad Sci USA* 78:4213–4217, 1981.

25. Donehower LA, Huang AL, Hager GL: Regulatory and coding potential of the mouse mammary tumor virus long terminal redundancy. *J Virol* 37:226–238, 1981.

26. Yamamoto T, Jay G, Pastan I: Unusual features in the nucleotide sequence of a cDNA clone derived from the common region of avian sarcoma virus messenger RNA. *Proc Natl Acad Sci USA* 77:176–180, 1980.

27. Panganiban AT, Temin HM: The terminal nucleotides of retrovirus DNA are required for integration but not virus production. *Nature* 306:155–160, 1983.

28. Varmus H: Retroviruses. *Science* 240:1427–1435, 1988.

29. Coffin J: Structure of the retroviral genome, in Weiss R, Teich N, Varmus H, Coffin J (eds): *RNA Tumor Viruses.* Cold Spring Harbor, NY, Cold Spring Harbor Laboratory, 1985, pp 17–73.

30. Shimotohno K, Takano M, Terunchi T, Miwa M: Requirement of multiple copies of a 21-nucleotide sequence in the U3 regions of human T-cell leukemia virus type I and type II long terminal repeats for trans-activation of transcription. *Proc Natl Acad Sci USA* 83:8112–8116, 1986.

31. Kitado H, Chen ISY, Shah NP, et al: U3 sequences from the HTLV-I and -II LTRs confer pX protein responsiveness to a murine leukemia virus LTR. *Science* 235:901–904, 1987.

32. Nabel G, Baltimore D: An inducible transcription factor activates expression of human immunodeficiency virus in T cells. *Nature* 326:711–714, 1987.

33. Siekevitz M, Josephs SF, Dukovich M, et al: Activation of the HIV-1 LTR by T cell mitogens and the trans-activator protein of HTLV-I. *Science* 238:1575–1578, 1987.

34. Tong-Starksen SE, Luciw PA, Peterlin BM: Human immunodeficiency virus long terminal repeat responds to T-cell activation signals. *Proc Natl Acad Sci USA* 84:6845–6849, 1987.

35. Rosen CA, Sodroski JG, Haseltine WA: The location of cis-acting sequences in the human T-cell leukemia virus III (HTLV-III/LAV) long terminal repeat. *Cell* 41:813–823, 1985.

36. Sodroski J, Rosen C, Wong-Staal F, et al: *Trans*-acting transcriptional regulation of human T-cell leukemia virus type III long terminal repeat. *Science* 227:171–173, 1985.

37. Ohtani K, Nakamura M, Saito S, et al: Identification of two distinct elements in the long terminal repeat of HTLV-I responsible for maximum gene expression. *EMBO J* 6:389–395, 1987.

38. Oroszlan S, Copeland TD, Kalyanaraman VS, et al: Chemical analyses of human T-cell leukemia virus structural proteins, in Gallo RC, Essex ME, Gross L (eds): *Human T-cell Leukemia/Lymphoma Viruses.* Cold Spring Harbor, NY, Cold Spring Harbor Laboratory, 1984, pp 101–110.

39. Hattori S, Kiyokawa T, Imagawa K-I, et al: Identification of *gag* and *env* gene products of human T-cell leukemia virus (HTLV). *Virology* 136:338–347, 1984.

40. Robey WG, Safai B, Oroszlan S, et al: Characterization of envelope and core structural gene products of HTLV-III with sera from AIDS patients. *Science* 228:593–595, 1985.

41. Veronese FD, Copeland TD, Oroszlan S, Gallo RC, Sarngadharan MG: Biochemical and immunological analysis of human immunodeficiency virus *gag* gene products p17 and p24. *J Virol* 62:795–801, 1988.

42. Dickson C, Eisenman R, Fan H: Supplement protein biosynthesis and assembly, in Weiss R, Teich N, Varmus H, Coffin J (eds): *RNA Tumor Viruses.* Cold Spring Harbor, NY, Cold Spring Harbor Laboratory, 1985, pp 135–145.

43. Allan JS, Coligan JE, Barin F, et al: Major glycoprotein antigens that induce antibodies in AIDS patients are encoded by HTLV-III. *Science* 228:1091–1094, 1985.

44. Barin F, McLane MF, Allan JS, et al: Virus envelope protein of HTLV-III represents major target antigen for antibodies in AIDS patients. *Science* 228:1094–1096, 1985.

45. Montagier L, Dauguet C, Axler C, et al: A new type of retrovirus isolated from patients presenting with lymphadenopathy and acquired immune deficiency syndromes: Structural and antigenic relatedness with equine infectious anemia virus. *Virology* 144:283–289, 1985.

46. Veronese FD, DeVico AL, Copeland TD, et al: Characterization of gp41 as the transmembrane protein coded by the HTLV-III/LAV envelope gene. *Science* 229:1402–1405, 1985.

47. McDougal JS, Kennedy MS, Sligh JM, et al: Binding of HTLV-III/LAV to T4+ cells by a complex of the 110K viral protein and the T4 molecule. *Science* 231:382–385, 1986.

48. Bishop JM: Cellular oncogenes and retroviruses. *Ann Rev Biochem* 52:301–354, 1983.

49. Bishop JM: Viral oncogenes. *Cell* 42:23–38, 1985.

50. Chen ISY, Quan SG, Golde DW: Human T-cell leukemia virus type II transforms normal human lymphocytes. *Proc Natl Acad Sci USA* 80:7006–7009, 1983.

51. Miyoshi I, Yoshimoto S, Kubonishi I, et al: Transformation of normal human cord lymphocytes by co-cultivation with a lethally irradiated human T-cell line carrying type C particles. *Gann* 72:997–998, 1981.

52. Popovic M, Lange-Wantzin G, Sarin PS, Mann D, Gallo RC: Transformation of human umbilical cord blood T cells by human T-cell leukemia/lymphoma virus. *Proc Natl Acad Sci USA* 80:5402–5406, 1983.

53. Yamamoto N, Okada M, Koyanagi Y, et al: Transformation of human leukocytes by cocultivation with an adult T cell leukemia virus producer cell line. *Science* 217:737–739, 1982.

54. Seiki M, Eddy R, Shows TB, Yoshida M: Nonspecific integration of the HTLV provirus genome into adult T-cell leukaemia cells. *Nature* 309:640–642, 1984.

55. Cann AJ, Rosenblatt JD, Wachsman W, et al: Identification of the gene responsible for human T-cell leukemia virus transcriptional regulation. *Nature* 318:571–574, 1985.

56. Felber BK, Paskalis H, Kleinman-Ewing C, et al: The pX protein of HTLV-I is a transcriptional activator of its long terminal repeats. *Science* 229:675–679, 1985.

57. Fujisawa J, Seiki M, Kiyokawa T, Yoshida M: Functional activation of the long terminal repeat of human T-cell leukemia virus type I by a *trans*-acting factor. *Proc Natl Acad Sci USA* 82:2277–2281, 1985.

58. Sodroski J, Rosen C, Goh WC, Haseltine W: A transcriptional activator protein encoded by the x-lor region of the human T-cell leukemia virus. *Science* 228:1430–1434, 1985.

59. Cross SL, Feinberg MB, Wolf JB, et al: Regulation of the human interleukin-2 receptor alpha promoter: Activation of a nonfunctional promoter by the transactivator gene of HTLV-I. *Cell* 49:47–56, 1987.

60. Greene WC, Leonard WJ, Wano Y, et al: *Trans*-activator gene of HTLV-II induces IL-2 receptor and IL-2 cellular gene expression. *Science* 232:877–880, 1986.

61. Inoue J, Seiki M, Taniguchi T, Tsuru S, Yoshida M: Induction of interleukin-2 receptor gene by p40^{xl} encoded by human T-cell leukemia virus type I. *EMBO J* 5:2883–2888, 1986.

62. Maruyama M, Shibuya H, Harada H, et al: Evidence for aberrant activation of the interleukin-2 autocrine loop by HTLV-I-encoded p40^{xl} and T3/Ti complex triggering. *Cell* 48:343–350, 1987.

63. Siekevitz M, Feinberg MB, Holbrook N, Wong-Staal F, Greene WC: Activation of interleukin 2 and interleukin 2 receptor (Tac) promoter expression by the trans-activator (tat) gene product of human T-cell leukemia virus, type I. *Proc Natl Acad Sci USA* 84:5389–5393, 1987.

64. Nerenberg M, Hinrichs SH, Reynolds RK, Khoury G, Jay G: The *tat* gene of human T-lymphotropic virus type I induces mesenchymal tumors in transgenic mice. *Science* 237:1324–1329, 1987.

65. Duc Dodon M, Gazzolo L: Loss of interleukin 2 requirement for the generation of T-cell colonies defines an early event of human T-lymphotropic virus infection. *Blood* 69:12–17, 1987.

66. Gazzolo L, Duc Dodon M: Direct activation of resting T lymphocytes by human T-lymphotropic virus type I. *Nature* 326:714–717, 1987.

67. Zack JA, Cann AJ, Lugo JP, Chen ISY: AIDS virus production from infected peripheral blood T cells following HTLV-I–induced mitogenic stimulation. *Science* 240:1026–1029, 1988.

68. Gallo R, Wong-Staal F, Montagnier L, Haseltine WA, Yoshida M: HIV/HTLV gene nomenclature. *Nature* 333:504, 1988.

69. Shimotohno K, Takahashi Y, Shimizu N, et al: Complete nucleotide sequence of an infectious clone of human T-cell leukemia virus type II: A new open reading frame for the protease gene. *Proc Natl Acad Sci USA* 82:3101–3105, 1985.

70. Slamon DJ, Shimotohno K, Cline MJ, Golde DW, Chen ISY: Identification of the putative transforming protein of the human T-cell leukemia viruses HTLV-I and HTLV-II. *Science* 226:61–65, 1984.

71. Seiki M, Hikikoshi A, Taniquchi T, Yoshida M: Expression of the px gene of HTLV-I: General splicing mechanism in the HTLV family. *Science* 228:1532–1535, 1985.

72. Wachsman W, Shimotohno K, Clark SC, Golde DW, Chen ISY: Expression of the 3′ terminal region of human T-cell leukemia viruses. *Science* 226:177–179, 1984.

73. Chen ISY, Slamon DJ, Rosenblatt JD, et al: The *x* gene is essential for HTLV replication. *Science* 229:54–58, 1985.

74. Seiki M, Inoue J-I, Takeda T, Yoshida M: Direct evidence that p40[xl] of human T-cell leukemia virus type I is a *trans*-acting transcriptional activator. *EMBO J* 5:561–565, 1986.

75. Sodroski JG, Rosen CA, Haseltine WA: *Trans*-acting transcriptional activation of the long terminal repeat of human T lymphotropic viruses in infected cells. *Science* 225:381–385, 1984.

76. Kiyokawa T, Seiki M, Iwashita S, et al: p27[xlll] and p21[xlll], proteins encoded by the pX sequence of human T-cell leukemia virus type I. *Proc Natl Acad Sci USA* 82:8359–8363, 1985.

77. Nagashima K, Yoshida M, Seiki M: A single species of pX mRNA of human T-cell leukemia virus type I encodes *trans*-activator p40x and two other phosphoproteins. *J Virol* 60:394–399, 1986.

78. Shima H, Takano M, Shimotohno K, Miwa M: Identification of p26[xb] and p24[xb] of human T-cell leukemia virus type II. *FEBS Lett* 209:289–294, 1986.

79. Inoue J, Seiki M, Yoshida M: The second pX product p27[xlll] of HTLV-I is required for *gag* gene expression. *FEBS Lett* 209:187–190, 1986.

80. Inoue JI, Yoshida M, Seiki M: Transcriptional (p40[x]) and post-transcriptional (p27[xlll]) regulators are required for the expression and replication of human T-cell leukemia virus type I genes. *Proc Natl Acad Sci USA* 84:3653–3657, 1987.

81. Rosenblatt JD, Cann AJ, Slamon DJ, et al: HTLV-II *trans*-activation is regulated by two overlapping nonstructural genes. *Science* 240:916–919, 1988.

82. Wong-Staal F, Shaw FM, Hahn BH, et al: Genomic diversity of human T-lymphotropic virus type III (HTLV-III). *Science* 229:759–762, 1985.

83. Feinberg MB, Jarrett RF, Aldovini A, et al: HTLV-III expression and production involve complex regulation at the levels of splicing and translation of viral RNA. *Cell* 46:807–817, 1986.

84. Sodroski J, Goh WC, Rosen C, et al: A second post-transcriptional *trans*-activator gene required for HTLV-III replication. *Nature* 321:412–417, 1986.

85. Rosen CA, Terwilliger EF, Dayton AI, et al: Intragenic cis-acting art gene responsive sequences of the human immunodeficiency virus. *Proc Natl Acad Sci USA* 85:2071–2075, 1988.

86. Heaphy S, Dingwall C, Ernberg I, et al: HIV-1 regulator of virion expression (Rev) protein binds to an RNA stem-loop structure located within the rev response element region. *Cell* 60:685–693, 1990.

87. Malim MH, Tiley LS, McCarn DF, et al: HIV-1 structural gene expression requires binding of the Rev *trans*-activator to its RNA target sequence. *Cell* 60:675–683, 1990.

88. Olsen HS, Nelbock P, Cochrane AW, Rosen CA: Secondary structure is the major determinant for interaction of HIV *rev* protein with RNA. *Science* 247:845–848, 1990.

89. Allan JS, Coligan JE, Lee T-H, et al: A new HTLV-III/LAV encoded antigen detected by antibodies from AIDS patients. *Science* 230:810, 1985.

90. Fisher AG, Ratner L, Mitsuya H, et al: Infectious mutants of HTLV-III with changes in the 3′ region and markedly reduced cytopathic effects. *Science* 233:655–659, 1986.

91. Luciw PA, Cheng-Mayer C, Levy JA: Mutational analysis of the human immunodeficiency virus: The *orf*-B region down-regulates virus replication. *Proc Natl Acad Sci USA* 84:1434–1438, 1987.

92. Guy B, Kieny MP, Riviere Y, et al: HIV F/3' *orf* encodes a phosphorylated GTP-binding protein resembling an oncogene product. *Nature* 330:266–269, 1987.

93. Ahmad N, Venkatesan S: *nef* protein of HIV-1 is a transcriptional repressor of HIV-1 LTR. *Science* 241:1481–1485, 1988.

94. Niederman TMJ, Thielan BJ, Ratner L: Human immunodeficiency virus type 1 negative factor is a transcriptional silencer. *Proc Natl Acad Sci USA* 86:1128–1132, 1989.

95. Hammes SR, Dixon EP, Malim MH, Cullen BR, Greene WC: Nef protein of human immunodeficiency virus type 1: Evidence against its role as a transcriptional inhibitor. *Proc Natl Acad Sci USA* 86:9549–9553, 1989.

96. Kim S, Ikeuchi K, Byrn R, Groopman J, Baltimore D: Lack of a negative influence on viral growth by the *nef* gene of human immunodeficiency virus type 1. *Proc Natl Acad Sci USA* 86:9544–9548, 1989.

97. Lee T-H, Coligan JE, Allan JS, et al: A new HTLV-III/LAV protein encoded by a gene found in cytopathic retroviruses. *Science* 231:1538–1546, 1986.

98. Sodroski J, Goh WC, Rosen C, et al: Replicative and cytopathic potential of HTLV-III/LAV with *sor* gene deletions. *Science* 231:1549–1553, 1986.

99. Kan NC, Franchini G, Wong-Staal F, et al: Identification of HTLV-III/LAV *sor* gene product and detection of antibodies in human sera. *Science* 231:1553–1555, 1986.

100. Strebel K, Daugherty D, Clouse K, et al: The HIV 'A' (*sor*) gene product is essential for virus infectivity. *Nature* 328:728–731, 1987.

101. Fisher AG, Ensoli B, Ivanoff L, et al: The *sor* gene of HIV-1 is required for efficient virus transmission in vitro. *Science* 237:888–893, 1987.

102. Wong-Staal F, Chanda PK, Ghrayeb J: Human immunodeficiency virus: The eighth gene. *AIDS Res Hum Retrov* 3:33–39, 1987.

103. Dedera D, Hu W, Vander Heyden N, Ratner L: Viral protein R of human immunodeficiency virus types 1 and 2 is dispensable for replication and cytopathogenicity in lymphoid cells. *J Virol* 63:3205–3208, 1989.

104. Cohen EA, Terwilliger EF, Sodroski JG, Haseltine WA: Identification of a protein encoded by the *vpu* gene of HIV-1. *Nature* 334:532–534, 1988.

105. Strebel K, Klimkait T, Martin MA: A novel gene of HIV-1, *vpu*, and its 16-kilodalton product. *Science* 24:1221–1223, 1988.

106. Henderson LE, Sowder RC, Copeland TD, Benveniste RE, Oroszlan S: Isolation and characterization of a novel protein (X-ORF product) from SIV and HIV-2. *Science* 241:199–201, 1988.

107. Bartholomew C, Saxinger WC, Clark JW, et al: Transmission of HTLV-I and HIV among homosexual men in Trinidad. *JAMA* 257:2604–2608, 1987.

108. Getchell JP, Heath JL, Hicks DR, et al: Detection of human T-cell leukemia virus type I and human immunodeficiency virus in cultured lymphocytes of a Zairian man with AIDS. *J Infect Dis* 155:612–616, 1987.

109. Kanner SB, Parks ES, Scott GB, Parks WP: Simultaneous infection with human T-cell leukemia virus type I and the human immunodeficiency virus. *J Infect Dis* 155:617–625, 1987.

110. Harper ME, Kaplan MH, Marselle LM, et al: Concomitant infection with HTLV-I and HTLV-III in a patient with T_8 lymphoproliferative disease. *N Engl J Med* 315:1073–1078, 1986.

111. Koyanagi Y, Kobayashi S, Harada S, Kikukawa R, Yamamoto N: Detection of antibodies to human T-lymphotropic viruses type I and III in Japanese hemophiliacs. *AIDS Res* 1:353–358, 1984.

112. Robert-Guroff M, Weiss SH, Giron JA, et al: Prevalence of antibodies to HTLV-I, -II, and -III in intravenous drug abusers from an AIDS endemic region. *JAMA* 255:3133–3137, 1986.

113. Bartholomew C, Blattner W, Cleghorn F: Progression to AIDS in homosexual men coinfected with HIV and HTLV-I in Trinidad. *Lancet* 2:1469, 1987.

4
Transfusion-Transmitted Human Immunodeficiency Virus Infection

Dennis M. Smith, Jr., MD

The scientific reality that blood transfusion transmits HIV and the public's fear of transfusion-associated AIDS have transformed blood banking from a laboratory science of little interest to most physicians into the clinical speciality of transfusion medicine.[1] While acknowledging the human tragedy involved with each case of transfusion-associated AIDS, we must recognize that the recent scientific and clinical advances in preventing all transfusion-transmitted infections would have undoubtedly taken much longer to develop if it had not been for the fact that transfusion transmits HIV. The current interests in inactivating viruses in blood components and derivatives, in preoperative autologous blood donation, in intraoperative and postoperative blood salvage, in minimizing the use of a homologous blood, and in informed consent spring directly from this fact. The present chapter focuses on issues related to transfusion-transmitted HIV infection and transfusion-associated AIDS that are not addressed elsewhere in this text.

Definition

Transfusion-associated AIDS is defined as AIDS occurring in a person who has received a transfusion since 1977 but who has no other risk factors for HIV infection.[2] The first suspicion that HIV could be transmitted by blood products arose with the description in 1982 of AIDS in three hemophiliacs.[3] It is now known that HIV occurs in both cellular and noncellular blood components and in nonsterilized derivatives.

Epidemiology and Demographic Characteristics

Through November 1990, 157,525 cases of AIDS were reported to the Centers for Disease Control (CDC).[4] Of these cases, 5,371 (3.4%) were associated with transfusion of blood components or coagulation factor concentrates. Of the transfusion-associated AIDS (TAA) cases, 1,498 (27.8%) occurred in patients who had congenital factor deficiency. The 3,623 cases of TAA reported in adults who did not have congenital factor deficiency represent 2.3% of the total; the 1,360 cases related to congenital factor deficiency are 0.9% of the adult total. Of the 2,734 cases of AIDS in children, 250 (9.1%) were transfusion-related; 138 (5.0%) occurred in children with congenital factor deficiency.

As with the AIDS epidemic in general, the number of reported transfusion-associated AIDS cases represents only a small portion of all persons infected with HIV by transfusion. Estimates suggest that approximately 12,000 persons with transfusion-transmitted HIV infection were alive in 1987.[5] Because up to 60% of transfusion recipients die of underlying disease within 1 year and because of the long incubation period for HIV infection, the number of currently infected individuals who will develop the syndrome is unknown.[5,6] Recent projections, based on the assumption that 40% of individuals infected with HIV from transfusion will develop AIDS within 8 years, indicate that approximately 15,000 cases of TAA will eventually be reported among 13 to 69-year-old persons who received transfusions before June 1985.[6] Kalbfleisch and Lawless[6] have discussed the difficulties in estimating the number of TAA cases; they suggest that these difficulties relate primarily to the facts that the actual number of persons infected via transfusion is unknown and that the distribution of the incubation period from the time of infection and the development of AIDS is also uncertain.

The demographic characteristics of transfusion-associated AIDS demonstrate several variances from those of the syndrome in general. As previously noted, a disproportionately high number of cases of transfusion-associated AIDS occur in the pediatric (3 to 12 years old) age group, a situation explained by the fact that sexual transmission and intravenous drug use are uncommon routes of exposure in this age group. Transfusion-associated disease is more commonly found in the greater than 59-year-old group and the 6- to 20-year-old group.[4] The former of these two groups contains the segment of the population most likely to receive transfusion and the latter group includes the hemophiliacs. Finally, transfusion-associated AIDS afflicts higher percentages of white persons in both adult (73% of adult transfusion-associated AIDS cases are white *v* 58% of all AIDS cases) and pediatric (56% of pediatric transfusion-associated cases are white *v* 24% of all AIDS cases) populations.[4]

Natural History of Transfusion-Transmitted HIV Infection

Transfusion appears to be a very efficient method of transmitting the virus; estimates indicate that up to 95% of persons receiving HIV-seropositive blood become infected.[7,8] Once infection occurs, clinical disease from transfusion-associated infection shows no significant deviation from that which occurs with the syndrome in general. An acute, flulike illness may develop in approximately one-third of those infected.[7] The asymptomatic incubation period varies greatly from 4.5 to 9 years in adults.[7] A recent study suggests that 50% of persons infected by transfusion will develop AIDS within 7 years.[7] In comparison, only 33% of non–transfusion-related HIV infections progress to AIDS within 7 years of infection.[7] Thus, transfusion-associated HIV infection may progress to AIDS more rapidly than HIV infection unrelated to transfusion. Some authors suggest that the incubation period may be shorter in children than in adults.[9-11] However, in hemophiliacs, the incubation period appears to be directly related to the age of the individual at the time of infection.[12] For example, among 1 to 17-year-old hemophiliacs, 13% will develop AIDS within 8 years, as compared with 27% of hemophiliacs 18 to 34 years old.[12] Only the 35 to 70-year-old category shows a conversion rate (44% within 8 years) similar to that of adults with non–transfusion-associated AIDS.[12] Once fully developed, the transfusion-associated syndrome closely parallels typical AIDS.

Ward et al[7] have noted other interesting facts concerning TAA. They found that AIDS is more likely to develop in a transfusion recipient if the donor also develops AIDS, in contrast to the donor being HIV-seropositive but not having AIDS.[7] The incubation time also shortens in this situation.[7] Proposed explanations include a heavier inoculum of HIV or more pathogenic strains of virus.[7] Ward et al[7] also demonstrated that transfusion recipients with AIDS received greater numbers of transfusions than recipients with only HIV infection. This observation may reflect the fact that transfusion itself induces a state of immunosuppression,[7,13-15] the possibility that transfusion introduces viral cofactors,[16] or the chance that the recipient had more substantial underlying disease.[7]

Current Risk of Transfusion-Transmitted Infection

The risks of transmitting HIV infection through blood transfusion has been decreasing steadily since the spring of 1985, when screening of blood donors for antibody to HIV was begun. Cumming et al[17] have documented a 30% per year decrease in risk through December 1987. This increased safety in the blood supply can be attributed to changes in the donor pool, including fewer HIV seropositive donors and larger numbers of tested, repeated donors.[17] This trend toward increased safety is expected to continue.

Estimates of the current risk of transfusion-transmitted HIV infection require numerous assumptions and utilization of complex mathematical models. Several studies are available in the literature.[17-19] Since the variables used in determining risk change with time, the most recently published study probably provides the most accurate current estimate.[17] The study by Cumming et al[17] indicates that, in 1987, 131 units of blood containing undetected HIV were transfused. Statistically, the number of infected units ranged between 67 and 227, with 131 being most likely. The risk of having 131 infected units in the blood supply yields odds of a patient becoming infected with HIV from transfusion of one chance per 153,000 units transfused. Because the average patient receives exposure to 5.4 units of blood, the odds per patient are approximately 1:28,000. Cumming et al[17] have illustrated that current donor deferral practices and testing for antibody to HIV are 99.9% effective in eliminating HIV-infected units.[17] In addition, these authors' analyses of preliminary data for 1988 suggest that the likelihood of infectious units entering the blood supply has decreased by one third for 1988, resulting in 87 infected units going undetected. This trend toward increasing safety in subsequent years is expected to continue as efforts to recruit low-risk donors and the sensitivity of screening tests improve.

An evaluation of the first 88 cases of possible TAA reported to the CDC since the implementation of screening of donated blood for antibodies to HIV provides additional evidence for the improving safety of blood transfusion.[20] Of these 88 patients, 82 (93%) have had other risk factors for HIV infection or have received previous transfusion with untested blood. Only 6 (7%) patients apparently contracted HIV infection through the transfusion of tested blood. All six individuals were adults. Through November 1990, an additional eight adults who only received blood products screened for antibody to HIV have been found to have TAA.

Even though transfusion-transmitted HIV infection has now been largely eliminated, the number of reported cases of TAA will continue to increase for several years because of the number of persons infected before testing was available. Because of this fact, one cannot assess trends in transfusion-related HIV infections based on trends in the number of reported TAA cases.[20]

Finally, the recent determination that HIV provirus can be present for up to 35 months before seroconversion yields yet another variable that may influence the accuracy of current estimates.[21] The reader is urged to review the current literature for more recent estimates of risk since the facts cited above will undoubtedly change with time.

Prevention of HIV Infection by Transfusion

Prevention of transfusion-transmitted HIV infection and, subsequently, transfusion-associated AIDS involves four separate processes, all of which independently add to the safety of blood transfusion. These processes include donor selection and recruitment, laboratory testing, conservative transfusion therapy, and blood product "sterilization."

Selection of safe blood donors is a primary responsibility of blood centers and other agencies collecting blood. The selection process begins with education of prospective donors about the risk factors for HIV infection. Persons at risk are asked not to donate. Signs and symptoms of AIDS, a medical history of risk factors for AIDS, or sex with another at-risk person exclude donation. Residency in an HIV-endemic area or sex with someone from such a region also results in donor deferral. Finally, each donor may confidentially indicate that his or her unit should not be transfused through a process generally referred to as confidential unit exclusion. Chapter 13, "Donor Screening Procedures and Their Role in Enhancing Transfusion Safety," presents a complete discussion of these procedures.

Recent reports indicate that these techniques of donor exclusion have not been completely satisfactory.[17,22] Apparently, some donors previously having a high-risk lifestyle but currently enjoying good health feel they are not in an at-risk category.[22,23] These people continue to donate.[17,22] A growing number of authors are recommending that the educational materials presented to donors be discussed verbally with the donor and that direct, explicit questions about risky behavior be asked.[7,22-25] A preliminary report demonstrates that such questioning is not offensive to donors and is effective in deferring at-risk persons.[24] Recently, the FDA has recommended direct questioning of donors about high-risk activities.

Refining current donor recruitment techniques may also improve the safety of the blood supply. Cumming et al[17] have demonstrated that blood from repeated female donors is nine times as safe as blood from a first-time male donor. These investigators also have demonstrated that the riskiest category of female donors is safer than the safest category of male donors.[17] Thus, recruitment and retention of female blood donors by blood collection agencies should be encouraged. In addition, their study clearly illustrates that repeated blood donors are safer than new ones, a fact that emphasizes the need for retaining donors and for having them donate more frequently.[17]

The second stage of ensuring collection of a safe unit of blood requires careful laboratory testing of that unit. Currently, regulations require that all plasma or blood donations be tested for antibody to HIV using a licensed assay. Units giving repeatedly reactive results must be discarded. Units having an initially reactive but not repeatedly positive result may be transfused and do not carry an increased risk of infectivity.[22] Current studies show that seropositivity rates among voluntary blood donors have fallen from 380 per million blood donations in 1985 to 130 per million donations in 1987.[17] Chapter 14, "Donor Testing and its Impact on Transfusion-Transmitted Infection," provides a complete description of testing blood donations for antibody to HIV.

Testing blood for HIV antigen will not improve the safety of the blood supply; two reports of over 500,000 donors showed no donors who were HIV antigen–positive in the absence of antibody to HIV.[26] One recent model estimates that testing donated blood for HIV antigen would prevent approximately one case of AIDS per year.[27]

Because the risk of HIV infection from blood transfusion is directly proportional to the number of donor exposures, the judicious use of homologous blood products remains a cornerstone in the prevention of posttransfusion HIV infections. The decision to transfuse must be based on a combination of clinical signs and symptoms and laboratory data, not on laboratory values alone. Recent NIH consensus conferences and reviews on red blood cell and whole blood usage, platelet utilization, and fresh-frozen plasma transfusion outline appropriate indications for transfusing these products.[28-31] Chapter 16,

"Decreasing the Incidence of Transfusion-Transmitted Infection," also discusses these concepts. Furthermore, recent advances in preoperative autologous donation, hemodilution, and intraoperative and postoperative blood salvage make it possible to avoid homologous transfusion even in major surgery.[32] Finally, newly developed genetically engineered Factor VIII concentrate, viral inactivation processes for factor concentrates, and the use of DDAVP provide attractive alternatives for treating persons with factor deficiencies.[33] Chapters 15 and 16 contain more information on these issues.

References

1. Klein HG: Transfusion medicine: The evolution of a new discipline. *JAMA* 258:2108–2109, 1987.

2. Dodd RY: Transfusion-associated AIDS, in Rapoza N (ed): *HIV Infection and Disease.* Chicago, American Medical Association, 1989, pp 23–33.

3. Possible transfusion-associated acquired immune deficiency syndrome (AIDS)—California. *MMWR* 31:653–654, 1982.

4. *HIV/AIDS Surveillance Report.* Centers for Disease Control, Atlanta, January 1990, pp 1–22.

5. Peterman TA, Lui KJ, Lawrence DN, Allen JR: Estimating the risks of transfusion-associated acquired immune deficiency syndrome and human immunodeficiency virus infection. *Transfusion* 27:371–374, 1987.

6. Kalbfleisch JD, Lawless JF: Estimating the incubation time distribution and expected number of cases of transfusion-associated acquired immune deficiency syndrome. *Transfusion* 29:672–676, 1989.

7. Ward JW, Bush TJ, Perkins HA, et al: Natural history of transfusion-associated infection with human immunodeficiency virus. *N Engl J Med* 321:947–952, 1989.

8. Ward JW, Deppe DA, Samson S, et al: Risk of human immunodeficiency virus infection from blood donors who later developed the acquired immunodeficiency syndrome. *Ann Intern Med* 106:61–62, 1987.

9. Medley GF, Anderson RM, Cox DR, Billard L: Incubation period of AIDS in patients infected via blood transfusion. *Nature* 328:719–721, 1987.

10. Medley GF, Billard L, Cox DR, Anderson RM: The distribution of the incubation period for the acquired immunodeficiency syndrome (AIDS). *Proc R Soc Lond Biol* 233:367–377, 1988.

11. Kalbfleisch JD, Lawless JF: Estimating the incubation period for AIDS patients (letter). *Nature* 333:504–505, 1988.

12. Goedert JJ, Kessler CM, Aledort LM, et al: A prospective study of human immunodeficiency virus type 1 infection and the development of AIDS in subjects with hemophilia. *N Engl J Med* 321:1141–1148, 1989.

13. Perkins HA: Transfusion-induced immunologic unresponsiveness. *Transfus Med Rev* 2:196–203, 1988.

14. Blumberg N, Heal JM: Evidence for plasma-mediated immunomodulation-transfusions of red cells are associated with a lower risk of AIDS than transfusions of plasma-rich blood components. *Transplant Proc* 20:1138–1142, 1988.

15. Blumberg N, Heal JM: Transfusion and recipient immune function. *Arch Pathol Lab Med* 113:246–253, 1989.

16. Webster A, Lee CA, Cook DG, et al: Cytomegalovirus infection and progression towards AIDS in haemophiliacs with human immunodeficiency virus infection. *Lancet* 2:63–66, 1989.

17. Cumming PD, Wallace EL, Schorr JB, Dodd RY: Exposure of patients to human immunodeficiency virus through the transfusion of blood components that test antibody-negative. *N Engl J Med* 321:941–946, 1989.

18. Kleinman S, Secord K: Risk of human immunodeficiency virus (HIV) transmission by anti-HIV negative blood: Estimates using the lookback methodology. *Transfusion* 28:499–501, 1988.

19. Ward JW, Holmberg SD, Allen JR, et al: Transmission of human immunodeficiency virus (HIV) by blood transfusion screened as negative for HIV antibody. *N Engl J Med* 318:473–478, 1988.

20. Peterman TA, Ward JW: What's happening to the epidemic of transfusion-associated AIDS? *Transfusion* 29:659–660, 1989.

21. Imagawa DT, Lee MH, Wolinsky SM, et al: Human immunodeficiency virus type 1 infection in homosexual men who remain seronegative for prolonged periods. *N Engl J Med* 320:1458–1462, 1989.

22. Leitman SF, Klein H, Melpolder JJ, et al: Clinical implications of positive tests for antibodies to human immunodeficiency virus type 1 in asymptomatic blood donors. *N Engl J Med* 321:917–924, 1989.

23. Menitove JE: The decreasing risk of transfusion-associated AIDS. *N Engl J Med* 321:966–968, 1989.

24. Silvergleid AJ, Leparc GF, Schmidt PJ: Impact of explicit questions about high-risk activities on donor attitudes and donor deferral patterns: Results in two community blood centers. *Transfusion* 29:362–364, 1989.

25. Zuck TF: Transfusion-associated AIDS reassessed. *N Engl J Med* 318:511–512, 1988.

26. Alter HJ, Epstein JS, Swenson SG, et al: Prevalence of human immunodeficiency virus type 1 p24 antigen in U.S. blood donors: an assessment of the efficacy of testing in donor screening. *N Engl J Med* 323:312–317, 1990.

27. Mendelson D, Sandler SG: A model for estimating incremental benefits and costs of testing donated blood for human immunodeficiency virus antigen. *Transfusion* 30:73–75, 1990.

28. National Institutes of Health Consensus Development Conference Statement: Perioperative red cell transfusion. *JAMA* 260:2700–2703, 1988.

29. Smith DM, Summers SH (eds): *Platelets.* Arlington, VA, American Association of Blood Banks, 1988.

30. Consensus Development Panel, National Institutes of Health: Fresh frozen plasma. Indications and risks. *JAMA* 253:551–553, 1985.

31. Summers SH, Smith DM (eds): *Transfusion Therapy: Guidelines for Practice.* Arlington, VA, American Association of Blood Banks, 1990.

32. Carlson KB, Golub AH (eds): *Limiting Homologous Exposure: Alternative Strategies.* Arlington, VA, American Association of Blood Banks, 1989.

33. Schwartz RS, Abildgaard CF, Aledort LM, et al: Human recombinant DNA-derived antihemophilic factor (Factor VIII) in the treatment of hemophilia. *N Engl J Med* 323:1800–1805, 1990.

5
Other Retroviruses Transmitted by Blood Transfusion

Alan E. Williams, PhD
Marian T. Sullivan, MS

Despite two decades of rapid research developments in transfusion medicine, no event occurring before 1983 could have matched the profound impact made upon the blood bank by AIDS. Many of the same advances in technology that allowed the isolation and characterization of HIV-1 as the causative agent of AIDS are now being applied to the detection and characterization of other human retroviruses. For those in the field of retrovirology this is an exciting time, since each newly discovered human retrovirus may provide answers to questions about poorly understood human diseases. Accompanying this exciting potential for rapid medical advances, however, are numerous burdens that these rapid advances in retrovirology have placed on the field of transfusion medicine. In addition to reviewing the epidemiology, disease associations, and virology of the known human retroviruses other than HIV-1, we will outline some of the effects these viruses have had on the practice of transfusion medicine.

The currently known human retroviruses can be broadly divided into three categories based on their structural and functional characteristics. The first category is the type C oncoviruses, including HTLV-I, HTLV-II, and HTLV-V. These viruses, which are typically lymphoproliferative, can be broadly characterized by their ability to induce cellular transformation, which may result in malignancy after a prolonged incubation period. Of the human oncoviruses, the most information is known about HTLV-I, which was isolated from the peripheral blood lymphocytes of a patient with cutaneous T-cell lymphoma.[1] A second human retrovirus, HTLV-II, was described 2 years later as an isolate from a patient with a variant form of hairy cell leukemia. Although distinct from HTLV-I, HTLV-II was found to have considerable nucleic acid homology and antigenic cross-reactivity with HTLV-I.[2,3] A third human oncovirus candidate, HTLV-V, has been the subject of only limited reports, but has also been characterized as a distinct human type-C retrovirus.[4]

The second category of human retroviruses is the lentiviruses, including HIV-1 and HIV-2, which ultimately have a cytolytic effect on infected lymphocytes producing a state of immunodeficiency. HIV-1 (and to a lesser extent HIV-2) are the causative agents of the current AIDS pandemic.[5]

The third category is the spumaretroviruses (foamy viruses), which contain the same structural elements as the more fully characterized retroviruses; but about which little else is known. These viruses are known to be frequent contaminants of primary human cell cultures.[6] Although no serologic tests for or epidemiologic data on these foamy viruses exist, it is reasonable to expect that they may be spread by homologous blood transfusion, with or without any resulting effect on the host.

Although quite varied in function and pathogenic potential, the exogenous human retroviruses do have several characteristics in common. All contain the essential structural genes *gag, pol,* and *env,* and all contain additional regulatory genes. In addition, each of these human retroviruses is characterized by a tropism for cells of both lymphoid and CNS origin, and is transmitted both parenterally and by the intimate exchange of body fluids. Although broad generalizations can be made about different biologic effects of infection with each type of virus, there is evidence that both the lentiviruses and the oncoviruses are capable of producing both lymphoproliferative and nonlymphoproliferative diseases in an infected host.

Human Type C Oncoviruses HTLV-I, HTLV-II, and HTLV-V

Epidemiology

Reports of HTLV-I seroprevalence in selected population samples now abound in the medical literature. Despite the number of such reports, an accurate picture of worldwide HTLV-I infection remains difficult to assemble for several reasons. Like HIV-1 and most other known human retrovirus agents, current knowledge about the prevalence and incidence of HTLV-I and HTLV-II infection in various human subpopulations is based on the detection of circulating antibodies made by the host in response to infection, rather than the detection of the virus itself.

HTLV-I and HTLV-II are known to be two distinct viruses that differ both at the genomic level and in the biology of their host interaction. Although there are known to be subtle differences in the provirus coding sequences and the molecular weights of the structural proteins of the two viruses, there is genome sequence homology of approximately 65% between the viruses, which results in major antigenic overlap and an inability, until recently, to distinguish them serologically. For this reason, the seroepidemiology of HTLV-I, as described in the literature, must be considered as a mixture of data on HTLV-I and HTLV-II unless proven otherwise. Throughout this chapter, references to serologically defined human T-lymphotropic viruses type I and II will be noted as HTLV-I/II.

A second limitation of current detection methods for HTLV-I and HTLV-II antibody is the wide variety of antibody detection methods that have been used for epidemiologic studies of HTLV-I/II. These methods include immunofluorescence, ELISA, ELISA plus neutralization, and gelatin particle agglutination. At present, only limited comparative evaluations of the sensitivity and specificity characteristics of these antibody detection methods have been performed.[7-9] Although, in some reports, serum found to be reactive by screening assays has been subjected to in-depth confirmation analysis such as protein immunoblot and radioimmunoprecipitation, here also, the standardization of methodology and interpretation has only recently been described.[10]

Third, the relationship between HTLV-I/II latency and the appearance of circulating viral antibodies remains largely unexplored. Antibody distribution patterns in many HTLV-I/II–endemic areas appear to reflect sexual transmission of the virus, ie, an age-dependent rise beginning at puberty.[11,12] While such a pattern is consistent with the appearance of anti-HTLV-I/II in all instances of infection, these reports can be contrasted with data showing that persons born in endemic areas of the world who relocate to nonendemic areas early in life also show age-specific increases in HTLV-I/II seroprevalence.[13] Therefore, an alternate explanation of the age dependence of HTLV-I/II antibody appearance consistent with the observed latency of animal retroviruses could be the acquisition of infection early in life followed by a delayed antibody response triggered by a later event. For these reasons, it should be kept in mind that the growing body of descriptive epidemiology based on serologically defined HTLV-I/II infection will be subject to revision as additional information about the serologic characterization of infection and latency of these viruses becomes available.

Worldwide seroprevalence.   HTLV-I/II infection is characterized by macroclustering and microclustering in several endemic areas of the world, particularly southern Japan, the Caribbean basin, and Africa. The earliest and most complete seroprevalence data for HTLV-I/II come from extensive studies of blood donors and other asymptomatically infected persons conducted in Japan over the past 10 years. The geographic pattern of HTLV-I/II antibody was also found to share a marked codistribution with recognized cases of adult T-cell leukemia, a newly recognized clinical entity first described in 1977.[14,15] It was during this same period that HTLV-I was first isolated and characterized in the United States. Since its initial description, HTLV-I has been implicated as the causative agent of adult T-cell leukemia by in vitro virologic studies,[16,17] and by the remarkable similarities in geographic distribution, particularly in the southern districts of Japan.[18-25]

Seroprevalence studies of HTLV-I in both the Japanese general population and Japanese blood donors have shown marked geographic variations, ranging from a high of 8.0% in the southern district of Kyushu to comparatively lower values in northern districts such as Hokkaido (1.2%), Tokyo (1.1%), and Shikoku (0.5%).[21,24] The island of Okinawa is now recognized as having hyperendemic levels of infection with seropositivity rates as high as 37.5% in men and 44.5% in women.[13]

Additional geographic clustering of HTLV-I infection is found at the village and household level within endemic areas of Japan. A logical explanation of such microclustering is the occurrence of intrafamilial transmission, or infection by close personal contact. However, these patterns of HTLV-I distribution have apparently been stable for many generations, and are likely to be the result of complex virus-host dynamics that are not yet fully understood. It has been estimated that currently over 1 million Japanese inhabitants are asymptomatically infected with HTLV-I.[25]

Based on several recent studies, populations native to the Caribbean basin exhibit HTLV-I seroprevalence levels of 2% to 12%.[26-28] Similar to the strong association seen between HTLV-I and adult T-cell leukemia in Japan, increased HTLV-I seroprevalence has been reported in both US patients with adult T-cell leukemia and Jamaican patients with non-Hodgkin's lymphoid malignancies.[29,30]

The presence of endemic HTLV-I/II infection, as well as an increased prevalence of the HTLV-I–associated lymphoid malignancies and myelopathies, has also been documented in the Caribbean, and in sub-Saharan Africa, where a 13.2% prevalence of HTLV-I/II antibodies was reported in random hospitalized Zairian patients.[31-36] Serologic evidence of the presence of HTLV-I/II infection has now also been reported for general population samples from South Africa, Nigeria, Egypt, Tunisia, and Ghana.[37,38] In South America, HTLV-I/II infection has now also been reported from Panama, Colombia, and Venezuela.[21,28]

There have not been extensive molecular epidemiology studies to distinguish HTLV-I from HTLV-II in Japan or the Caribbean basin. Although molecular characterization of isolates from patients with HTLV-I–related disease has not revealed the presence of HTLV-II and it has been generally assumed that the endemic infection in Japan and the Caribbean is due to HTLV-I, there are no data with which to estimate the differential distribution of these two agents worldwide.

Seroprevalence in the United States. Although rare cases of HTLV-I–associated lymphoid neoplasias and neurologic disease have been described in the United States and Europe, the magnitude of HTLV-I–associated disease does not approach that seen in the endemic areas of Japan and the Caribbean. Seroepidemiologic and virologic studies of HTLV-I/II infection in the United States have been targeted largely at selected population samples, including users of illicit intravenous drugs, blood donors, blood recipients, and various other patient categories. The best conservative estimate of overall HTLV-I/II infection in the United States is provided by current seroprevalence data for US blood donors, of whom 0.02% are found to be seropositive nationwide.[39] When seropositive donors are questioned about risk factors that may be associated with infection, approximately two thirds of them admit having risk factors that parallel the known epidemiology of the infection.[39,40] These include a history of intravenous drug use, sexual contact with an intravenous drug user, birth in the Caribbean, sexual contact with a Caribbean native, or a history of blood transfusion. Although persons of Japanese ancestry have been identified within the seropositive donor population, this risk accounts for only about 3% of the observed donor seroprevalence nationwide.[39]

Estimates of HTLV-I seroprevalence in the general population are certain to exceed the levels found in blood donors who are all in good health and have been carefully selected for an absence of AIDS risk factors. For instance, hyperendemic foci of infection are known to exist in US urban intravenous drug abusers, in whom HTLV-I/II seroprevalence has generally been found to range from 2% to 10%,[41,42] but has also been reported to be as high as 49.3% and 30.2% in selected minority intravenous drug users in New Orleans and New Jersey, respectively.[43,44] Although the seroprevalence estimates have been based on HTLV-I viral antigens, several recent reports based on advanced molecular virologic techniques have shown that HTLV-II may be the infecting agent in many US intravenous drug users.[45]

Although representative estimates of HTLV-I/II worldwide seroprevalence remain limited, it is likely that human infection with HTLV-I and HTLV-II occurs globally. As indicated below, endemic infection is sustained by complex mechanisms of virus transmission, and is etiologically related to at least two unique human diseases.

Modes of Transmission

Unlike the relatively recent appearance of HIV-1 infection, HTLV-I/II is generally considered to have been present in the world's populations for at least several generations. This view arises, in part, from the breadth of HTLV-I/II distribution and the appearance of HTLV-I associated disease in persons, now in their second or third decade, who appear to have been infected at birth. Despite a lengthy human experience with HTLV-I/II however, infection with these agents exhibits a remarkable degree of microclustering, both geographically and within individual family units. Although an understanding of human retrovirus epidemiology is still at an early stage, the distribution patterns of HTLV-I/II infection, and associated diseases are currently believed to represent a complex interrelationship of the following transmission modes, which appear to result in static patterns of infection in some parts of the world and rapidly spreading infection in others.

Perinatal infection.   Clustering of HTLV-I infection in families has repeatedly been observed in Japan. It has been reported that 50% of children born to HTLV-I–infected mothers in Japan seroconvert by the age of 2 years, making this the most important means of virus transmission in areas of the world with endemic infection.[46-48] The principal means of familial transmission appears to be perinatal transmission via HTLV-I/II–infected lymphocytes present in an infected mother's breast milk. Although the mechanisms of infection through the oral route are not fully understood, there has been no evidence for true vertical (germ cell) or transplacental infection from mother to child based on seroconversion studies.[46] In light of recent observations regarding seronegative infections, the absence of infant infection based on serologic findings alone needs to be verified by gene probe analysis. Preliminary data from an experimental study of breast-feeding intervention being conducted in Japan indicates that the risk of infection declined with the decreased duration of breast-feeding. Furthermore, at 1 year after birth, eight of 285 children not breast-fed (3%) were seropositive, in contrast with 34 of 205 children who were breast-fed (17%).[47]

Blood transfusion. The first description of transfusion-associated HTLV-I transmission was provided by cross-sectional and prospective studies conducted in Japan early in the 1980s. Evidence for posttransfusion seroconversion was reported for leukemia, cardiac surgery, and hemodialysis patients who had received homologous whole blood transfusions from unscreened donors. This initial series of papers, as well as several later Japanese reports detailing the success of donor screening for HTLV-I antibody, established several key observations about the transmission of HTLV-I/II from a seropositive infected donor to an uninfected recipient.[49-53]

1. HTLV-I transmission is limited to cellular products.
2. Infected recipients generally seroconvert within 2 months of exposure.
3. The efficiency of HTLV-I transmission by infected cellular products is approximately 63% and appears to decrease with advancing product age.
4. The acquisition of HTLV-I by transfusion is rarely associated with a pathologic outcome because of the long incubation period between infection and disease.
5. Screening of blood donors is an effective means of reducing the transmission of HTLV-I infection to seronegative recipients.

These observations, considered together with the known reservoir of HTLV-I/II infection in the intravenous drug–using population and the 0.025% prevalence of HTLV-I/II infection found in a large cross-sectional study of US blood donors,[40] led to the recommendation for screening of all US blood product donations for HTLV-I/II antibody. In November 1988, HTLV-I screening assays from three commercial manufacturers were licensed by the US Food and Drug Administration.[54] Phase-in of blood donor screening began immediately, and testing of all US blood products became the standard as of March 1989.

The extent to which blood recipients in the United States have been infected with HTLV-I as a result of transfusion is currently unknown. It has been predicted, however, that approximately 2000 HTLV-I/II seropositive blood donors will be detected during the first year of screening in the United States, and that their prior donations will have been received by approximately 6000 living blood recipients.[39] Preliminary studies of such recipients indicate that 13% to 17% are seropositive. Transmission of both HTLV-I and HTLV-II has been documented and, thus far, only cellular blood products have been implicated.[55,56]

Needle sharing. Intravenous drug users who share needles are recognized as major reservoirs of parenterally transmitted infections such as hepatitis B and HIV, both of which are easily transmitted by cell-free virus. Because cellular transfer appears to be necessary to produce new HTLV-I/II infection, such transmission by blood contamination of a syringe and needle may be somewhat less efficient. Despite this, however, intravenous drug users in the United States show moderate to high rates of HTLV-I/II infection and appear to serve as a major reservoir of secondary infection via sexual contact. An increase in the severity of HIV-related disease has been reported in individuals who are dually infected with HIV and HTLV-I/II,[57] but few instances of diseases known to be associated with HTLV-I alone have been observed in intravenous drug users in the United States. The absence of such disease may reflect a predominance of HTLV-II, or the fact that HTLV-I/II infection has been recently introduced to this population.

Sexual transmission.   Worldwide HTLV-I/II seroepidemiologic data have primarily been obtained through cross-sectional studies of convenience samples of patients or other population subgroups of particular epidemiologic interest. Although few prospective studies have been undertaken to study directly the sexual transmission dynamics of HTLV-I/II, several key epidemiologic observations confirm this route of transmission. The first is the marked age-specific increase in antibody prevalence beginning at puberty that is seen in population-based samples from HTLV-I/II–endemic areas such as Japan and Jamaica.[11,12] The slope of the age-specific prevalence curves is usually steeper for females, indicating a more efficient transmission from male to female, or more frequent exposure of females to HTLV-I/II. Additional observational data are available from retrospective studies of long-term sexual partners of infected individuals who were not born in an endemic area. These include 0.076% seroprevalence in US marines stationed in Okinawa,[58] and studies of seropositive married couples identified through blood donor screening in the US, where approximately 30% of individuals have no defined risk of infection other than a long-term sexual relationship with a spouse infected through a different route.[39]

Results of a 10-year study of married couples in Japan indicate that male-to-female transmission of HTLV-I (60.8%) is far more efficient than female-to-male transmission (0.4%).[59] However, there is growing evidence that in other parts of the world sexual transmission in both directions is an important means of HTLV-I/II spread, particularly during a long-term sexual relationship.[39]

The Agents

This section will summarize current understanding of the human oncoviruses and their interaction with host cells. Detailed reviews of HTLV-I and HTLV-II virology are available and the reader is referred to these for additional details.[60,61]

HTLV-I was first isolated from a patient with cutaneous T-cell lymphoma as a highly cell-associated type C retrovirus with $Mg^{(2+)}$–dependent reverse transcriptase activity. Morphologically, HTLV-I is a type-C retrovirus with a

Table 5–1   Recognized Genes and Polypeptides of HTLV-I and HTLV-II

	HTLV-I	HTLV-II
gag	p55/24/19	p53/24/19
pol	p~100	p~100
env	gp61/gp46,gp21	gp61/gp46,gp21
tax	p40	p37
rex	p27,p21	p26,p24
pro	Undetermined	

central core surrounded by an envelope. HTLV-I exhibits a primary tropism for CD4(+) cells, including lymphocytes and astrocytes, and appears to bind cells through a unique protein receptor coded by human chromosome 17.[62,63] The genome of HTLV-I is 9.03 kb long, with an organization that resembles other known animal retroviruses and contains *gag* (group antigen), *pro* (protease), *pol* (reverse transcriptase), and *env* (envelope) genes for the production of virus structural proteins. These structural genes are flanked by LTR sequences at each end of the genome that together regulate proviral gene expression, and a nonstructural coding region "x" at the 3′ end. The size and functions of the gene products are indicated in Table 5–1.[60]

The proteins encoded by the *tax* and *rex* genes within the *x* region of the HTLV-I genome have been the subject of intense study during the past several years because of their *trans*-activation properties. These proteins are not found in the virion, but are expressed in the host cell and provide regulation of viral replication.[64] In addition to inducing the IL-2 receptor promoter gene that results in IL-2R expression on the surface of infected cells, the *tax* protein has also been found to induce the production of other cellular gene products that may be associated with some of the clinical manifestations found in HTLV-I disease (Table 5–2).[65] Attempts to demonstrate the HTLV-I *tax* protein directly in adult T-cell leukemia or tumor tissue have been largely unsuccessful, however, and it is currently believed that the *tax* protein acts through a "hit and run" mechanism by activation of cellular promoter genes and subsequent disappearance.[66]

The *rex* gene of HTLV-I regulates the production of HTLV-I structural proteins by promoting the transport of unspliced mRNA into the cytoplasm where the viral proteins are translated. The rex protein of HTLV-I is functionally equivalent to the rev protein of HIV-1 and is capable of rescuing rev-deficient mutants of HIV in vitro.[65]

It has also been recently found that purified HTLV-I and HTLV-II virions are capable of both inducing uninfected T-cell proliferation, and stimulating HIV-infected T lymphocytes to increase production of HIV-1 p24 antigen.[64] In light of recent clinical observations that the clinical course of patients dually infected with HIV and HTLV-I is one of rapid deterioration, this latter observation may be of value in relating HIV-1 pathologic outcome to specific cellular activation events.

Table 5–2 Proteins Induced In Vitro by the HTLV-I *tax* Transcriptional Activation

Protein	Possible In Vivo Outcome
IL-1	Encephalopathy
IL-3,4,5,6	?
GM-CSF	?
IL-2R	T-cell proliferation
Gamma IFN	?
TNF (LT)	Hypercalcemia

HTLV-II is morphologically identical and structurally very similar to HTLV-I. Although the 8.95-kb genome of HTLV-II is slightly smaller than that of HTLV-I and has only approximately 35% sequence homology with HTLV-I in both the LTR sequences and at the 3' end, there is approximately 60% overall homology between the two viruses, with particular conservation of the genes required for regulation of proviral gene expression.[66] The viral structural proteins are similar in molecular weight and function, and are highly cross-reactive antigenically (Table 5–2). Although not as well studied as HTLV-I, many biologic properties of HTLV-II, such as transformation potential via the *trans*-acting tax protein, appear to be shared between the two viruses.

Associated Diseases

The presence of HTLV-I/II antibody can generally be equated with the concurrent presence of integrated HTLV-I or HTLV-II provirus and the ability to transmit infection by the transfer of infected cells. Although direct examination of peripheral blood without some means of provirus amplification will generally produce negative results, infection can be demonstrated by the production of HTLV-I in cultures of peripheral blood cells derived from asymptomatic carriers. More recently, the polymerase chain reaction has been used to amplify selected HTLV-I proviral gene sequences directly from peripheral blood of asymptomatic carriers. Despite the presence of integrated provirus, the vast majority of HTLV-I–seropositive persons remain asymptomatic. Although HTLV-I is strongly associated with both the hematologic and neurologic disorders described below, these diseases are manifested only after prolonged incubation periods, and only in a small proportion of infected individuals. Although both HTLV-II and HTLV-V have been isolated from patients with oncologic disease, no causative role in human disease has yet been attributed to these agents.

HTLV-I and adult T-cell leukemia.　　The clinical stages of adult T-cell leukemia include a preleukemic state, chronic or smoldering adult T-cell leukemia, and acute adult T-cell leukemia, which are reviewed in detail elsewhere.[60,67] Acute adult T-cell leukemia is a rapidly progressive fatal illness and is generally accompanied by eosinophilia, lymphadenopathy, hepatosplenomegaly, and elevated serum calcium, bilirubin, and lactate dehydrogenase levels, in addition to increases in the white blood cell count. The tumors of adult T-cell leukemia are generally monoclonal, with cells that contain integrated HTLV-I provirus. Interestingly, however, there does not appear to be a consistent provirus integration site, implying that a *trans-acting* gene (such as *tax*) may be producing a diffusible product that is capable of inducing tumor formation without dependence on its location within the cellular genome. Although *tax* protein has not been directly observed in tumor cells or tissues, transgenic mouse models carrying the HTLV-I *tax* gene have developed similar hematologic disorders.[68]

Approximately 600 cases of adult T-cell leukemia are reported annually in Japan. Current estimates predict a 1% to 3% chance of adult T-cell leukemia development in individuals infected with HTLV-I at birth; however, the incidence of adult T-cell leukemia in those who acquire infection later in life is unknown.[69] Based on family studies, however, there is some evidence that genetic cofactors may lead to a familial predisposition to adult T-cell leukemia.[69-71] Approximately 11% of adult T-cell leukemia cases diagnosed in Japan are negative for HTLV-I infection by serologic and virologic assessment. Similarly, only a fraction of those persons with HTLV-I infection progress to leukemia. Since HTLV-I is now generally considered to be the causative agent of adult T-cell leukemia, the explanation for these observations is unknown, but is likely to be related to the need for genetic or environmental cofactors for disease development.

HTLV-I and neuromuscular disease.   A second clinical syndrome that roughly parallels the worldwide distribution of HTLV-I is HTLV-I–associated myelopathy and its Caribbean equivalent, tropical spastic paraparesis. These two designations refer to the same slowly progressing myelopathy, which is characterized by weakness of the lower trunk and legs, resulting in an inability to walk and eventual lower limb paralysis. Mild sensorimotor neuropathy is sometimes observed, but the upper body and cognitive functions are generally not affected.[72]

The association of HTLV-I/II infection with endemic myelopathy was first made in Martinique, where two HTLV-I–seropositive patients with tropical spastic paraparesis were identified in the course of a retrospective serosurvey of hospitalized patients and controls. In addition, 15 of 22 patients with tropical spastic paraparesis were found to be HTLV-I/II–seropositive.[31] Similar reports of HTLV-I/II associated with tropical spastic paraparesis have been made from Trinidad and Jamaica, in which 60% to 85% of patients diagnosed as having tropical spastic paraparesis were found to be HTLV-I/II–seropositive.[32,33,72-75] Similarly, in a large study of 230 myelopathy patients from Japan, 100% were found to be HTLV-I/II–seropositive.[34] A comparison of the clinical and pathologic characteristics of Caribbean tropical spastic paraparesis and

Japanese HTLV-I–associated myelopathy indicated that these two designations refer to the same disease, now called HAM/TSP.[35]

Although there appears to be a close relationship between HTLV-I infection and HAM/TSP, the virus-host interactions that may directly result in myelopathy are not understood, although the finding of intrathecal HTLV-I antibody and viral proteins in these patients supports the hypothesis that viral proliferation is occurring within the blood-brain barrier.[76,77] It has been the practice in Japan to include HTLV-I seropositivity as part of the diagnostic criteria for HTLV-I–associated myelopathy.

There is some clinical and radiologic overlap between the diagnosis of HAM/TSP and the progressive spinal form of multiple sclerosis, and it is sometimes difficult to distinguish HAM/TSP from multiple sclerosis and other progressive myelopathies.

The question of an etiologic involvement of HTLV-I with multiple sclerosis has been controversial for several years, since the first report of HTLV-I p24 antibody in approximately 30% of multiple sclerosis patients from Sweden and the United States.[78] Although several conflicting reports have since appeared regarding this association, recent genome amplification studies have provided evidence of HTLV-I *pol* and *env* gene sequences in the peripheral blood cells of a proportion of thoroughly studied, HTLV-I–seronegative multiple sclerosis patients.[79,80] The extent to which the HTLV-I–multiple sclerosis association can be extended to an etiologic relationship is unknown, but is currently under intense investigation.

Unknown role of HTLV-II in disease. Before 1987, only a limited number of HTLV-II isolates had been described. Two of these viruses were obtained from patients with atypical forms of hairy cell leukemia.[2,3,81] Similar to findings with tumors induced by HTLV-I, HTLV-II genome could be found integrated monoclonally into the genome of the patient's tumors. Although HTLV-I and HTLV-II are generally thought to exhibit tropism for CD4(+) cells, one of the patients from whom HTLV-II was isolated had a CD8(+) tumor, and subsequently developed a fatal B-cell leukemia. Although HTLV-II genome was not seen in the B-cell tumor by hybridization analysis, and there is no direct evidence to suggest that HTLV-II was etiologically related to these malignancies, HTLV-II has been shown to transform human peripheral blood lymphocytes in vitro, and it has been hypothesized that HTLV-II may induce in vivo cellular transformation by indirect mechanisms similar to those of HTLV-I. At present, further information regarding potential disease associations of HTLV-II is restricted by the lack of a screening assay capable of serologically distinguishing this virus from HTLV-I.

Diagnosis

Initial screening methods. A variety of methods are currently in use for the initial detection of natural antibodies to HTLV-I viral proteins (Table 5–3). These include the commercial enzyme-linked immunoassays, indirect immunofluorescence assay,[16] ^{125}I-labeled p24 radioimmunoassay,[82] competitive

Table 5–3   Methods of HTLV-I Antibody Screening and Confirmation

Test Method*	Commonly Used Cell Lines	Preparation	Protein Products Reliably Present	Criteria for HTLV-I(+)
ELISA	HUT102.B2	Banded virus	p19,p24,p55	Not confirmatory
125I-p24 ELISA	HUT102.B2	Gel filtration	p24	Not confirmatory
PPA	TCL-Kan	Banded virus	p19,p24,p55	Not confirmatory
IFA	HUT102.B2, MT-2	Fixed, antigen-positive cells		Not confirmatory
Competitive ELISA	HUT102.B2	Banded virus	p19,p24,p55	Not confirmatory
Protein Immunoblot	HUT102.B2, MT-2	Banded virus	p19,p24,(p28)	Not confirmatory unless anti-p24 and an *env*-specific band appear
		Whole-cell	p19,p24,(p28), gp46,p55,gp61/68	
Radioimmuno-precipitation	SLB-1,MT-2	Whole-cell	p19,p24,p55, gp61/68,p40X	Antibody to 2 gene products by RIP +/or blot, including p24
PCR/hybridization		Synthetic DNA probes		Hybridization to 2 HTLV-I–specific probes

*ELISA indicates enzyme-linked immunosorbent assay; PPA, passive particle agglutination assay; IFA, indirect immunofluorescence assay; RIP, radioimmunoprecipitation; and PCR, polymerase chain reaction.

ELISA,[83] and passive particle agglutination assay.[84] These methods primarily employ the HUT102, HUT102.B2, and MT-2 cell lines. HUT102 is the prototype HTLV-I–infected T-cell culture established from an American patient, and MT-2 is a standard HTLV-I–infected T-cell line established with virus from a Japanese patient.[62,85]

A problem inherent to the descriptive epidemiology of HTLV-I is the unknown sensitivity and variable specificity of these assays in reference to the presence of HTLV-I infection. Like the widely used assays for HIV-1 antibody, screening assays for HTLV-I depend on antiviral antibodies produced by the infected host in response to infection. Antibody response in the host can be to any or all of the HTLV-I antigens, including p40x, and the levels of reactivity to individual viral polypeptides are variable both in patients with HTLV-I–specific diseases, and in asymptomatic carriers.

All currently licensed assays for HTLV-I antibody utilize virus lysate preparations from the long-term human T lymphocyte cell lines described above. Because of a close association between the virus and the host cell, the amount of HTLV-I proteins that can be harvested from these producer cell lines is low, and the proteins must be meticulously purified away from host contaminants. The result of this purification is that the representation of viral antigens available to react in a test system becomes somewhat selective, and favors the more stable *gag* proteins. The amount of *env*-encoded protein in such a preparation is likely to be variable; however, the surface glycoproteins of 46 and 61 kd encoded by the *env* gene are the most immunogenic of the HTLV-I proteins,[86] and anti-*env* is probably the earliest serologic marker for seroconversion.[87] The p40x (*tax*) protein, because of its close association with the host cell nucleus, is not retained. Although no extensive comparison testing has been performed between these methods, reports from various investigators have noted the relative sensitivity of the indirect immunofluorescence assay, the passive protein agglutination assay, and the competitive ELISA.[10,88,89]

Other recently developed ELISA tests, which employ synthetic peptides, provide the advantage of minimizing the incidence of nonspecific reactions resulting from antibody cross-reactivities to cellular antigens.[90] Such assays typically employ synthetic envelope peptides that correspond to a highly antigenic, conserved segment of the transmembrane protein of either HTLV-I or HTLV-II. The combined use of two such ELISAs, therefore, may allow for the distinction of virus type by the interpretation of the ratio of absorbance values from each assay.[91,92]

HTLV-I antibody confirmation methods

Protein immunoblot. Reactivity demonstrated by an initial screening test such as ELISA must be confirmed by a secondary procedure, which in most laboratories is a protein immunoblot (Western blot) (Figure 5–1) or radioimmunoprecipitation assay, or a combination of the two. The immunoblot allows for the detection of HTLV-I–specific antibodies in serum that bind to viral antigens immobilized on a nitrocellulose membrane. The antigens are trans-blotted onto the membrane after resolution based on molecular weight by polyacrylamide gel electrophoresis following protein dissociation by the detergent sodium dodecyl sulfate (SDS).[93]

Cell lines commonly used in the preparation of viral antigen impregnated strips are MT-2 and HUT102.B2. The antigen preparation is generally the same type of (banded-virus) lysate used in the screening assay. This procedure favors detection of the *gag* encoded polypeptides p19, p24, and the p55 precursor. A *gag-tax* fusion protein, p28, is also commonly observed in MT-2 viral antigen preparations.[94] Carefully purified antigen preparations and whole-cell lysates may retain the gp46 *env* component, which appears as a broad glycoprotein band; however, cellular membrane proteins often contaminate any of these preparations and may be the source of nonspecific cross-reactivities. Alternatively, purified gp46 or p21e can be added to such preparations to enhance anti-*env* detectability.

At present, a conservative approach is applied to HTLV-I/II antibody confirmation that requires the detection of antibodies to the *gag* (p24) and *env* (gp46 or gp61/68) viral proteins. This may be achieved by any combination of results from immunoblot or radioimmunoprecipitation assays.[10] In practice, a viral lysate Western blot appears to be insufficient for confirmation purposes in most cases, and further testing by radioimmunoprecipitation is required in about 70% of such samples. It has been the experience of this laboratory that solo p24 reactive samples are more likely than solo p19 reactive samples to be confirmed positive by radioimmunoprecipitation assay. A possible explanation for nonspecific reactions with p19 is cross-reactivity with anti-thymus antibodies. This is supported by the observation that monoclonal antibody to p19 will stain normal human thymus.[95] Nonspecific antibody reactions have also been recognized in the region of gp46, due primarily to actin. Actin, with a molecular weight of approximately 43 kd, is ubiquitous in eukaryotic cells. Interference from anti-actin also occurs in the radioimmunoprecipitation assay. However, using an SLB-1 cell lysate, the primary *env* gene product has a molecular weight of 61 kd.[96]

Data from routine blood donor screening indicate that, analogous to testing for HIV-1, a proportion of persons with indeterminate test results is likely to be identified, ie, those who have reactive screening tests but do not meet the full criteria for confirmation. Using the Abbott HTLV-I ELISA, approximately one third of reactive serum specimens are confirmed positive, one third remain indeterminate, and one third are negative.[39] Thirty-seven blood donors with indeterminate HTLV-I status were identified by the American Red Cross during the initial phase of a large cross-sectional, case-control study of 39,898 donors.[40] Follow-up of eight (21.6%) of these persons disclosed no seroconversions, and the indeterminate band patterns showed no significant fluctuations after 2 years. While the importance of indeterminate findings is not currently known, with the exception of p24, the specificity of solitary *gag*-related reactions in the immunoblot is suspect.

Radioimmunoprecipitation assay.   The radioimmunoprecipitation assay, while considerably more labor-intensive, demonstrates greater specificity for

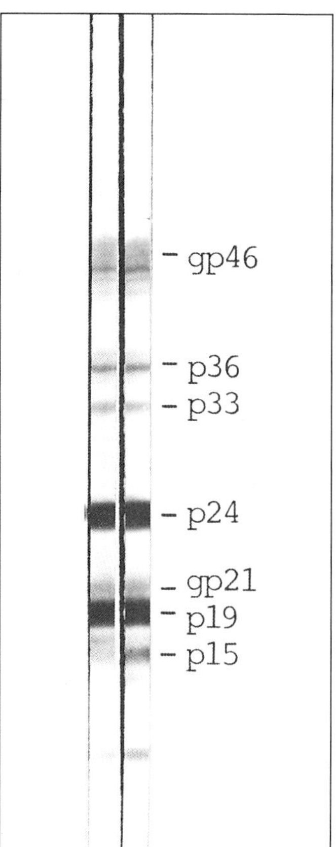

Figure 5–1   Protein immunoblot assay for confirmation of HTLV-I antibody reactivity. Both lanes contain samples that are confirmed positive based on reactivity against p24 and gp46.

HTLV-I viral proteins. Because of its reliance on a whole-cell lysate, it also has increased sensitivity for anti-*env* proteins, although the size of the *env* gene product most commonly observed often depends on the cell line used for expression, eg, MT-2=gp68, SLB-1=gp61, and HUT102=gp46.[94] The *gag*-specific reactivities (p24 and particularly p19) are less consistent from preparation to preparation. Sensitivity to anti-*tax* protein (p40x) is variable, depending primarily on the cell line employed. The SLB-1 cell line is a high producer of p40x antigen, whereas MT-2 cells are not.

While highly specific, the radioimmunoprecipitation assay requires 5 to 6 days for completion (Figure 5–2). The HTLV-I–infected cell line is labeled with a radioactive amino acid, typically ^{35}S-cysteine, after which the cells are lysed. Lysate is incubated overnight with 5 to 10 μL of each sample to be tested, at which time soluble labeled antigen-antibody complexes will form. These complexes are precipitated away from unbound labeled antigen by the addition of protein A-Sepharose™. The protein A from *Staphylococcus aureus*

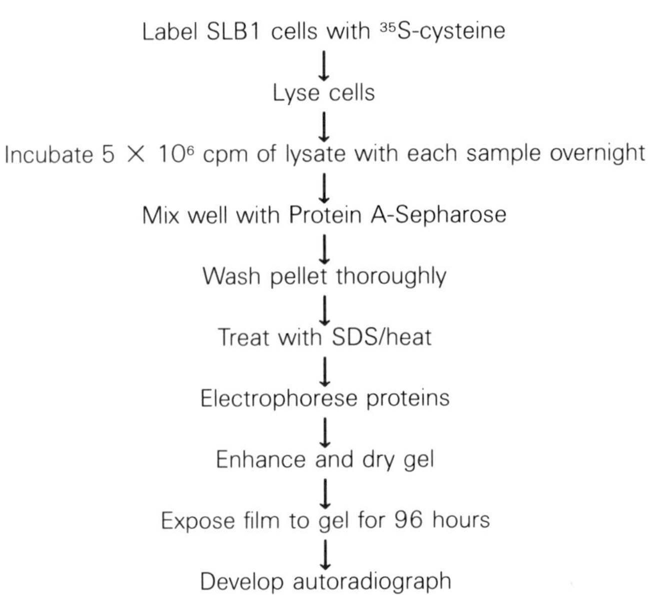

Figure 5–2   Procedure for the confirmation of HTLV-I antibodies by radioimmunoprecipitation.

binds preferentially to IgG, while the solid-phase Sepharose™ facilitates the separation of the immunoprecipitate.

After repeated washing, each immunoprecipitate pellet is boiled in the presence of SDS and loaded onto an SDS polyacrylamide gel that enables the separation of the labeled viral antigens by molecular weight. The gel is treated with a fluor and dried, and is then exposed to XAR film for 2 to 3 days at −70 °C to produce the autoradiograph.

Using the SLB-1 cell line, we have found that the viral gene products p24, p40x, p55, and gp61 appear reliably (Figure 5–3). The percentage frequency of seroreactivity to the respective proteins in the sum total of confirmed positive samples evaluated by our laboratory is 83%, 88%, 63%, and 83%. These samples represent populations of healthy Japanese and American blood donors, intravenous drug users, and leukemia patients. With the exception of the Japanese samples, which commonly display full antibody profiles, no significant differences in band frequencies are evident between populations.

Studies we have conducted on more than 650 intravenous drug users from Connecticut yielded the observation that five (0.77%) of these subjects may have seroreactivity solely to p40x. None of these samples tested positive by initial screening methods (ELISA) and all were immunoblot-negative. The significance of this observation is not known.

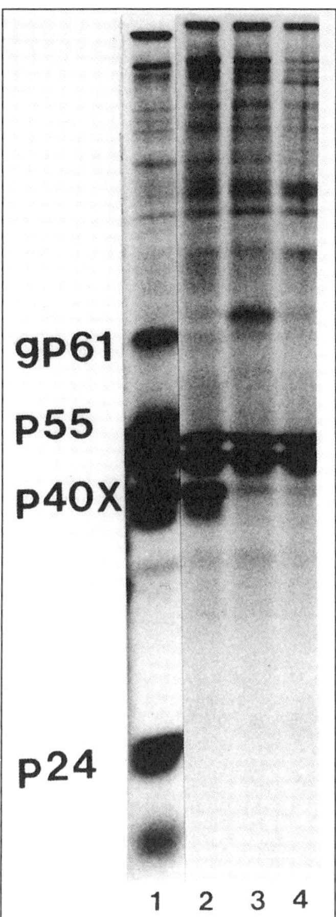

Figure 5–3   Radioimmunoprecipitation assay for confirmation of HTLV-I antibody reactivity. Each sample was reacted with 5 × 10⁶ cpm of ³⁵S-cysteine–labeled lysate of SLB-1 cells. Lane 1 is a sample positive for HTLV-I antibodies exhibiting reactivity against p24, p40X, p55, and gp61. Lane 2 is a sample from an intravenous drug user found to be negative by standard ELISA and immunoblot methods, and considered "indeterminate" as a result of p40X reactivity by radioimmunoprecipitation. Lanes 3 and 4 are negative samples.

We have made numerous attempts to enhance the sensitivity of the radioimmunoprecipitation assay, including using a double-labeled lysate incorporating both ³⁵S-cysteine and ³⁵S-methionine. The observed lack of substantial improvement of detectability with the addition of ³⁵S-methionine is explainable by HTLV-I sequence analysis, since Cys residues outnumber methionine by a factor of three in the coding regions of the genome.[97]

Leucine, on the other hand, is more prevalent than Cys, particularly in the Leu-rich *env* glycoprotein. When a ³H-leucine–labeled lysate was used, a slight improvement in the detection of anti-gp61 was apparent. In fact, preliminary data on two of the five intravenous drug user serum samples with apparent solo p40x reactivity indicate that very low levels of *env* antibody are present in these samples.

The recent development of other research level assays for HTLV-I has yielded a wealth of comparative information and increased the possibility of creating a simplified confirmatory algorithm. The use of a genetically engineered HTLV-I *env* gene–derived peptide, p21e, expressed in *Escherichia coli,* has yielded a highly sensitive and specific recombinant assay that has been used successfully in the American Red Cross confirmation algorithm.[90]

Genome amplification by PCR.   Many factors influence the yield of viral proteins, and hence the quantity of circulating antibodies in the serum. Therefore, direct detection of HTLV-I–integrated and proviral DNA is of use when analyzing samples with atypical or negative serologic reactions. In addition, nucleic acid hybridization with highly characterized sequences allows for the distinction of similar retroviruses, such as HTLV-I and HTLV-II, as well as the comparison of isolates from different geographic populations and risk groups.

Southern blotting and dot blotting techniques, in the absence of gene amplification, minimally require one copy of virus per 100 cells. Such a high number of copies is found only in leukemia patients, and most HTLV-I–infected persons would have too few infected cells to be detected by these methods. In such cases, in vitro enzymatic gene amplification, or the PCR,[98] has been employed to multiply both the proviral DNA and the viral RNA of discreet regions of retroviral genomes present in peripheral blood.[99-104]

Genome amplification permits the replication of a specific sequence or target region within a complex template, provided that the nucleic acid sequence is known (Figure 5–4). Primers, or short pieces of synthetic DNA with sequences complementary to the DNA flanking the target region, define the ends of the DNA to be duplicated. The DNA to be tested is extracted and purified from lymphocytes isolated from 15 mL of fresh peripheral blood by Ficoll-Hypaque™ gradient and treated with sodium dodecyl sulfate and proteinase K. Standard techniques are followed for the preparation of high molecular weight DNA, taking care to inhibit degradation and prevent contamination (Figure 5–5). Additionally, the quantity and quality of the DNA can be verified by the use of an HLA-DQa primer pair.[104]

Rapid, repetitive cycles of DNA denaturation, primer hybridization, and polymerase extension are made possible by the use of a heat-stable DNA polymerase from *Thermus aquaticus.*[105,106] Each reaction step takes approximately 2 minutes, at temperatures of 94°, 37°, and 72 °C, respectively. Automation and standardization of the amplification protocol is provided by the GeneAmp™ DNA Amplification Reagent Kit and the DNA Thermal Cycler, an automated heating and cooling block (Perkin Elmer Cetus, Norwalk, CT).

Because each cycle of the PCR results in a doubling of the DNA target region the amount of amplified nucleic acid accumulates geometrically. Twenty cycles, for example, can theoretically amplify a single sequence of target DNA by a factor of approximately 1×10^6. For this reason, it is im-

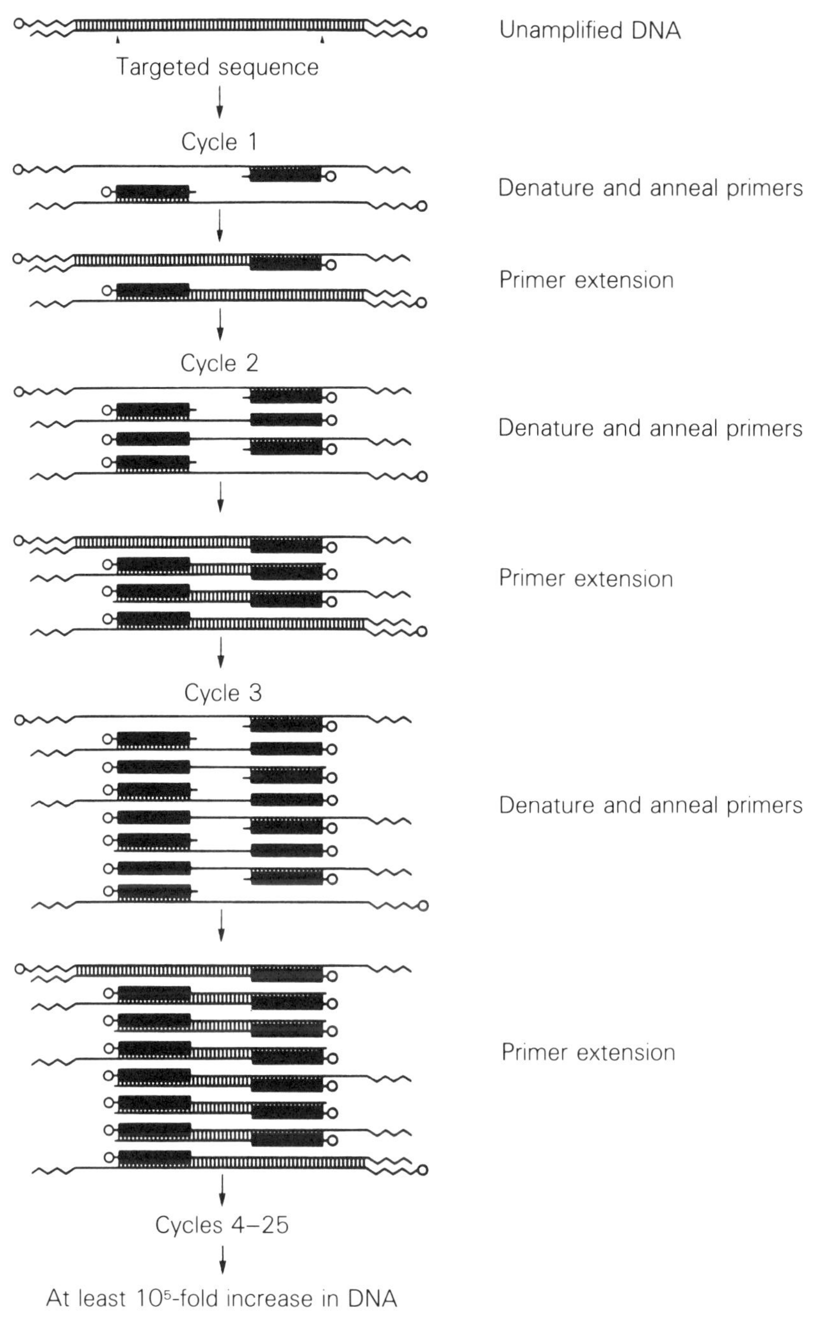

Figure 5–4 Principle of the enzymatic amplification of DNA by the PCR.[106]

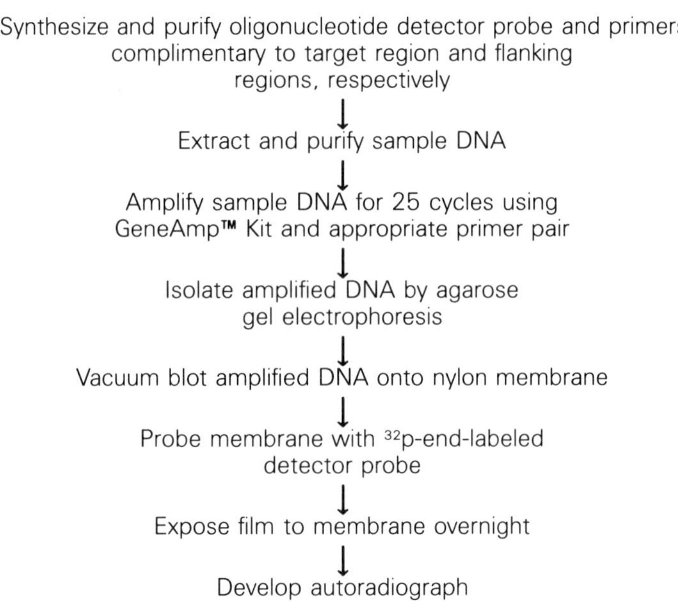

Figure 5–5   Procedure for the detection of HTLV-I integrated and proviral DNA by gene amplification and hybridization.

perative to eliminate any opportunity for sample contamination, including prevention of aerosolization and the use of dedicated reagents and pipettes. Furthermore, controls for each reagent should be included in every amplification run.

Sequence information is available for each of the human retroviruses. Selection of primer pairs homologous to specific regions of the HTLV-I, HIV-1, or HTLV-II genomes is determined by their intended application. The amplified product is transferred onto a nylon or nitrocellulose membrane and probed with the appropriate synthetic detector oligomer.[107] The amount of ^{32}P end-labeled probe that hybridizes to the nucleic acid on the membrane can be visualized by autoradiography and quantitated by densitometry.

Probes can be selected to perform a variety of tasks, such as distinguishing between HTLV-I and HTLV-II. Current radioimmunoprecipitation methodology, like the serologic assays mentioned thus far (with the exception of type-specific synthetic peptide assays), cannot make this distinction. For this purpose, numerous primer pairs are used, beginning with a generic pair such as a *pol* gene primer pair homologous to regions within both viruses. If hybridization occurs with the *pol* probe the amplified material is rehybridized separately with *pol* probes specific to type I and type II. Under stringent hybridization conditions two detector oligonucleotides, located within the region defined by the primer pair, enable the identification of samples positive for HTLV-I *v* HTLV-II DNA.[108,109]

Although ^{32}P-labeled probes are commonly used in research laboratories, the use of biotinylated and other nonradioactive probes will likely become routine, allowing for early and specific detection of retroviral infections by clinical laboratories.[110]

Viral culture. Routine isolation of virus from HTLV-I–infected individuals has proven relatively simple since infected cells express elevated levels of the IL-2 receptor.[111] Such cells then have a distinct growth advantage over uninfected cells when cultured in the presence of IL-2. Typically, peripheral blood mononuclear cells, isolated from whole blood by Ficoll-Hypaque™ density gradient centrifugation, are grown in suspension culture. Although HTLV-I is not cytopathic and causes no obvious cell damage, the periodic addition of fresh phytohemagglutinin-stimulated peripheral blood mononuclear cells from normal persons improves the outgrowth of infected cells.

The standard technique for detecting retroviruses in cell culture fluids is to assay for reverse transcriptase activity.[112] The RNA-dependent DNA polymerase of HTLV-I is unique among mammalian retroviruses by virtue of its very large size (100 kd) and its preference for the divalent cation $Mg^{(2+)}$ instead of $Mn^{(2+)}$.[1,62] This latter characteristic can be used to help distinguish the source of polymerase activity observed in infected cultures.

Monoclonal and polyclonal antibodies to all of the major structural proteins of HTLV-I are available, making it possible to probe cultured cells for the production of specific viral proteins. Fixed cells can be analyzed with indirect immunosandwich assays that tag the infected cells with fluorescein isothiocyanate. The cells can then be examined on a fluorescence microscope.[113] The expression of the p19 and p24 proteins of HTLV-I may be evident by immunofluorescence as soon as 2 days after culture initiation, and reverse transcriptase activity is detectable, routinely, in 14-day-old cell culture media.[101,113] Even in patients with a relatively low percentage of infected cells (<1:100), it is possible to detect virus after 1 month in culture.[114] To confirm that a population of cells is infected with HTLV-I, the DNA is typically isolated, digested with EcoRI (HTLV-I contains no EcoRI sites in the proviral genome), and analyzed by Southern blot hybridization for sequences complementary to an HTLV-I DNA probe. Autoradiography permits recognition of sites of integration of the virus, as well as sites containing HTLV-I nucleic acid smaller than the entire proviral genome (9.03 kbp).[101]

Human Lentiviruses: HIV-2

HIV-2 was isolated and characterized by investigations first conducted in 1985 at the Pasteur Institute in Paris.[115] This discovery was made based upon studies of two West African patients with AIDS who were HIV-1–seronegative by HIV-1 enzyme immunoassay. When tested by protein immunoblot using purified HIV-1 antigens, serum from these patients showed atypical antibody band patterns. A virus with reverse transcriptase activity and cytopathic effects similar to HIV-1 was subsequently isolated from the peripheral blood lymphocytes of these patients. Electron microscopy of infected cells showed the presence of mature virions and budding viral particles morphologically identical to those of HIV-1. Nucleic acid sequences from the new isolate subsequently showed approximately 60% homology with the *gag* and *pol* regions of known HIV-1 isolates, but somewhat less homology with the other HIV-1 genes.[115] Several additional strains of HIV-2 have now been isolated from West African patients with immunodeficiency disease,[116] and serologic assays have been developed to measure worldwide seroprevalence. As described below, HIV-2 is more limited in geographic distribution than HIV-1 and is also potentially less virulent. However, HIV-2 is associated with the production of serious human immunodeficiency disease and its potential threat to the safety of the blood supply should be carefully monitored.

Epidemiology

Several isolates of HIV-2 have been used as sources of viral antigens for serologic screening tests. These include HIV-2$_{rod}$ (LAV-2), and SBL-6669.[115-117] As indicated below, considerable serologic data have also been accumulated, with assays based on a closely cross-reactive simian retrovirus that has also been described as a human isolate (HTLV-IV).[118,119] Current seroprevalence data indicate that HIV-2 infection is highly focused and its worldwide distribution is considerably different from that of HIV-1. West Africa is the only area where HIV-2 infection is endemic. Countries known to be foci of infection include Burkina Faso, Ghana, Guinea Bissau, Guinea, Ivory Coast, Mali, Senegal and the Cape Verde Islands, Gambia, Benin, Angola, Mozambique, and the Central African Republic. Seroprevalence estimates in these countries range from 0.3% to 17% in healthy adults in the general population.[120-122]

Recent data from studies conducted in Senegal, Guinea-Bissau, and other West African countries indicate that HIV-2 seropositivity rises with increased age, and can be as high as 65% in persons who have had greater sexual exposure to infectious disease-causing agents, such as patients being treated for sexually transmitted disease and female prostitutes. These observations support the hypothesis that heterosexual transmission is an important means of HIV-2 transmission in these endemic areas.[123]

While a low-level presence of HIV-2 infection has been documented in Central Africa, Western Europe, the United States, and Canada,[124-129] in a recent cross-sectional study 1508 persons from six Central African nations with high rates of HIV-1 seroprevalence showed no evidence of HIV-2 infection.[130] In areas of the world where HIV-2 infection is rare, such infections can ultimately be traced to birth, residence, or sexual contact within the endemic focus of West Africa. It therefore appears that HIV-2 constitutes a relatively recent infection in humans, one which is just beginning to spread across the world.

The seroprevalence of HIV-2 in the United States was assessed in 1986 and 1987 in a large cross-sectional study of 14,196 persons considered to be at increased risk, and in 8503 healthy blood donors. Although reactivity was observed with HIV-2 enzyme immunoassays in these populations, none of the reactions could be confirmed as representing true HIV-2.[131] At this writing, two published and several unpublished cases of HIV-2 infection had been identified in the United States.[132,133] Most of these infections have been identified in individuals of West African origin, and have been found as a result of HIV-2 screening tests conducted on HIV-1 "indeterminate" serum from high-risk populations, or from virologic follow-up of HIV-1–seronegative patients with AIDS.

In direct response to the possibility that a healthy HIV-2–infected individual from West Africa could present as a blood donor, US blood banks now exclude all blood donors from countries of West Africa where HIV-2 infection is endemic. In April 1990 the FDA licensed the first HIV-2 ELISA, manufactured by Genetic Systems Corp, Seattle. Although specific HIV-2 blood screening does not appear to be indicated, it is anticipated that existing HIV-1 enzyme immunoassays used in the blood bank will eventually be reconfigured to provide dual specificity for HIV-1 and HIV-2 antibody detection.

Agent

HIV-2 virus isolates have many features in common with HIV-1. The viruses are morphologically indistinct by electron microscopy. Both have a tropism for human T lymphocytes expressing the CD4 antigen on their surfaces, and are cytopathic for other cells bearing the CD4 cell surface receptor. In addition, both viruses possess regulatory genes capable of transactivating both viral structural genes and cellular genes.

Although HIV-1 and HIV-2 share a similar genomic organization, they differ considerably with respect to their nucleotide sequences. Genomic analysis of cloned HIV-2 isolates reveals 60% homology with HIV-1 for the more conserved *gag* and *pol* genes, and approximately 30% to 40% for the other viral genes and LTRs.[134] The *gag* gene products of HIV-2 are designated p55, p16, p26, and p12. The *pol* gene codes for the reverse transcriptase, p68, and an endonuclease, p34. The envelope protein precursor, gp130/140, is processed into an external glycoprotein, gp105/120, and a transmembrane component, gp36/41 (Table 5–4).[131] It is estimated that antigenic cross-reaction is sufficient to allow the detection of approximately 60% of HIV-2–positive serum by an HIV-1 ELISA. An HIV-1 immunoblot with HIV-2–positive serum generally produces an indeterminant result.

In addition to the above-mentioned genes, HIV-1 and HIV-2 possess six additional genes that function to regulate viral replication or infectivity.[134] There appear to be some dissimilarities between the viruses with respect to this group of regulatory genes, particularly the *vpu* region, found only in HIV-1, and the *vpx* region, exclusive to HIV-2.[135] The *vpx* region is an open reading frame that codes for a protein of unknown function with a molecular weight of 16 kd.

Table 5–4   Recognized Genes and Polypeptides of HIV-1 and HIV-2

	HIV-1	HIV-2
gag	p55/p24,p15,p9	p57/p26/p16/p12
pol	p68/p34	p64/p36
env	gp160/gp120,gp41	gp160/gp120,gp40
tat	p14	p<27
trs	p19	p<27
ORF Q (sor)	p23	~p23
ORF F (3'ORF)	p27	~p27

Several early seroepidemiologic studies were based on purified viral antigens of HTLV-IV, the virus isolate reported in 1986 as a human retrovirus with little or no associated pathology.[118,119] As mentioned above, it has since been determined that HTLV-IV does not represent a new human retrovirus, but is essentially indistinguishable from isolates of the simian immunodeficiency virus (formerly called STLV-III).[136] Despite the temporary confusion in nomenclature, published seroepidemiologic studies based on HTLV-IV viral antigens are considered to be an accurate reflection of HIV-2 infection due to the high degree of serologic cross-reactivity between human HIV-2 and simian immunodeficiency virus.

Disease

Many isolations of HIV-2 have now been made from HIV-1–seronegative patients with AIDS, and there appears to be adequate epidemiologic and clinical evidence to link this agent causally with the development of AIDS and related illnesses in some individuals. A recent report on 30 highly selected HIV-2–infected West African patients documented a pathologic spectrum very similar to that caused by HIV-1, including 17 cases of frank AIDS (resulting in seven deaths), four cases of AIDS-related complex, three cases with other associated illnesses, and six asymptomatic cases. Each of these patients was shown serologically to be free of HIV-1 infection. In several patients, nucleic acid hybridization analysis of isolated virus indicated that HIV-2 was present.[137]

Although the spectrum of possible HIV-2 pathology appears to parallel that of HIV-1, there are only preliminary data from longitudinal studies that can be applied to a quantitative assessment of disease risk in infected persons. Prospective data that are available, however, appear to reflect a lower disease potential for HIV-2 compared with HIV-1. Recent reports from ongoing studies in infected female prostitutes from Dakar, Senegal, indicate that much less disease is observed in HIV-2–infected individuals over a 2-year period than would be observed in HIV-1–infected individuals.[138,139] This may be a function of lower disease frequency, or a longer incubation period between infection and disease. While a precise estimation of HIV-2 disease incidence remains to be determined, there is cautious optimism that HIV-2 may not pose the threat of widespread immunodeficiency disease in West Africa that has been realized in Central Africa because of HIV-1 infection.

Several instances of dual HIV-1 and HIV-2 infection in a single person have been reported, particularly from the Ivory Coast, but the prevalence and biologic effect of such dual infections remains unknown.

Diagnosis

As a result of the high degree of antigenic cross-reactivity between HIV-1 and HIV-2, currently licensed HIV-1 assays will detect from 40% to 90% of HIV-2–seropositive individuals, depending on the assay used.[131] For this reason, future blood screening tests will most likely be designed to enhance the simultaneous detection of both agents.

Enzyme immunoassays specific for HIV-2 antibody are available commercially. These assays are based on gradient-purified viral antigen bound to microplate wells, and subsequently exposed to the test serum and a suitable reaction detection system. As with HIV-1, adequate confirmation assays are needed to confirm the antibody specificity contained in any test sample.[140,141]

In many ways, confirmation testing for HIV-2 infection is similar to HIV-1 testing. The first step for serologic confirmation of HIV-2 is the protein immunoblot, with confirmed reactivity based on the presence of antibody to defined viral polypeptides. Protein immunoblot assays for HIV-2 are typically capable of detecting the p16, p26, p55, p56, and p68 core proteins of HIV-2, as well as the p34 polymerase and the viral glycoproteins gp36 and gp140.

Confirmation of HIV-2 reactivity is currently based on the presence of specific antibody to the gp140 and gp36 *env* glycoproteins. The ability to serologically distinguish HIV-1 and HIV-2 infection remains problematic however, because of the serologic cross-reactivity and similar molecular weights of the *gag-* and *pol*-encoded viral proteins.[131]

Since documentation of HIV-2 infection in any member of the US general population will carry major implications for public health policy, serologically defined HIV-2 infections should be further investigated by radioimmunoprecipitation and by virologic studies to verify the presence of HIV-2 gene sequences after culture, or after amplification of DNA extracted from peripheral blood lymphocytes by the PCR. A synthetic peptide immunoassay capable of distinguishing HIV-1 and HIV-2 antibodies has also been recently described.[142]

Conclusion

The advent of AIDS has caused all aspects of transfusion medicine to be opened to reexamination. Effects already realized include targeted donation by autologous and directed donors, and the limited extent to which logical cost-benefit analyses are allowed to dictate the implementation of screening procedures that might incrementally improve the safety of the nation's blood supply.

The trend toward more and more blood screening is complicated further by the discovery of new human retroviruses, and the fact that our ability to detect these agents and make tests to screen for their presence readily surpasses our ability to define their natural history. For blood bankers, this has become a frustrating time. Within a very short period, the blood-banking community has found itself responding to a seemingly endless array of operational and laboratory initiatives, all designed to bring transfusion closer to a mythical "no-risk" status. Consequently, the threat of legal liability is frequently weighed against the prospect of screening the blood supply (at a cost of up to $15 million) for a rare agent with unknown or limited disease potential for exposed recipients.

These issues are now getting increased attention at the national level. In addition, efforts are currently underway to effectively inactivate etiologic agents contained in blood and blood products. Until definitive answers are available, however, it is likely that each new virus discovery will begin a round of test development, surveillance, and difficult decisions.

References

1. Poiesz BJ, Ruscetti FW, Gazdar AF, et al: Detection and isolation of type C retrovirus particles from fresh and cultured lymphocytes of a patient with cutaneous T-cell lymphoma. *Proc Natl Acad Sci USA* 77:7415–7419, 1980.

2. Rosenblatt JD, Golde DW, Wachsman W, et al: A second isolate of HTLV-II associated with atypical hairy-cell leukemia. *N Engl J Med* 315:32–35, 1986.

3. Kalyanaraman VS, Sarngadharan MG, Robert-Guroff M, et al: A new subtype of human T-cell leukemia virus (HTLV-II) associated with a T-cell variant of hairy cell leukemia. *Science* 218:571–573, 1982.

4. Manzari V, Gismondi A, Barillari G, et al: HTLV-V: A new human retrovirus isolated in a Tac-negative T-cell lymphoma/leukemia. *Science* 238:1581–1583, 1987.

5. Courouce AM, Barin F, Baudelot J, et al: HIV-2 infection among blood donors and other subjects in France. *Transfusion* 29:368–370, 1989.

6. Maurer B, Flugel RM: Genomic organization of the human spumaretrovirus and its relatedness to AIDS and other retroviruses. *AIDS Res Hum Retrovir* 4:467–473, 1988.

7. Saxinger C, Gallo RC: Application of the indirect enzyme-linked immunosorbent assay microtest to the detection and surveillance of human T-cell leukemia-lymphoma virus (HTLV). *Lab Invest* 49:317–379, 1983.

8. Kobayashi S, Yoshida T, Yamamoto K, et al: Evaluation of a new agglutination test kit for ATLA antibody detection. *J Med Tech* 30:1143–1146, 1986.

9. Fang CT, Williams AE, Sandler SG, et al: Detection of antibodies to human T-lymphotropic virus type 1 (HTLV-1). *Transfusion* 28:179–183, 1988.

10. Anderson DW, Lee T-HL, Lairmore M, et al: Serologic confirmation of human T-lymphotropic virus type I infection in healthy blood and plasma donors. *Blood* 74:2585–2591, 1989.

11. Tajima K, Tominaga S, Suchi T, et al: Epidemiological analysis on distribution of antibody to adult T-cell leukemia virus associated antigen (ATLA): Possible horizontal transmission of adult T-cell leukemia virus. *Gann* 73:893–901, 1982.

12. Clark JW, Saxinger C, Gibbs WN, et al: Seroepidemiologic studies of human T-cell leukemia/lymphoma virus type I in Jamaica. *Int J Cancer* 42:7–12, 1985.

13. Blattner WA, Nomura A, Clark JW, et al: Modes of transmission and evidence for viral latency from studies of human T-cell lymphotropic virus type 1 in Japanese migrant populations in Hawaii. *Proc Natl Acad Sci USA* 83:4895–4898, 1986.

14. Takatsuki K, Uchiyama T, Sagawa K, Yodoi J: Adult T-cell leukemia in Japan, in Seno F, Takaku F, Irino S (eds): *Topics in Hematology.* Amsterdam, Excerpta Medica, 1977, pp 73–77.

15. Uchiyama T, Yodoi J, Sagawa K, et al: Adult T cell leukemia: Clinical and hematologic features of 16 cases. *Blood* 50:481–492, 1977.

16. Hinuma Y, Nagata K, Hanaoka M, et al: Adult T-cell leukemia: Antigen in an ATL cell line and detection of antibodies to the antigen in human sera. *Proc Natl Acad Sci USA* 78:6476–6480, 1981.

17. Gallo RC, Kalyanaraman VS, Sarngadharan MG, et al: Association of the human type-C retrovirus with a subset of adult T-cell cancers. *Cancer Res* 43:3892–3899, 1983.

18. Robert-Guroff M, Nakao T, Notake T, et al: Natural antibodies to human retrovirus HTLV in a cluster of Japanese patients with adult T-cell leukemia. *Science* 215:975–978, 1982.

19. Robert-Guroff M, Gallo RC: Establishment of an etiologic relationship between the human T-cell leukemia/lymphoma virus (HTLV) and adult T-cell leukemia. *Blut* 47:1–12, 1983.

20. Sarin PS, Aoki T, Shibata A, et al: High incidence of human type-C retrovirus (HTLV) in family members of a HTLV-positive Japanese T-cell leukemia patient. *Proc Natl Acad Sci USA* 80:2370–2374, 1983.

21. Blattner WA, Gallo RC: Human T-cell leukemia/lymphoma viruses: Clinical and epidemiological features. *Curr Top Microbiol Immunol* 115:68–88, 1985.

22. Takatsuki K, Yamaguchi K, Kawano F, et al: Clinical aspects of adult T-cell leukemia/lymphoma, in Vogt PX (ed): *Current Topics in Microbiology and Immunology.* Berlin, Springer-Verlag, 1985, 89–98.

23. Tajima K, Tominaga S, Kuroishi T, et al: Geographical features and epidemiological approach to endemic T-cell leukemia/lymphoma in Japan. *Jpn J Clin Oncol* 9(suppl):495–504, 1979.

24. The T-Cell and B-Cell Malignancy Study Group. Statistical analyses of clinicopathological, virological and epidemiological data on lymphoid malignancies with special reference to adult T-cell leukemia/lymphoma: A report of second nationwide study of Japan. *Jpn J Clin Oncol* 15:517–535, 1985.

25. Hinuma Y: Seroepidemiology of adult T-cell leukemia virus (HTLV-I/ATLV): Origin of virus carriers in Japan. *AIDS Res* 2:517–522, 1986.

26. Catovski D, Rose M, Goolden AWG, et al: Adult T-cell lymphoma-leukemia in blacks from the West Indies. *Lancet* 1:61–63, 1982.

27. Blattner WA, Kalyanaraman VS, Robert-Guroff M, et al: The human type C retrovirus, HTLV, in blacks from the Caribbean region and relationship to adult T-cell leukemia/lymphoma. *Int J Cancer* 30:257–264, 1982.

28. Blattner WA, Blayney DW, Robert-Guroff M, et al: Epidemiology of human T-cell leukemia/lymphoma virus. *J Infect Dis* 147:406–416, 1983.

29. Jaffe ES, Blayney DW, Blattner WA, et al: HTLV and associated T-cell malignancies in the United States. *Am J Surg Pathol* 8:263–275, 1984.

30. Blattner WA, Clark JW, Gibbs WN, et al: HTLV: Epidemiology and relationship to human malignancy, in Gallo RC, Essex ME, Gross L (eds): *Human T-cell Leukemia/Lymphoma Virus.* Cold Spring Harbor, NY, Cold Spring Harbor Press, 1984, pp 267–274.

31. Gessain A, Barin F, Vernant JC, et al: Antibodies to human T-lymphotropic virus type-I in patients with tropical spastic paraparesis. *Lancet* 2:407–410, 1985.

32. Bartholomew C, Cleghorn F, Charles W, et al: HTLV-I and tropical spastic paraparesis. *Lancet* 2:227–228, 1986.

33. Rodgers-Johnson P, Morgan OS, Mora C, et al: The role of HTLV-I in tropical spastic paraparesis in Jamaica. *Ann Neurol* 23(suppl):S121–126, 1988.

34. Osame M, Igata A, Usuku K, et al: Mother-to-child transmission in HTLV-I associated myelopathy. *Lancet* 1:106, 1987.

35. Roman GC, Osame M: Identity of HTLV-I-associated tropical spastic paraparesis and HTLV-I-associated myelopathy. *Lancet* 1:651, 1988.

36. Gazzolo L, Robert-Guroff M, Jennings A, et al: Type-I and type-III HTLV antibodies in hospitalized and out-patient Zairians. *Int J Cancer* 36:373–378, 1985.

37. Fleming AF, Yamamoto N, Bhusnurmath SR, et al: Antibodies to ATLV (HTLV) in Nigerian blood donors and patients with chronic lymphatic leukemia or lymphoma. *Lancet* 1:334–335, 1983.

38. Saxinger W, Blattner WA, Levine PH, et al: Human T-cell leukemia virus (HTLV-I) antibodies in Africa. *Science* 225:1473–1476, 1984.

39. Williams AE, Fang CT, Sandler SG: HTLV-I/II and blood transfusion in the United States, in Blattner WA (ed): *Human Retrovirology: HTLV.* New York, Raven Press, 1990, pp 349–362.

40. Williams AE, Fang CT, Slamon DJ, et al: Seroprevalence and epidemiological correlates of HTLV-1 infection in U.S. blood donors. *Science* 240:643–646, 1988.

41. Williams AE, Sullivan MT, D'Aquila RT, et al: Prevalence of HTLV-1 antibodies among intravenous drug users in Connecticut. in Abstracts of the IVth International Conference on AIDS, Stockholm, 1988.

42. Saxinger C, Moore J, Weiss S, et al: Retrospective study of HTLV1/HTLV2-related antibody reactivity in U.S. drug abusers, in *Abstracts of the IVth International Conference on AIDS.* Stockholm, 1988.

43. Weiss SH, Ginzberg HM, Saxinger WC, et al: Emerging high rates of human T-cell lymphotropic virus type 1 (HTLV-1) and HIV infection among U.S. drug abusers, in *Abstracts of the IIIrd International Conference on AIDS.* Washington, DC, 1987, p 211.

44. Robert-Guroff M, Weiss SH, et al: Prevalence of antibodies to HTLV-I, -II, and -III in intravenous drug abusers from an AIDS endemic region. *JAMA* 255:3133–3137, 1986.

45. Lee H, Swanson P, Shorty VS, et al: High rate of HTLV-II infection in seropositive IV drug abusers in New Orleans. *Science* 244:471–475, 1989.

46. Sugiyama H, Doi H, Yamaguchi K, et al: Significance of postnatal mother-to-child transmission of human T-lymphotropic virus type-I on the development of adult T-cell leukemia/lymphoma. *J Med Virol* 20:253–260, 1986.

47. Hino S, Kubota K, Doi H, Miyamoto T: Preliminary follow-up survey of children born to HTLV-I carrier mothers who refrained from breast-feeding. Presented at 3rd Annual Retrovirology Conference, Maui, HI, 1990.

48. Kinoshita K, Hino S, Amagasaki T, et al: Demonstration of adult T-cell leukemia virus antigen in milk from three seropositive mothers. *Gann* 75:103–105, 1984.

49. Okochi K, Sato H: Adult T-cell leukemia virus, blood donors and transfusion: Experience in Japan, in Dodd RY, et al (eds): *Infection, Immunity, and Blood Transfusion.* New York, Alan R Liss Inc, 1984, pp 245–258.

50. Hino S, Kawamichi T, Funakoshi M, et al: Transfusion mediated spread of the human T-cell leukemia virus in chronic hemodialysis patients in a heavily endemic area, Nagasaki. *Gann* 76:1075–1080, 1984.

51. Okochi K, Sato H, Hinuma Y: A retrospective study on transmission of adult T cell leukemia virus by blood transfusion: Sero-conversion in recipients. *Vox Sang* 46:245–253, 1984.

52. Okochi K, Sato H: Blood transfusion related transmission of HTLV-I (ATLV), in *Proceedings of XIXth Congress of the International Society of Blood Transfusion.* Sydney, Australia, 1986, pp 13–15.

53. Kamihira S, Nakasima S, Oyakawa Y, et al: Transmission of human T-cell lymphotropic virus type I by blood transfusion before and after mass screening of sera from seropositive donors. *Vox Sang* 52:43–44, 1987.

54. Licensure of screening tests for antibody to human T-lymphotropic virus type I. *MMWR* 37:736–747, 1988.

55. Donegan E, The Transfusion Safety Study Group: Comparison of HTLV-I/II with HIV-1 transmission by component type and shelf storage before administration. Presented at the American Association of Blood Banks Annual Meeting, New Orleans, 1989.

56. Sullivan MT, Williams AE, Fang CT, et al: Transmission of HTLV-I and HTLV-II to Prior Recipients of Blood Products from HTLV-I/II Seropositive Donors. *Arch Intern Med* In press.

57. Akao M, Yorifuji H, Koike K, Hada M, Ikematsu S, Fujimaki M: Hemophiliacs doubly infected by HIV-1 and HTLV-I. Presented at the Vth International Conference on AIDS, Montreal, 1989.

58. Brodine, S, Oldfield EC, Corwin AL, et al: Seroprevalence of HTLV-I among US Marines stationed in a hyperendemic area. Presented at the Vth International Conference on AIDS, Montreal, 1989.

59. Kajiyama W, Kashiwagi S, Iketmatsu H, et al: Intrafamilial transmission of adult T-cell leukemia virus. *J Infect Dis* 154:851–857, 1986.

60. Rosenblatt JD, Chen ISY, Wachsman W: Infection with HTLV-I and HTLV-II: Evolving concepts. *Semin Hematol* 25:230–246, 1988.

61. Sarngadharan MG, Markham PD, Gallo RC: Human T-cell leukemia viruses, in Fields BN, Knipe DM, Melnick JL, et al (eds): *Virology*. New York, Raven Press, 1985.

62. Poiesz BJ, Ruscetti FW, Reitz MS, et al: Isolation of a new type C retrovirus (HTLV) in primary uncultured cells of a patient with Sézary T-cell leukemia. *Nature* 294:268–271, 1981.

63. Sommerfelt MA, Williams BP, Clapham PR, et al: Human T cell leukemia viruses use a receptor determined by human chromosome 17. *Science* 242:1557–1559, 1988.

64. Slamon DJ, Shimotohno K, Cline MJ, et al: Identification of the putative transforming protein of the human T-cell leukemia viruses HTLV-I and HTLV-II. *Science* 226:61–65, 1984.

65. Greene W: HTLV-I and human T-cell activation, in Blattner WA (ed): *Human Retrovirology: HTLV.* New York, Raven Press, 1990, pp 35–43.

66. Rosenblatt JD, Cann AJ, Slamon DJ, et al: HTLV-II transactivation is regulated by the overlapping *tax/rex* nonstructural genes. *Science* 240:916–919, 1988.

67. Wachsman W, Golde DW, Chen ISY: HTLV and human leukemia: Perspectives 1986. *Semin Hematol* 23:246–256, 1986.

68. Nerenberg M, Hinrichs SH, Reynolds RK, et al: The *tat* gene of human T-lymphotropic virus type 1 induces mesenchymal tumors in transgenic mice. *Science* 237:1324–1329, 1987.

69. Tajima K, Kuroishi T: Estimation of rate of incidence of ATL among ATLV (HTLV-I) carriers in Kyushu, Japan. *Jpn J Clin Oncol* 15:423–430, 1985.

70. Kondo T, Nonaka H, Miyamoto N, et al: Incidence of adult T-cell leukemia-lymphoma and its familial clustering. *Int J Cancer* 35:749–751, 1985.

71. Murphy EL, Hanchard B, Figueroa B, et al: Modeling the risk of adult T-cell leukemia/lymphoma in persons infected with human T-lymphotropic virus type I. *Int J Cancer* 43:250–253, 1989.

72. Osame M, Usuku K, Izumo S, et al: HTLV-I associated myelopathy, a new clinical entity. *Lancet* 1:1031–1032, 1986.

73. Gessain A, Francis H, Sonan T, et al: HTLV-I and tropical spastic paraparesis in Africa. *Lancet* 2:698, 1986.

74. Newton M, Cruickshank K, Miller D, et al: Antibody to human T-lymphotropic virus type 1 in West-Indian–born UK residents with spastic paraparesis. *Lancet* 1:415–416, 1987.

75. Roman GC, Schoenberg BS, Madden DL, et al: Human T-lymphotropic virus type I antibodies in the serum of patients with tropical spastic paraparesis in the Seychelles. *Arch Neurol* 44:605–607, 1987.

76. Ceroni M, Piccardo P, Rodgers-Johnson P, et al: Intrathecal synthesis of IgG antibodies to HTLV-I supports an etiological role for HTLV-I in tropical spastic paraparesis. *Ann Neurol* 23(suppl):s188–191, 1988.

77. Bhagavati S, Ehrlich G, Kula RW, et al: Detection of human T-cell lymphoma/leukemia virus type-I DNA and antigen in spinal fluid and blood of patients with chronic progressive myelopathy. *N Engl J Med* 318:1141–1147, 1988.

78. Koprowski H, DeFreitas EC, Harper ME, et al: Multiple sclerosis and human T-cell lymphotropic retrovirus. *Nature* 318:154–160, 1986.

79. Reddy EP, Sandberg-Wollheim M, Mettus RV, et al: Amplification and molecular cloning of HTLV-I sequences from DNA of multiple sclerosis patients. *Science* 243:529–533, 1989.

80. Greenberg SJ, Ehrlich GD, Abbott MA, et al: Detection of sequences homologous to human retroviral DNA in multiple sclerosis by gene amplification. *Proc Natl Acad Sci USA* 86:2878–2882, 1989.

81. Saxon A, Stevens RH, Golde DW: T-lymphocyte variant of hairy-cell leukemia. *Ann Intern Med* 88:323–326, 1978.

82. Schupbach J, Kalyanaraman VS, Sarngadharan MG, et al: Antibodies against three purified proteins of the human type C retrovirus, human T-cell leukemia-lymphoma virus, in adult T-cell leukemia-lymphoma patients and healthy blacks from the Caribbean. *Cancer Res* 43:886–891, 1983.

83. Kannagi M, Sugamura K, Sato H, et al: Establishment of human cytotoxic T-cell lines specific for human adult T-cell leukemia virus bearing cells. *J Immunol* 130:2942, 1983.

84. Kimura I, Miyamoto K, Sato J: A novel T-cell line derived from adult T-cell leukemia. *Gann* 71:155, 1980.

85. Miyoshi I, Kubonishi I, Yoshimoto S, et al: Detection of type-C virus particles in a cord T-cell line derived by co-cultivation of normal human leukocytes and human leukemic T-cells. *Nature* 296:770–771, 1981.

86. Lee T, Coligan JE, Homma T, et al: Human T-cell leukemia virus-associated antigens: Identity of the major antigens recognized after infection. *Proc Natl Acad Sci USA* 81:3856–3860, 1984.

87. Chen YA, Gomez-Lucia E, Okayama A, et al: Antibody profile of early seroconverters to human T-cell leukemia virus type I infection. Presented at 3rd Annual Retrovirology Conference, Maui, HI, 1990.

88. Gallo D, Hoffmann MN, Cossen CK, et al: Comparison of immunofluorescence, immunoassay, and western blot (immunoblot) methods for detection of antibody to human T-cell leukemia virus type I. *J Clin Microbiol* 26:1487–1491, 1988.

89. Yoshida T, Kobayashi S, Yamamoto N: Discrepancy between gelatin particle agglutination assay and indirect immunofluorescence assay for antibodies to adult T-cell leukemia associated antigen (ATLA). *J Clin Exp Med* 134:377–378, 1985.

90. Fang CT, Akins R, Sandler SG: An HTLV-I EIA using recombinant *env*-encoded peptides. Presented at the American Association of Blood Banks Annual Meeting, New Orleans, 1990.

91. Fang CT, Williams AE, Sandler SG, the American Red Cross HTLV-I/II Study Group: Seroprevalence and geographical distribution of anti-HTLV among blood donors in the US. Presented at 3rd Annual Retrovirology Conference, Maui, HI, 1990.

92. Blomberg J, Pipkorn R, Robert-Guroff M: Type and group specific antigenic determinants of HTLV: Use of synthetic peptides for serotyping of HTLV-I and -II infection. Presented at 3rd Annual Retrovirology Conference, Maui, HI, 1990.

93. Towbin H, Staehelin T, Gordon J: Electrophoretic transfer of proteins from polyacrylamide gels to nitrocellulose sheets: Procedure and some applications. *Proc Natl Acad Sci USA* 76:4350–4354, 1979.

94. Kobayashi N, Yamamoto N, Koyanagi Y, et al: Translation of HTLV (human T-cell leukemia virus) RNA in a nuclease-treated rabbit reticulocyte system. *EMBO J* 3:321–325, 1984.

95. Palker TJ, Scearce RM, Ho W, et al: Monoclonal antibodies reactive with human T cell lymphotropic virus I (HTLV-I) p19 internal core protein: Cross-reactivity with normal tissues and differential reactivity with HTLV types I and II. *J Immunol* 135:247–254, 1985.

96. Koeffler H, Chen ISY, Golde DW: Characterization of a novel HTLV-infected cell line. *Blood* 64:482–490, 1984.

97. Seiki M, Hattori S, Hirayama Y, Yoshida M. Human adult T-cell leukemia virus: Complete nucleotide sequence of the provirus genome integrated in leukemia cell DNA. *Proc Natl Acad Sci USA* 80:3618–3622, 1983.

98. Mullis K, Faloona F, Scharf S, et al: Specific enzymatic amplification of DNA in vitro: The polymerase chain reaction. *Cold Spring Harbor Symp Quant Biol* 51:263–272, 1986.

99. Murakawa G, Zaia JA, Spallone PA, et al: Direct detection of HIV-1 RNA from AIDS and ARC patient samples. *DNA* 7:287–295, 1988.

100. Kwok S, Mack DH, Mullis KB, et al: Identification of human immunodeficiency virus sequences by using in vitro enzymatic amplification and oligomer cleavage detection. *J Virol* 61:1690–1694, 1987.

101. Poiesz BJ, Ehrlich GD, Papsidero D, Sninsky JJ. Detection of human retroviruses, in DeVita VT, Hellman S, Rosenberg SA (eds): *AIDS: Etiology, Diagnosis, Treatment and Prevention*, ed 2. Philadelphia, JB Lippincott Co, 1988.

102. Duggan D, Ehrlich GD, Davey FP, et al: HTLV-1-induced lymphoma mimicking Hodgkin's disease: Diagnosis by polymerase chain reaction amplification of specific HTLV-1 sequences in tumor DNA. *Blood* 71:1027–1032, 1988.

103. Loche M, Mach B: Identification of HIV-infected seronegative individuals by a direct diagnostic test based on hybridization to amplified viral DNA. *Lancet* 2:418–421, 1988.

104. Jackson JB, Kwok SY, Hopsicker JS, et al: Absence of HIV-1 infection in antibody negative sexual partners of HIV-1 infected hemophiliacs. *Transfusion* 29:265–267, 1989.

105. Saiki R, Gelfand DH, Stoffel S, et al: Primer-directed enzymatic amplification of DNA with a thermostable DNA polymerase. *Science* 239:487–491, 1988.

106. Oste C: Polymerase chain reaction. *Biotechniques* 6:162–167, 1988.

107. Southern EM: Detection of specific sequences among DNA fragments separated by gel electrophoresis. *J Mol Biol* 98:503–517, 1975.

108. Abbott MA, Poiesz BJ, Byrne BC, et al: Enzymatic gene amplification: Qualitative and quantitative methods for detecting proviral DNA amplified in vitro. *J Infect Dis* 158:1158–1169, 1988.

109. Kwok S, Ehrlich G, Poiesz B, Kalish R, Sninsky JJ: Enzymatic amplification of HTLV-I viral sequences from peripheral blood mononuclear cells and infected tissues. *Blood* 72:1117–1123, 1988.

110. Bugawan T, Saiki RK, Levenson CH, Watson RM, Erlich HA: The use of non-radioactive oligonucleotide probes to analyze enzymatically amplified DNA for prenatal diagnosis and forensic HLA typing. *Biotechnology* 6:943–947, 1988.

111. Kronke M, Leonard WJ, Depper JM, Greene WC: Deregulation of interleukin-2 receptor gene expression in HTLV-1-induced adult T-cell leukemia. *Science* 228:1215–1217, 1985.

112. Yoshida M, Miyoshi I, Hinuma Y: Isolation and characterization of retrovirus from cell lines of human adult T-cell leukemia and its implication in the disease. *Proc Natl Acad Sci USA* 79:2031–2035, 1982.

113. Robert-Guroff M, Ruscetti FW, Posner LE, Poiesz BJ, Gallo RC: Detection of the human T-cell lymphoma virus p19 in cells of some patients with cutaneous T-cell lymphoma and leukemia using a monoclonal antibody. *J Exp Med* 154:1957–1964, 1981.

114. Chen I, Quan SG, Golde DW: Human T-cell leukemia virus type II transforms normal human lymphocytes. *Proc Natl Acad Sci USA* 80:7006–7009, 1983.

115. Clavel F, Guetard D, Brun-Vezinet F, et al: Isolation of a new human retrovirus from West African patients with AIDS. *Science* 233:343–346, 1986.

116. Albert J, Bredberg U, Chiodi F, et al: A new human retrovirus isolate of West African origin (SBL-6669) and its relationship to HTLV-IV, LAV-II, and HTLV-IIIB. *AIDS Res Hum Retrovir* 3:3–10, 1987.

117. Brun-Vezinet F, Rey MA, Katlama C, et al: Lymphoadenopathy-associated virus type 2 in AIDS and AIDS-related complex. *Lancet* 1:128–132, 1987.

118. Kanki PJ, Barin F, M'Boup S, et al: New human T-lymphotropic retrovirus related to simian T-lymphotropic virus type III (STLV-III$_{AGM}$). *Science* 232:238–243, 1986.

119. Kanki PJ, M'Boup S, Ricard D, et al: Human T-lymphotropic virus type 4 and the human immunodeficiency virus in West Africa. *Science* 236:827, 1987.

120. Biberfeld G, Bottiger B, Bredberg-Raden U, et al: Findings in four HTLV-IV seropositive women from West Africa. *Lancet* 2:1330–1331, 1986.

121. Denis F, Gershy-Damet G, Lhuillier M, et al: Prevalence of human T-lymphotropic retroviruses type III (HIV) and type IV in Ivory Coast. *Lancet* 1:408–411, 1987.

122. Horsburgh CR Jr, Holmberg SD: The global distribution of human immunodeficiency virus type 2 (HIV-2) infection. *Transfusion* 28:192–195, 1988.

123. M'Boup S, N'Doye I, Samb N, et al: HIV and related viruses in Senegal, in *Proceedings of IVth International Conference on AIDS.* Stockholm, 1988, pp 320.

124. Rey F, Salaun D, Lesbordes JL, et al: HIV-1 and HIV-2 double infection in Central African Republic. *Lancet* 2:1391–1392, 1986.

125. Werner A, Staszewski S, Helm EB, et al: HIV-2 (West Germany, 1984). *Lancet* 1:868–869, 1987.

126. Ferroni P, Tagger A, Lazzarin A, Moroni M: HIV-1 and HIV-2 infections in Italian AIDS/ARC patients. *Lancet* 1:869–870, 1987.

127. Saal F, Sidibe S, Alves-Cardos E, et al: Anti-HIV-2 serological screening in Portuguese populations native from or having had close contact with Africa. *AIDS Res Hum Retrovir* 3:341–342, 1988.

128. Rey MA, Girard PM, Harzic M, et al: HIV-1 and HIV-2 double infection in French homosexual male with AIDS-related complex (Paris, 1985). *Lancet* 1:388–389, 1987.

129. Neumann PW, O'Shaughnessy MV, Lepine D, et al: Laboratory diagnosis of the first cases of HIV-2 infection in Canada. *CMAJ* 140:125, 1989.

130. Kanki PJ, Allan J, Barin F, et al: Absence of antibodies to HIV-2/HTLV-4 in six central African nations. *AIDS Res Hum Retrovir* 3:317–322, 1988.

131. Cabrian K, Shriver K, Goldstein L, Krieger M: Human immunodeficiency virus type-2: A review. *J Clin Immunoassay* 11:107–114, 1988.

132. AIDS due to HIV-2 infection—New Jersey. *MMWR* 37:33–35, 1988.

133. Ruef C, Dickey P, Schable CA, et al: Acquired immunodeficiency syndrome due to human immunodeficiency virus type 2, in the United States: A case report. *Am J Med* 86:709–712, 1989.

134. Guyader M, Emerman M, Sonigo P, et al: Genome organization and transactivation of the human immunodeficiency virus type 2. *Nature* 326:662–669, 1987.

135. Franchini G, Collati E, Arya SK, et al: Genetic analysis of a new subgroup of human and simian T-lymphotropic retroviruses: HTLV-IV, Lav-2, SBL-6669, and STLV III$_{agm}$. *AIDS Res Hum Retrovir* 3:11–17, 1987.

136. Kestler HW, Li Y, Naidu YM, et al: Comparison of simian immunodeficiency virus isolates. *Nature* 331:619–622, 1988.

137. Clavel F, Mansinho K, Chamaret S, et al: Human immunodeficiency virus type 2 infection associated with AIDS in West Africa. *N Engl J Med* 316:1180–1185, 1987.

138. Kanki PJ, M'Boup S, Romieu I, et al: Epidemiology of HIV-2 in female prostitutes in Senegal, in *Abstracts of the Vth International Conference on AIDS*. Montreal, 1989, p 47.

139. Marlink R, Thior I, Siby T, et al: Observations on the natural history of HIV-2, in *Abstracts of the Vth International Conference on AIDS*. Montreal, 1989, p 47.

140. Handsfield HH, Wandell M, Goldstein L, Shriver K, The Cooperative Study Group: Screening and diagnostic performance of enzyme immunoassay for antibody to lymphadenopathy associated virus. *J Clin Microbiol* 25:879–884, 1987.

141. Denis F, Leonard G, Mounier M, et al: Efficacy of five enzyme immunoassays for antibody to HIV in detecting antibody to HTLV-IV. *Lancet* 1:324–325, 1987.

142. Gnann JW Jr, McCormick JB, Mitchell S, et al: Synthetic peptide immunoassay distinguishes HIV type 1 and type 2 infections. *Science* 237:1346–1349, 1987.

6
Transfusion-Associated Hepatitis

Robert L. Randell, MD
Paul V. Holland, MD

Transfusion-associated hepatitis is the most common infectious complication of blood transfusion. However, the current risk of transfusion-associated hepatitis is substantially less than in the early days of transfusion therapy. This reduction is due to a better understanding of its causes and the corresponding actions taken to make the blood supply safer. The changes have occurred in four principal areas: the development of new assays and testing schemes, the switch to predominantly volunteer blood donors, the evolution of donor educational materials and medical history questionnaires, and the retrospective identification and deferral of donors implicated in posttransfusion infections.

The evidence that these changes have resulted in decreased transfusion-associated hepatitis is compelling. The discovery of HBsAg and the implementation of blood donor testing in the early 1970s substantially decreased the incidence of transfusion-associated hepatitis. However, investigators soon realized that hepatitis B probably accounted for only 20% to 25% of the cases of icteric hepatitis.[1] The residual cases did not have the serologic or epidemiologic characteristics of hepatitis A. This led to additional investigation and the description of another kind of hepatitis that was termed non-A, non-B hepatitis because of the inability of investigators to define the agent(s) serologically. It soon was recognized that non-A, non-B hepatitis was the most common transfusion-associated hepatitis, accounting for over 90% of the cases.[2] More recently, blood banks have implemented various measures for screening blood donors and their blood, including routine tests for antibodies to the HIV-1 and HTLV-I as well as two ''surrogate'' tests for non-A, non-B hepatitis, ALT, and anti-HB$_c$. Most recently, a specific test for carriers of non-A, non-B transfusion-associated hepatitis, antibody to the hepatitis C virus, was introduced. These all directly or indirectly have decreased the risk of transfusion-associated hepatitis.

In the 1960s and 1970s, numerous investigators confirmed that transfusion-associated hepatitis occurred with greater frequency in recipients of multiple transfusions of blood from paid donors as compared with volunteer donors. The incidence of non-A, non-B hepatitis in recipients of blood entirely donated by volunteers ranged from 4.8% to 12.8%, as documented by serial laboratory follow-up. In contrast, the incidence of non-A, non-B hepatitis ranged from 24.7% to 53.8% in recipients who received at least 1 unit of blood from a paid donor.[3] This first led to a decision in many areas of the United States to draw primarily volunteer blood donors and then to a requirement to label all blood as either "paid" or "volunteer."[4]

The evolution of the educational materials and the medical history questionnaire given to prospective blood donors pertaining to transfusion-transmitted diseases has undoubtedly increased the safety of the blood supply. Increasingly stringent criteria for donor deferral and exclusion of individuals at high risk for AIDS, which are also often high-risk populations for hepatitis, have probably had the most important impact. Guidelines for donor educational materials and the medical history questionnaire are outlined in *Standards for Blood Banks and Transfusion Services of The American Association of Blood Banks.*[5] There are a number of criteria for donor suitability that are intended to decrease the potential for hepatitis transmission. Unsuitable, prospective donors include those who have a history of hepatitis after 10 years of age, have a reactive test for HBsAg, or have donated the only unit of blood or blood component transfused to a patient who within 6 months developed transfusion-associated hepatitis and received no other blood component or derivative known to transmit viral hepatitis (and there was no other probable source of infection). Prospective donors who have been tattooed or have had close contact with an individual with viral hepatitis in the preceding 12 months must be deferred. Individuals who have received hepatitis B immune globulin are deferred for 12 months because of the possibility of delayed development of disease due to this therapeutic intervention. There is a requirement for visual inspection of both arms of the donor for signs of intravenous drug use (needle tracks),[5] and the donor is questioned about any history of intravenous drug use.

The overall strategy to reduce the risk of transfusion-associated hepatitis also includes a surveillance system to identify and defer blood donors implicated in cases of transfusion-transmitted diseases. However, there is substantial underreporting of even clinical cases of hepatitis because of the requirement for great vigilance on the part of the physicians responsible for transfusing blood or blood components. Optimal follow-up of transfusion recipients really includes serial liver enzyme and hepatitis serologic studies to identify those recipients with asymptomatic hepatitis. There may be 100-times more transfusion-associated hepatitis cases occurring than are actually reported.[6] Nonetheless, evaluation of donors implicated in reported cases of transfusion-associated hepatitis provides another means of identifying individuals who can transmit viral hepatitis despite meeting all blood donation criteria.

With all the changes that have occurred, the risk of transfusion-associated hepatitis has continually decreased during the past 15 to 20 years. The current risk to recipients of multiple transfusions is difficult to quantitate but is probably 2% to 4%, with the risk per unit transfused being less than 1%. Unfortunately, despite our efforts, transfusion-associated hepatitis due to a variety of etiologic agents continues to occur. The types of transfusion-associated hepatitis addressed in this chapter include hepatitis A, B, non-A, non-B hepatitis (now C), and delta (D).

Hepatitis A

Epidemiology

Hepatitis A is spread primarily by person-to-person contact, usually by the fecal-oral route. In the United States, transmission is associated with crowding, poor personal hygiene, improper sanitation, and intimate (sexual) contact. Consequently, hepatitis A is a virus most often implicated in water-borne, food-handler–related, and institutional hepatitis outbreaks. Hepatitis A has recently been shown to be transmitted between intravenous drug users. Possible routes of infection in drug users include sexual, parenteral, or oral transmission.[7]

The hepatitis A virus is rarely transmitted by blood transfusion because no chronic carrier state occurs. The disease must be in its incubation phase for a blood donor to spread this virus to a recipient; this phase is confined to a limited period of 2 to 6 weeks. Furthermore, many adults who require a transfusion are immune to reinfection because of exposure (and immunity) to hepatitis A virus earlier in life. Additional evidence that hepatitis A virus rarely spreads by parenteral routes comes from serologic studies of patients who have received multiple transfusions, eg, those with hemophilia, thalassemia, and persons undergoing chronic renal dialysis.[8,9] These patients show the same prevalence of antibody to hepatitis A virus as healthy blood donors and other comparable nonpatient populations.

There have been a small number of reported cases of transmission of hepatitis A virus through blood transfusions.[10-15] The donors were not symptomatic but on follow-up were shown to be incubating hepatitis A. The length of survival of hepatitis A virus under normal storage conditions is unknown, but transfusion-associated infections have occurred from blood stored for up to 14 days.[10] Fresh-frozen plasma has also been implicated.[12] The attack rate in recipients of blood from hepatitis A virus–infected donors is very high (100% in some reports). A number of these transfusion-associated cases have occurred in neonatal care units, sometimes with secondary transmission of hepatitis A virus to staff or family members.[11]

Agent

Hepatitis A is caused by a 27-nm (diameter) RNA virus that is categorized as an enterovirus within the picornavirus family. Hepatitis A virus is very stable and at physiologic pH retains its physical integrity and biologic activity at 60 °C for 30 minutes.[16] It also has enhanced resistance to chlorine compared with other enteroviruses. These characteristics facilitate its spread through contaminated food or water.

Disease

Hepatitis A virus infection usually has an incubation period of 2 to 6 weeks. The virus typically is shed in the stool during the final week of the incubation period, at which time there is also transient viremia. Viral shedding in the stool decreases as antibodies to hepatitis A virus develop. The initial antibody response is predominantly of the IgM subclass; IgG antibodies develop soon thereafter and IgM antibody disappears within several weeks to months. Therefore, the presence of IgM antibody to hepatitis A virus almost always is an indication of current or recent infection.

The illness caused by hepatitis A virus is quite diverse in both clinical manifestations and course. It is characterized by the sudden onset of fever, anorexia, nausea, malaise, easy fatigability, weakness, and jaundice. Typically, patients have dark urine and light-colored stools. Severity is related to age; the illness is usually asymptomatic in children but most adults are symptomatic and exhibit jaundice. Symptoms normally subside in 3 to 4 weeks but may persist for months. Acute cholestatic hepatitis has accompanied hepatitis A virus infection. Acute fulminant hepatitis and massive hepatic necrosis are rare, with fatalities occurring in about 0.6% of cases. Pregnant women are more likely to develop severe, life-threatening disease.

Diagnosis

If hepatitis A virus infection is suspected in those patients who are symptomatic or in the early convalescence phase of the illness, a laboratory test for IgM antibody to hepatitis A virus is performed. In the absence of anti–hepatitis A virus IgM, a positive test result for total anti–hepatitis A virus (IgG and IgM) indicates remote infection with, and immunity to, the virus.

Prevention

The prevention of transfusion-associated hepatitis A depends on obtaining a thorough medical history of the blood donor to rule out recent exposure to individuals with hepatitis. Since the test for ALT now is performed routinely on all blood donations, it offers an extra margin of safety in those individuals who have been recently infected with hepatitis A virus. Even if a person is not overtly symptomatic because of hepatitis A virus infection, a mild to moderate elevation of the ALT level may be present. If blood is transfused from a donor who subsequently develops hepatitis A, the recipient of the blood should receive immune globulin. The recommended intramuscular dose is 0.02 mL/kg, and it is 80% to 90% effective in modifying hepatitis A infection if given early in the incubation period.[17] Immune globulin does not actually prevent hepatitis A infection but decreases its clinical severity, making some clinical cases milder or even totally asymptomatic. Vaccines for hepatitis A are being developed and may eventually play a role in preventing the disease.

Hepatitis B

Epidemiology

Worldwide, most hepatitis B virus infections are transmitted perinatally from infected mother to newborn infant. Hepatitis B virus is also transmitted parenterally and sexually. In many cases in the United States, however, there is no apparent route of infection. Despite very sensitive third-generation tests for HBsAg, hepatitis B virus still accounts for approximately 5% to 10% of transfusion-associated hepatitis.[2] Overall, however, transfusions account for a minute fraction of hepatitis B virus infections.

There is a marked variation in frequency of infection and patterns of transmission of hepatitis B virus. In the United States and Western Europe, it is a disease of low endemicity: 0.1% to 0.5% of the population are virus carriers. Certain subpopulations have higher endemic rates of infection because of increased exposure or impaired immunity. These include intravenous drug users, renal dialysis patients, medical care professionals such as laboratory workers and dialysis nurses, sexual partners of infected persons, promiscuous male homosexuals, institutionalized individuals with Down's syndrome, and patients with lymphoproliferative disorders. In other areas of the world such as China, Southeast Asia, and sub-Saharan Africa, the disease is highly endemic, with 5% to 15% of the population carrying hepatitis B virus; most of these individuals acquire their infection at birth or during childhood. The epidemiologic association between hepatocellular carcinoma and chronic hepatitis B virus infection makes hepatocellular carcinoma one of the most common fatal malignant neoplasms worldwide.[18] Recent estimates of deaths caused by hepatocellular carcinoma range from 250,000 to 1,000,000 per year.[19] The progression to malignancy is slow, averaging 40 years.

Agent

Hepatitis B virus is a 42-nm (diameter) particle (the Dane particle) comprising a 3.2-kb, partially double-stranded DNA genome enclosed in a 27-nm nucleocapsid of the HBcAg, surrounded by a surface coat (HBsAg). The surface and core components of the virus are antigenically and structurally distinct. The surface coat is composed of lipid and protein. HBsAg can be serologically separated into different subtypes (adr, adw, ayr, ayw), which can be useful epidemiologic markers. The viral core consists of DNA, DNA polymerase, and the determinants for HBcAg) and hepatitis B e (HBeAg) antigens. The virus is sensitive to heat and to chemicals such as sodium hypochlorite. Heat-treated albumin and plasma protein fraction (10 hours, 60 °C) as well as cold ethanol–fractionated immune globulin preparations

(Cohn method) do not transmit infectious hepatitis B virus. The hepatitis B virus in unfractionated serum may not be inactivated by heat (10 hours, 60 °C) because of the protective function of other serum proteins. Additionally, there may not be the same physical separation of hepatitis B virus that occurs for albumin and immune globulin during the fractionation process.[20]

Disease

The onset of hepatitis B virus infection is often insidious and characterized by fever, anorexia, malaise, weakness, vomiting, and abdominal pain, although, in some patients, obvious clinical findings of jaundice, dark urine, and light-colored stools may be apparent. The incubation period varies between 2 weeks and 6 months, with an average of 7 weeks. The usual clinical presentation is indistinguishable from that of non-A, non-B hepatitis. However, with hepatitis B infection, extrahepatic manifestations such as skin rashes, arthritis, and, much less commonly, vasculitis and glomerulonephritis may occur. Glomerulonephritis is usually secondary to immune complex deposition. Characteristic elevation of levels of liver enzymes aspartate aminotransferase (AST) and ALT ensues. Development of chronic hepatitis occurs in 5% to 10% of infected persons; fulminant hepatitis and death may occur in 1% to 3%. The chronic carrier state is much more likely to occur in perinatally infected individuals, with 70% to 90% of infants born of HBeAg/HBsAg-positive mothers themselves becoming chronic hepatitis B virus carriers.[21]

Diagnosis

A diagnosis of acute hepatitis B infection in the appropriate clinical setting is confirmed by the laboratory test results for HBsAg and antibody to the core antigen (anti-HBc). HBsAg may appear in the serum of infected individuals as early as 2 weeks after infection and persist for variable periods. Since the presence of HBsAg in acute cases is usually transitory, it is important also to test for anti-HBc. Assays for anti-HBc of the IgM subclass are a reliable indicator of recent infection if performed semiquantitatively. It should be noted, however, that low levels of anti-HBc IgM may be present in chronic HBV infection.[22] Hepatitis B viral DNA can be detected in serum; its presence is the most sensitive indicator of infective virus. Methodologies for HBV DNA detection include molecular hybridization and the PCR. Hepatitis B e antigen (HBeAg) is usually detected early in the acute phase of the illness and is a marker of viral replication and high infectivity. With disappearance of HBeAg, antibody to HBeAg (anti-HBe) usually develops, and may herald the appearance of antibody to HBsAg (anti-HBs). Anti-HBe in the presence of HBsAg correlates with lower infectivity. After loss of HBsAg, anti-HBs is found weeks to months later. Anti-HBs is an indicator of resolution of infection and immunity, and may persist for years along with anti-HBc.

Prevention

The prevention of transfusion-transmitted hepatitis B starts with obtaining a blood donor history, as outlined in the introduction. Hepatitis occurring before age 10 is most likely to be due to hepatitis A virus that does not result in a chronic carrier state; however, after this age, hepatitis B virus or non-A, non-B hepatitis virus(es) are the more likely cause, so such persons are indefinitely deferred as blood donors. Detection of carriers of hepatitis B virus primarily depends on the routine testing of all units of blood and components for HBsAg. Testing for anti-HBc, currently used in blood banks as a surrogate marker for non-A, non-B hepatitis, will identify a small subset of blood donors with subdetectable levels of HBsAg who might otherwise be missed.

A very effective hepatitis B vaccine has been developed and is available either as a serum-derived or recombinant DNA product.[21] The vaccine is definitely indicated for patients who are likely to require multiple transfusions of blood or components during their lifetimes, eg, those with hemophilia or thalassemia. The hepatitis B virus vaccine is also important for those individuals who are sexual partners of chronic HBsAg carriers, medical care workers exposed to blood from patients who thus are at risk of acquiring hepatitis B virus infection, and offspring of mothers with HBsAg. The younger the patient, the more likely he or she will respond to the vaccine and be immune upon exposure to hepatitis B virus. In conjunction with hepatitis B immune globulin, the hepatitis B vaccine is 90% effective in preventing infection of neonates born to mothers who are infected with hepatitis B virus.[21] For acute needlestick injuries with HBsAg-positive blood, both hepatitis B immune globulins and the hepatitis B vaccine should be given to those who are susceptible (no anti-HBs and/or anti-HBc in their serum).

Non-A, Non-B Hepatitis: Now Hepatitis C, E, and ?

Epidemiology

At least three non-A, non-B hepatitis viruses have been epidemiologically characterized. Two of the viruses are transmitted parenterally, similar to the hepatitis B virus, and the third is transmitted enterically, similar to the hepatitis A virus.[23,24] One of the parenterally acquired non-A, non-B hepatitis viruses appears to be responsible for 90% to 95% of transfusion-associated hepatitis. The other virus has not been established to be epidemiologically important; its existence also has not been serologically verified. The enterically transmitted non-A, non-B virus has been responsible for a number of hepatitis outbreaks in the past 10 to 15 years in India, the Soviet Union, Africa, Mexico, and parts of Southeast Asia.[24,25] As with hepatitis A, enterically transmitted non-A, non-B hepatitis is associated with poor hygiene and sanitation. The current designation for this form of hepatitis is *E*. The genome of hepatitis E has been identified and preliminary research on serologic tests has been described.[26,27] To date, hepatitis E is not believed to be transmitted by transfusion.

The transmission routes of most of the sporadic cases of non-A, non-B hepatitis in the United States are unknown. Recent data from the CDC Sentinel Counties Studies show an absence of commonly recognized risk factors for acquiring non-A, non-B hepatitis in 52% of clinical cases.[28] Surveys of urban hospitals have shown that non-A, non-B hepatitis accounts for 6% to 46% of sporadic cases of viral hepatitis, with the latter figure probably being more accurate because of significant underreporting of this usually clinically mild disease.[2] The blood components and derivatives implicated in transmission of non-A, non-B hepatitis include whole blood, red blood cells (liquid or previously frozen), fresh-frozen plasma, cryoprecipitate, platelets, factor VIII concentrates, and factor IX concentrates. Newer, heat-treated factor concentrates do not appear to transmit non-A, non-B hepatitis. It seems to occur much less frequently in homosexuals than does hepatitis A or B. Non-A, non-B hepatitis also seems to be, at best, infrequently spread through heterosexual sex.[29]

Agent

The search for the causative agent of transfusion-associated non-A, non-B hepatitis has been a very long and difficult one spanning the past 15 years. Recently, it appears that substantial progress has been made. Michael Houghton and colleagues at Chiron Corp, in collaboration with Daniel Bradley at the CDC, using elegant molecular biology techniques, were able to identify a single-stranded RNA virus containing a genome of approximately 10,000 nucleotides that has been named hepatitis C virus.[30] It appears to be related to flaviviruses (arthropod-borne viruses such as yellow fever and dengue). Using large quantities of highly infectious plasma obtained from an experimentally infected chimpanzee, the genome of hepatitis C virus was cloned and a protein encoded by this virus was expressed. This protein reacts with antibodies present in serum from a high proportion of patients with chronic non-A, non-B transfusion-associated hepatitis[31] and blood donors implicated in the transmission of non-A, non-B hepatitis to recipients of their blood.[32] The ability to express non-A, non-B viral proteins in vitro has made it possible to develop enzyme-linked immunoassays to detect antibody to hepatitis C virus during the convalescent phase of non-A, non-B hepatitis. In addition, the PCR can be used to identify viral gene products in hepatitis C virus–infected individuals.[33]

The major parenterally transmitted non-A, non-B agent, hepatitis C virus, is an enveloped 30- to 60-nm virus, is sensitive to chloroform, and has the ability to induce the formation of characteristic cytoplasmic tubular ultrastructures in the liver of experimentally infected chimpanzees. Whether a second non-A, non-B hepatitis virus besides hepatitis C virus exists is not clear. Physicochemical studies and cross-challenge experiments in chimpanzees have yielded evidence for a second non-A, non-B agent.[34,35] However, no serologic test has been developed for what must be, at best, a minor cause of non-A, non-B hepatitis. Furthermore, studies with the hepatitis C virus assays could explain almost all cases of non-A, non-B hepatitis as being due to hepatitis C virus.

The enterically transmitted non-A, non-B agent (hepatitis E virus) has been successfully transmitted to nonhuman primates.[26,27] Pooled fecal specimens from infected animals contain 27- to 38-nm viruslike particles that are serologically and physically distinct from the hepatitis A virus. Immune electron microscopy has demonstrated antibodies against these viruslike particles in the acute-phase serum of individuals with enterically transmitted non-A, non-B hepatitis.[27] The genome of hepatitis E virus has been cloned[26] and immunoassays developed to begin to characterize the clinical, epidemiologic, and serologic features of this epidemic viral hepatitis.[27]

Disease

The natural history of transfusion-associated hepatitis C infections (non-A, non-B hepatitis) recently has been more fully elucidated. Disease due to hepatitis C virus appears to be much more serious than was initially appreciated. The incubation period is usually 5 to 12 weeks with a mean of 8 weeks and a range of 2 to 26 weeks. In the acute phase, symptoms are mild; 75% of the infections are anicteric and ALT levels are below 800 IU/L. Widely fluctuating ALT levels are characteristic and up to 50% of individuals show persistent elevation of ALT levels for more than 1 year. Most patients with elevated liver enzyme levels show chronic active hepatitis on liver biopsy. As many as 10% may go on to develop cirrhosis, usually after 10 to 20 years, but sometimes as early as 4 years. Some individuals with non-A, non-B hepatitis have developed hepatocellular carcinoma, typically 20 years or more after the onset of chronic infection. It was because of the long-term consequences of hepatitis C virus disease, along with its occurrence in up to 5% to 10% of prospectively followed up recipients of multiple transfusions, that led to the widespread implementation of "surrogate" testing (ALT and anti-HBc) for this agent by the blood-banking community in 1987. However, the implementation of testing for anti-hepatitis C virus in 1990 provided a more specific, and yet more effective, means to decrease the risk of transfusion-associated hepatitis C virus infection.

Diagnosis

The diagnosis of posttransfusion non-A, non-B hepatitis in the appropriate clinical setting initially depended on the documentation of at least two elevated ALT values (within 14 days) occurring 2 to 26 weeks after transfusion. The other important viral causes of hepatitis (hepatitis A virus, hepatitis B virus, CMV, and EBV) plus liver toxins, metabolic diseases, and hereditary disorders affecting the liver must be ruled out before classifying a case of hepatitis as non-A, non-B. With a specific antibody test, anti-hepatitis C virus, the diagnosis of non-A, non-B hepatitis is now much more certain. However, anti-hepatitis C virus may take a mean of 22 weeks to appear,[32] so convalescent-phase testing may be necessary to verify the diagnosis of hepatitis C virus infection (whether due to transfusions, which account for only about 5% of cases, or other identified or unknown routes of infection).

Prevention

The prevention of hepatitis C virus transmission through blood transfusion has relied on the use of volunteer (unpaid) blood donors, expanded donor screening and unit exclusions, plus the use of the surrogate markers ALT and anti-HBc. The association between an elevated ALT level or the presence of anti-HBc in blood donors and the development of non-A, non-B hepatitis in recipients of their blood has been well documented in the Transfusion Transmitted Viruses Study (TTVS) and studies conducted at the NIH.[36-39] The NIH studies were conducted as part of an ongoing hepatitis prevention research effort.[37,38] Both the TTVS and NIH groups followed up patients who had and had not received transfusions and looked for evidence of viral hepatitis using frequent sampling for serologic assays and chemical tests. Their results and conclusions are remarkably similar. Both TTV and NIH studies showed that the presence of anti-HBc and/or an elevated ALT level in donor blood correlated with an increased risk of transfusion-associated hepatitis, primarily of the non-A, non-B type. The two tests, when applied to blood donor samples, appeared to be independently associated with an increased risk of transfusion-transmitted hepatitis in recipients.[37]

Both study groups calculated a predicted efficacy if surrogate tests were implemented for blood donor screening. Using anti-HBc, the NIH study predicted a 43% reduction in transfusion-associated hepatitis, while the TTVS predicted a 33% reduction. The estimated loss of donors in the two studies was 4% and 5%, respectively. Using an elevated ALT level as a marker for non-A, non-B hepatitis carriers, the NIH study predicted a 29% efficacy for hepatitis reduction, while the TTVS predicted a 31% hepatitis reduction. The estimated donor loss in these two studies was 1.6% and 2.9%, respectively. The estimated efficacy of the two tests used together was in excess of 50%. Based on these findings, the AABB *Standards* require the use of anti-HBc and ALT testing as "interim" surrogate markers to reduce the risk of transfusion-associated non-A, non-B hepatitis.[5] Using the predicted efficacy of surrogate testing for non-A, non-B hepatitis from the data in the TTVS and NIH study, the risk of transfusion-associated non-A, non-B hepatitis per unit of tested blood can be calculated: 1:143 (TTV) and 1:500 (NIH); these figures are corrected for the "background" risk of non-A, non-B hepatitis that occurred in those studies' untransfused controls in the same hospitals.

Since the publication of the TTVS and NIH study, Sugg and colleagues[40] from the Federal Republic of Germany predicted a fivefold decrease in non-A, non-B hepatitis in blood transfusion recipients (from 10.1% to 2.1%) if anti-HBc was used as a surrogate marker of non-A, non-B hepatitis. In their study, blood had already been screened for an elevated ALT level. The estimated efficacy for reduction of cases of non-A, non-B hepatitis was 42%. On the other hand, two smaller European studies failed to demonstrate that anti-HBc would be useful as a surrogate marker for blood donors capable of transmitting non-A, non-B hepatitis.[41,42]

There are indications that the use of the surrogate tests, along with donor screening procedures, has resulted in a decrease in transfusion-associated non-A, non-B hepatitis in the United States. The most convincing evidence comes from the intensive surveillance for viral hepatitis conducted in four sentinel counties by the CDC.[28,43] From 1981 to 1985, 150 to 200 patients per year with clinically diagnosed non-A, non-B hepatitis were interviewed; a history of blood transfusion was reported by an average of 16% (range, 15% to 20%). In 1986, transfusions were reported as the risk factor for non-A, non-B hepatitis by only 8% of 185 patients, and in 1987, by only 4.6% of 151 patients. In contrast, intravenous drug use was reported by an average of 20% of patients from 1981 to 1985, 38% in 1986, and 42% in 1987. The percentage of patients with clinical non-A, non-B hepatitis and no identified risk factor remained constant throughout this time (about 50%). The proportion of cases of non-A, non-B hepatitis attributable to transfusion decreased by 50% in the year *before* institution of surrogate testing but has subsequently decreased by another 43%. The reported cases of transfusion-associated hepatitis caused by hepatitis B virus also decreased dramatically during this time.[44]

Even with the encouraging data to support the efficacy of surrogate testing for non-A, non-B hepatitis, surrogate markers have substantial deficiencies. The majority of blood donors have an elevated ALT level for reasons unrelated to non-A, non-B hepatitis. For example, alcohol consumption, strenuous exercise, obesity, and certain medications may cause mild to moderate elevation of the ALT level. In the TTVS and NIH study, viral hepatitis did not occur in almost 70% of recipients of blood from donors with an elevated ALT level. Likewise, the presence of anti-HBc is unrelated to non-A, non-B hepatitis in the majority of blood donors. This was also shown in the TTVS and NIH study, in which the majority of recipients of blood from anti-HBc–positive donors did not develop transfusion-associated hepatitis. There is evidence to suggest that 30% to 50% of the positive anti-HBc tests in blood donors may be falsely positive as a marker for hepatitis B virus infection, much less non-A, non-B infection.[45,46] Further, in a hepatitis B virus vaccination study by Lok and coworkers[47] in Hong Kong, 56% of individuals who were positive for anti-HBc by ELISA and negative for other markers of hepatitis B infection showed a primary immune response. Thus, these individuals appeared to have had a false-positive anti-HBc test by ELISA. The study group consisted of family members of patients at a liver disease clinic. This population is dramatically different from US blood donors. Therefore, the study needs to be repeated in the United States to confirm these findings.

There is a close correlation between the finding of an elevated ALT level or the presence of anti-HBc in blood donor serum and anti-hepatitis C virus.[48] However, while some donors with anti-hepatitis C virus have been deferred because of the surrogate tests, the majority are missed. Implementation of anti-hepatitis C virus testing, in addition to the other measures to decrease transfusion-associated non-A, non-B hepatitis, should effect at least a further

50% reduction in the residual cases of non-A, non-B hepatitis due to transfusions. ALT and anti-HBc testing of donor blood will likely remain in place to identify (1) carriers of hepatitis C virus before seroconversion, (2) HBsAg-negative carriers of hepatitis B virus, and (3) possible carriers of non-A, non-B, non-C hepatitis viruses. It can be estimated that 20,000 to 100,000 cases of transfusion-transmitted non-A, non-B hepatitis will be prevented each year with the introduction of anti-hepatitis C virus testing in blood banks.

Delta Agent

Epidemiology

Infection with the delta agent, hepatitis D virus, may occur concurrently with hepatitis B virus infection (coinfection) or it may occur in a carrier of HBsAg (superinfection). Transmission of the delta virus appears to occur by routes similar to those for the hepatitis B virus, ie, primarily through blood and body fluids. Delta infection is endemic in southern Italy, where it was first reported, but more recent studies have shown a global distribution. Delta infection in North America is largely limited to intravenous drug users and hemophiliacs. In hemophiliacs whose primary treatment was with factor concentrates produced from large donor pools, 47% to 85% were positive for antibody to hepatitis D virus.[49] There have been case reports of nosocomial transmission of delta hepatitis from patient to patient and patient to staff in dialysis units, presumably by parenteral transmission.

Agent

The delta agent is a 36-nm spherical particle comprising HBsAg coating a 1.75-kb RNA genome and a specific delta antigen. It is a naturally occurring defective virus of humans and is dependent on the helper function of hepatitis B virus for replication.

Disease

In persons who are simultaneously infected with hepatitis D and B viruses, an acute, self-limited illness occurs and there is no apparent increase in the likelihood of developing chronic hepatitis. In those cases in which superinfection occurs, hepatitis D virus infection usually becomes chronic and is associated with histopathologic findings of chronic active hepatitis. In a study that compared patients with hemophilia that were HBsAg carriers with and without anti-hepatitis D virus, 17 of 20 individuals with HBsAg and anti-hepatitis D virus had evidence of chronic liver disease.[50] Acute hepatitis D virus infection occasionally may cause a fulminant icteric hepatitis.

Diagnosis

The diagnosis of delta infection depends on the demonstration of antibodies to hepatitis D virus (IgM acutely or IgG chronically) in patients also infected with hepatitis B virus. Anti-hepatitis D virus test kits are commercially available. With research tests, hepatitis D virus RNA may also be detected in the serum. Almost invariably, evidence of hepatitis D virus is accompanied by reactive tests for HBsAg, anti-HBc, and anti-HBe.

Prevention

Prevention of transmission of the delta agent through blood transfusion is accomplished by testing for HBsAg and anti-HBc. Delta infection requires active hepatitis B replication; therefore, HBsAg-negative persons should not transmit hepatitis D virus. Anti-HBc testing offers added protection since it may identify and screen out a small number of donors who have subdetectable levels of HBsAg but nonetheless are capable of transmitting hepatitis B virus along with the delta agent. ALT testing of donors might also be helpful since subclinical cases of hepatitis D virus hepatitis occur and elevated ALT levels may be the only marker of infection. The ALT and anti-HBc surrogate tests for non-A, non-B hepatitis are of added importance when giving transfusions to chronic carriers of HBsAg since they are at much greater risk of infection with hepatitis D virus.

An effective way to avert hepatitis D virus infection is through immunization with hepatitis B vaccine, before exposure to the D virus. Prevention of hepatitis B virus infection remains the best way of preventing hepatitis D virus infection.

Conclusion

Transfusion-associated hepatitis continues to be a major problem in transfusion medicine. Steady progress has been made in the past 15 to 20 years and it appears that we are on the threshold of additional significant advances in the detection and prevention of transfusion-associated non-A, non-B hepatitis (now hepatitis C virus). With the addition of hepatitis C virus antibody testing, there should be an overall reduction of 80% to 90% in cases of transfusion-associated non-A, non-B hepatitis compared with the rate experienced in 1985; the residual risk should be on the order of 0.1% to 0.5% per unit of blood transfused.

Exciting work is also progressing in other areas. Viral inactivation offers the hope of ridding blood and blood products of all viruses. Methods of inactivation relevant to blood banking include heat inactivation, cold inactivation with ultraviolet light and beta propriolactone, membrane-active lipid solvents and detergents, and photochemical inactivation.[51] Progress has been made by Matthews and coworkers[52] using photodynamic inactivation of viral contaminants in blood. The challenge in this area is to maintain the integrity and functional capability of the components of blood while at the same time killing infectious agents.

Concern about transfusion-transmitted diseases, fueled primarily by the AIDS epidemic, has transformed blood banking and transfusion medicine and markedly influenced transfusion practices. Fortunately, there have been many positive changes. Challenges have been made to old dogma regarding indications for transfusion of blood and its components. For example, it is now suggested that 5.0 mmol/L (80 g/L) of hemoglobin may be a more appropriate "standard" for red blood cell transfusion than the traditional 6.2 mmol/L (100 g/L).[53]

Intense interest in autologous transfusion practices is being shown by patients and physicians alike. This has translated into a substantial increase in utilization of preoperative donation, intraoperative hemodilution, and salvage of the patient's own blood.[43] The use of heat-treated coagulation factor concentrates has virtually eliminated viral transmission to patients with hemophilia. Careful use of blood and its components and derivatives will serve to decrease the rate of infection with transfusion-associated hepatitis along with other transfusion-transmitted diseases.

At a time when transfusions have never been safer, there is heightened concern among patients in need of blood and components. Some avoid transfusions at all costs, while others seek their own donors in the mistaken belief they can select "safer" blood. Other patients may refuse transfusion because of religious convictions. Avoiding blood transfusions may result in increased morbidity, especially in the perioperative setting.[54]

The challenge for the future is to continue to work toward making the blood supply as safe as possible, realizing that it is not possible to achieve zero risk for transfusion-transmitted viral hepatitis or other potentially adverse consequences of a transfusion.

References

1. Seeff LB: Transfusion-associated hepatitis B: Past and present. *Trans Med Rev* 2:204–214, 1988.
2. Shih WK, Esteban Mur JI, Alter HJ: Non-A, Non-B hepatitis: Advances and unfulfilled expectations of the first decade. *Prog Liver Dis* 8:433–452, 1986.
3. Hollinger FB, Alter HJ, Holland PV, Aach RD: Non-A, non-B posttransfusion hepatitis in the United States, in Gerety R (ed): *Viral Hepatitis.* New York, Academic Press, 1981, pp 49–70.
4. Blood and blood product donor classification labeling requirements. 606.120b(2). *CFR.* 1980, p 29.
5. Holland PV (ed): *Standards for Blood Banks and Transfusion Services*, ed 13. Arlington, VA, American Association of Blood Banks, Arlington, VA, 1989.
6. Bove JR: Transfusion-associated hepatitis and AIDS: What is the risk? *N Engl J Med* 317:242–245, 1987.
7. Hepatitis A among drug abusers. *MMWR* 37:297–305, 1988.
8. Szmuness W, Dienstag JL, Purcell RH, et al: Hepatitis type A and hemodialysis: A seroepidemiologic study in 15 US centers. *Ann Intern Med* 87:8–11, 1977.
9. Papaevangelou G, Frosner G, Economidou J, et al: Prevalence of hepatitis A and B infections in multiply transfused thalassaemic patients. *Br Med J* 1:689–691, 1978.

10. Noble RC, Kane MA, Reeves SA, Roeckel I: Posttransfusion hepatitis A in a neonatal intensive care unit. *JAMA* 252:2711–2715, 1984.

11. Azimi PH, Roberto RR, Guralnik J, et al: Transfusion-acquired hepatitis A in a premature infant with secondary nosocomial spread in an intensive care nursery. *AJDC* 140:23–27, 1986.

12. Sherertz RJ, Russsell BA, Reuman PD: Transmission of hepatitis A by transfusion of blood products. *Arch Intern Med* 144:1579–1580, 1984.

13. Seeberg S, Brandberg A, Hermodsson S, et al: Hospital outbreak of hepatitis A secondary to blood exchange in a baby. *Lancet* 1:1155–1156, 1981.

14. Skidmore SJ, Boxall EH, Ala F: A case report of post-transfusion hepatitis A. *J Med Virol* 10:223, 1982.

15. Hollinger FB, Khan NC, Oefinger PE, et al: Posttransfusion hepatitis type A. *JAMA* 250:2313–2317, 1983.

16. Siegl G: Virology of hepatitis A, in Zuckerman AJ (ed): *Viral Hepatitis and Liver Disease*. New York, Alan R Liss Inc, 1988, pp 3–7.

17. Recommendations for protection against viral hepatitis. *MMWR* 34:313–335, 1985.

18. Beasley RP, Hwang LY: Epidemiology of hepatocellular carcinoma, in Vyas GN, Dienstag JL, Hoofnagle JH (eds): *Viral Hepatitis and Liver Disease*. Orlando, FL, Grune & Stratton, 1984, pp 209–224.

19. Popper H: Pathobiology of hepatocellular carcinoma, in Zuckerman AJ (ed): *Viral Hepatitis and Liver Disease*. New York, Alan R Liss Inc, 1988, pp 719–722.

20. Holland PV: Hepatitis B surface antigen and antibody (HBsAg/Anti-HBs), in Gerety RJ (ed): *Hepatitis B*. New York, Academic Press, 1985, pp 5–25.

21. Stevens CE, Taylor PE, Liu P: Hepatitis B virus infection: Epidemiology and immunoprophylaxis, in Moore SB (ed): *Transfusion-Transmitted Viral Diseases*. Arlington, VA, American Association of Blood Banks, 1987, pp 1–18.

22. Decker RH, Kuhns MC, Brawner TA, Mimms LT: Future advanced diagnostic techniques for hepatitis B, in Zuckerman AJ (ed): *Viral Hepatitis and Liver Disease*. New York, Alan R Liss Inc, 1988, pp 231–236.

23. Alter HJ, Prince AM: Transfusion-Associated non-A, non-B hepatitis: An assessment of the causative agent and its clinical impact. *Trans Med Rev* 2:288–293, 1988.

24. Ramalingaswami V, Purcell RH: Waterborne non-A, non-B hepatitis. *Lancet* 1:571–573, 1988.

25. Enterically transmitted non-A, non-B hepatitis—East Africa. *MMWR* 36:10–16, 1987.

26. Reyes GR, Purdy MA, Kim JP, et al: Isolation of a cDNA from the virus responsible for enterically transmitted non-A, non-B hepatitis. *Science* 247:1335–1339, 1990.

27. Krawczynski K: Antigens and antibodies of HEV infection in experimental models and man. The 1990 International Symposium on Viral Hepatitis and Liver Disease, Houston, April 4–8, 1990.

28. Alter MJ, Hadler SC, Margolis HS, et al: The changing epidemiology of non-A, non-B hepatitis in the United States: Relationship to transfusions. Transfusion-Associated Infections and Immune Response Seminar, University of California, San Francisco. March, 1988.

29. Everhart JE, DiBisceglie AM, Murray IM, et al: Risk for non-A, non-B hepatitis through sexual or household contact with chronic carriers. *Ann Intern Med* 112:544–545, 1990.

30. Choo QL, Kuo G, Weiner AJ, et al: Isolation of a cDNA clone derived from a blood-borne non-A, non-B viral hepatitis genome. *Science* 244:359–361, 1989.

31. Kuo G, Choo QL, Alter HJ, et al: An assay for circulating antibodies to a major etiologic virus of human non-A, non-B hepatitis. *Science* 244:362–364, 1989.

32. Alter HJ, Purcell RH, Shih JW, et al: Detection of antibody to hepatitis C virus in prospectively followed transfusion recipients with acute and chronic non-A, non-B hepatitis. *N Engl J Med* 321:1494–1500, 1989.

33. Weiner AJ, Kuo G, Bradley DW, et al: Detection of hepatitis C viral sequences in non-A, non-B hepatitis. *Lancet* 1:1–3, 1990.

34. Bradley SW, Maynard JE, Popper H, et al: Posttransfusion non-A, non-B hepatitis: Physiochemical properties of two distinct agents. *J Infect Dis* 148:254–265, 1983.

35. Yoshizawa H, Itoh Y, Iwakiri S, et al: Demonstration of two different types of non-A, non-B hepatitis by reinjection and cross-challenge studies in chimpanzees. *Gastroenterology* 81:107–113, 1981.

36. Stevens CE, Aach RD, Hollinger FB, et al: Hepatitis B virus antibody in blood donors and the occurrence of non-A, non-B hepatitis in transfusion recipients. *Ann Intern Med* 101:733–738, 1984.

37. Koziol DE, Holland PV, Alling DW, et al: Antibody to hepatitis B core antigen as a paradoxical marker for non-A, non-B hepatitis agents in donated blood. *Ann Intern Med* 104:488–495, 1986.

38. Alter HJ, Purcell RH, Holland PV, et al: Donor transaminase and recipient hepatitis: Impact on blood transfusion services. *JAMA* 246:630–634, 1981.

39. Aach RD, Szmuness W, Mosley JW, et al: The transfusion-transmitted virus study: Serum alanine aminotransferase of donors in relation to the risk of non-A, non-B hepatitis in recipients. *N Engl J Med* 304:989–994, 1981.

40. Sugg U, Schenzle D, Hess G: Antibodies to hepatitis B core antigen in blood donors screened for alanine aminotransferase level and hepatitis non-A, non-B in recipients. *Transfusion* 28:386–388, 1988.

41. Aymard P, Janot C, Gayet S, et al: Prospective analysis of donor blood anti-HBc antibody as a predictive indicator of the occurrence of non-A, non-B hepatitis in recipients. *Vox Sang* 51:236–238, 1986.

42. Van der Poel CL, Reesink HW, Lelie PN, et al: Anti-hepatitis C antibodies and non-A, non-B posttransfusion hepatitis in the Netherlands. *Lancet* 2:297–298, 1989.

43. Autologous Blood Transfusions: Principles, Policies, and Practices. *American Blood Commission Forum Focus Newsletter* Spring, 1988.

44. Alter MJ, Hadler SC, Margolis HS, et al: The changing epidemiology of hepatitis B in the United States: Need for alternative vaccination strategies. *JAMA* 263:1218–1222, 1990.

45. Schmidt PJ, Leparc GF, Samia CT: Comparison of assays for anti-HBc in blood donors. *Transfusion* 28:389–391, 1988.

46. Hanson MR, Polesky HF: Evaluation of routine anti-HBc screening of volunteer blood donors: A questionable surrogate test for non-A, non-B hepatitis. *Transfusion* 27:107–108, 1987.

47. Lok ASF, Lai CL, Wu PC: Prevalence of isolated antibody to hepatitis B core antigen in an area endemic for hepatitis B virus infection: Implications in hepatitis B vaccination programs. *Hepatology* 8:766–770, 1988.

48. Stevens CE, Taylor PE, Pindyck J, et al: Epidemiology of hepatitis C virus. A preliminary study in volunteer blood donors. *JAMA* 263:49–53, 1990.

49. Rizzetto M, Ponzetto A, Marinucci G: Transfusion-related delta hepatitis. *Trans Med Rev* 2:224–228, 1988.

50. Rosina F, Saracco G, Rizzetto M: Risk of post-transfusion infection with the hepatitis delta virus. *N Engl J Med* 312:1488–1491, 1985.

51. Alter HJ: You'll wonder where the yellow went: A 15-year retrospective of post-transfusion hepatitis, in Moore SB (ed): *Transfusion-Transmitted Viral Diseases*. Arlington, VA, American Association of Blood Banks, 1987, pp 53–86.

52. Matthews JL, Newman JT, Sogandares-Bernal F, et al: Photodynamic therapy of viral contaminants with potential for blood banking applications. *Transfusion* 28:81–83, 1988.

53. Consensus Conference: Perioperative Red Blood Cell Transfusion. *JAMA* 260:2700–2703, 1988.

54. Carson JL, Poses RM, Spence RK, Bonavita G: Severity of anaemia and operative mortality and morbidity. *Lancet* 1:727–729, 1988.

7
Post-Transfusion Cytomegalovirus Infection

Nancy L. Dock, PhD

The human herpesvirus family includes seven large, enveloped, species-specific DNA viruses that cause infections that last for the lifetime of the host. The hallmark of herpesvirus infections is the complicated life cycle of the virus that initiates primary disease followed by long periods of latency and intermittent reactivation. During acute primary infection, the virus disseminates throughout the body to specific tissues, with each herpesvirus exhibiting unique cellular tropism. At some point, the viral genome becomes latent or persistently maintained in a quiescent state that can continue for years. Prompted by unknown conditions related to the host, the environment, or the virus itself, reactivation occurs. Although reactivation can be influenced by a variety of factors, the exact mechanisms are unknown. Clinical manifestations of viral reactivation may only vaguely resemble the primary disease. For example, varicella-zoster virus (VZV), which causes chickenpox, later manifests as the reactivation disease, shingles. Sometimes shingles is a result of immunosuppression of the host, but it also occurs in apparently healthy persons for unknown reasons. Induction of different clinical symptoms by the same virus may be, in part, a consequence of the host's immunity or other host factors that are still undefined.

The cells and tissues where the latent herpesvirus persist appear to be either neural or lymphoid. Three members, herpes simplex virus types 1 and 2 (HSV-1, HSV-2) and VZV, are neurotropic and generally establish latency in sensory ganglia. Three other members have been isolated from lymphoid cells; EBV from B lymphocytes, and the two newest members, human herpesvirus type 6 and type 7 (HHV-6, HHV-7) from T lymphocytes. HHV-6 (originally named human B-lymphotrophic virus) and HHV-7 have been described recently,[1-3] and events surrounding latency and reactivation are beginning to be described. Finally, for CMV, which has been widely studied for many years, the site of latency is still unknown. Although transmission of CMV by transfusion has been thoroughly documented and is a strong indication that the virus is found in peripheral blood, there is conflicting evidence regarding which of the peripheral blood leukocytes is latently infected with CMV.

Each of the herpesviruses is described as being ubiquitous in the human population with varying prevalences worldwide. Most individuals who are infected at an early age develop lasting immunity to reinfection; thus, infection through blood transfusion would rarely cause disease. For example, HHV-6 causes the common childhood disease exanthem subitum (commonly called roseola infantum) that is so widespread during childhood that nearly everyone becomes infected.[4] Therefore, based on prevalence alone, consideration of transmission of herpesviruses by blood transfusion or organ transplantation would not seem to warrant special prevention efforts; with the exception of CMV, in effect this is true. The viremic state of primary herpesvirus infection is usually symptomatic, thus precluding blood donation during the illness. After resolution of the primary illness, if the site of viral latency is not in peripheral blood, as with the neurotropic herpesviruses HSV-1, HSV-2, and VZV, there would be no mechanism for transfusion transmission, explaining why there have been no reports of these viruses being transmitted by blood transfusion. However, when latent virus is maintained in peripheral blood cells and the genome is not eliminated, as is the case with EBV, the virus could be transmitted to uninfected transfusion recipients.[5] Whether this happens with HHV-6 and HHV-7 remains to be seen. Of all the herpesviruses then, the one repeatedly and convincingly linked to transfusion and transplantation transmission is CMV. The reasons for this are unclear at present but could include lower prevalence, the virus' ability to take opportunistic advantage of the immunosuppressed state of the host receiving a transplant or transfusion, or mechanisms of the host-virus interaction that may suppress the host's immune system that may be controlling viral latency.

Epidemiology

CMV is a ubiquitous virus in the human population, and is spread by a number of well-recognized routes: congenital, perinatal, venereal, and iatrogenic (by transfusion and transplantation). All routes of transmission require close contact with infectious body secretions, including urine, oropharyngeal secretions, breast milk, blood, semen, and cervical secretions. CMV is the most common cause of congenital viral infection in the United States, with an estimated 1% of neonates infected. Perinatal acquisition of CMV occurs via contact with infected cervical secretions during delivery or ingestion of breast milk containing infectious virions. During early childhood years, CMV can be spread through close contact with body secretions from children who are shedding the virus, as has been reported in day care settings.[6] In the adult years, the primary mode of spread is through sexual contact. Finally, CMV transmission by blood transfusion and organ transplantation has been well documented and can occur in any age group.[7-9]

Human CMV infection is pandemic and nonseasonal. Although there are no occupational, racial, or genetic predisposing factors for CMV infection, prevalence increases with age and is inversely proportional to socioeconomic status. Acquisition of CMV can be enhanced by crowded living conditions, poor hygiene, and extended family living situations in which all members participate in infant care.[7] Among individuals within a given age group, CMV antibody titers are significantly higher in women than in men and among sexually active individuals with multiple sexual partners. CMV prevalence in adults is high, with significant geographic variability ranging from about 40% to nearly 100%.[10]

Agent

The pathologic effects of CMV were recognized over 100 years ago and first reported in the scientific literature in 1904.[11] The term "cytomegalia" was coined to describe the appearance of greatly enlarged cells long before it was recognized that these cells were virally infected.[12] Isolation of the virus in cell culture as reported in 1956[13] was the first real breakthrough toward understanding the biology of CMV, which has been shown in the ensuing years of investigation to be exceedingly complex. CMV is morphologically indistinguishable from the other herpesviruses in tissue. In cell culture, however, characteristic cytopathic effects seen as clusters of enlarged, refractile cells represent foci of CMV infection. This typical cytopathology requires 3 to 6 weeks to develop, as CMV is highly cell-associated and spreads slowly from one infected cell to an adjacent cell in culture.

CMV is the largest of the herpesviruses, with a particle diameter of approximately 0.2 μm. The virus is composed of a core of double-stranded DNA enclosed by an icosahedral capsid surrounded by an envelope derived from the host cell nuclear membrane. The virus is readily inactivated by lipid solvents and by storage at a pH of less than 6.0, exposure to ultraviolet light for 5 minutes, and high heat (1 hour at 37 °C or 30 minutes at 56 °C). While studies have shown that CMV is labile at conventional freezing temperatures, minimal loss of infectivity can be achieved by storage in liquid nitrogen.[14,15]

This virus is not only large but has a highly regulated, complex replicative cycle that has been studied in vitro.[16,17] The mechanism for viral entry into host cells and specific requirements for recognition molecules or cell receptors are not known, although after entering the cell the virus quickly traverses the cytoplasm and can be localized in the nucleus within 5 minutes.[18] During infection of a permissive cell line in vitro, the viral genome is slowly transcribed in a regulated manner, resulting in the serial production of three classes of mRNAs and proteins: IE (immediately early), E (early), and L (late). Viral protein production is sequential: first it is regulatory, then nonstructural, and finally viral structural proteins are produced.[19] The IE phase begins within the first hour after infection when IE mRNA is transcribed in the nucleus and cytoplasmic translation of IE proteins becomes detectable. The IE products rapidly accumulate back in the nucleus, where they bind DNA and regulate CMV gene expression. The E phase occurs from approximately 4 hours after infection, when the first E mRNA can be detected, until approximately 16 to 24 hours after infection, when DNA replication begins. During the E phase, a perinuclear cytoplasmic inclusion develops and infected cells begin to enlarge, perhaps in part because of E protein stimulation of a burst of host cell macromolecular synthesis. One of the E proteins is the viral DNA polymerase required for viral DNA replication, the event that initiates the L phase. In the L phase, approximately 90% of the CMV genome is transcribed into stable, polyribosome-associated mRNA encoding viral structural proteins. Abundant amounts of at least 35 viral structural proteins are then produced during the next 48 hours. Nuclear inclusions appear and increase in size during this time. In addition, virus-induced Fc receptors develop in the perinuclear region of the cell. By 72 hours after infection, virus particles assemble in the nucleus and then bud through the nuclear membrane, acquiring an envelope of host-cell origin. Some virus particles acquire an additional envelope by budding into cytoplasmic vacuoles while crossing the cytoplasm to exit the cell. Finally, the accumulated infectious virions are released during cell lysis and can then infect other cells.

The CMV genome is the largest of the herpesviruses, consisting of approximately 235 kbp of DNA with a relative molecular weight of 150 Md, and the capacity to encode about 150 proteins.[20,21] Like the other herpesviruses, the genome is linear and double-stranded with nicks and gaps. Unlike other DNA viruses, the herpesviruses contain repeat sequences that, in the case of CMV, can invert, allowing the DNA molecule to adopt four isomeric forms. The CMV genome can be divided into long and short unique regions (82% and 18%, respectively) connected by internal repeating units and bound by terminal repeating units. DNA sequence homology among all of the human CMV isolates studied is approximately 80%, although each strain has a unique pattern when analyzed by restriction endonucleases. Since individual strains can be distinguished by restriction patterns, CMV DNA analysis has become a very useful epidemiologic tool for studying CMV transmission.[22-24]

CMV has marked species specificity. Although several mammals harbor CMV and the murine CMV model has been particularly useful in studying CMV biology, there are distinct features to each virus-host system that cannot be applied directly to humans and human CMV. Therefore, human CMV infection has been studied with human clinical samples and human cell cultures. CMV can be demonstrated in a variety of epithelial cell types, in vivo, but replication in vitro is reliable only in diploid fibroblasts, and occurs most efficiently in certain cell lines (human foreskin fibroblasts, HFF; embryonic lung fibroblasts, WI-38 and MRC-5). In addition, the majority of investigational work with CMV has been performed with laboratory-adapted strains of CMV, namely AD169, Towne, and Davis. Recognition that these strains may not fully represent wild-type CMV isolates has prompted a recent trend toward the use of clinical viral isolates for in vitro experiments that are examining functional activities of the virus such as growth enhancements, efficacy of therapeutic agents, and viral effects on immune cells.[25,26] Laboratory strains of CMV have been the source of antigens for production of monoclonal antibodies directed against specific viral proteins and for viral nucleic acid probes. Despite the functional differences in viral strains, these antibody and nucleic acid tools have been completely successful in identifying both clinical isolates and laboratory strains of CMV.

Disease

The complex biologic interaction between human CMV and the infected host is a dynamic lifelong process that includes primary infection, prolonged viral shedding, and long periods of latency which may be interrupted by reactivation or reinfection. The vast majority of primary CMV infections proceed unnoticed by the host, completely without symptoms. However, when a host's immune response is impaired, clinically severe disease can result. Generally, CMV reactivation and reinfection episodes do not result in symptoms, but exceptions occur in cases of severe immunosuppression. Consequently, the most serious clinical disease occurs in immunocompromised patients experiencing their primary CMV disease (which in some cases was transmitted by transfusion or transplantation) and in congenitally infected infants.

When a primary CMV infection occurs during pregnancy, the congenitally infected infant may experience severe disease and may even die. Of the 0.5% to 2.0% of infants congenitally infected with CMV, only 5% to 10% are symptomatic. Symptoms of fever, rash, jaundice, thrombocytopenia, cerebral calcifications, motor disability, and deafness have been described.[27,28] While many congenitally infected infants are asymptomatic at birth, some suffer significant sequelae such as deafness and mental retardation in early childhood. CMV infection remains as the major congenital infection causing mental retardation and deafness.[29,30]

Serious clinical disease can be seen when immunosuppressed CMV seronegative individuals become infected with CMV. In bone marrow transplant recipients, CMV is associated with death more frequently than any other infectious agent. In CMV-seronegative renal transplant recipients, the transplanted kidney is presumed to be the major source of CMV transmission, whereas CMV seropositive recipients can either reactivate endogenous virus or be reinfected by exogenous virus from a CMV-seropositive donor's kidney.[9,22] Low birth weight premature neonates, splenectomized patients, and patients receiving immunosuppressive chemotherapy are also at increased risk for serious CMV disease and long-term sequelae. Furthermore, evidence that CMV might contribute to the progression of HIV infection is accumulating: (1) more than 90% of individuals with HIV infection are seropositive for CMV; (2) CMV and HIV can infect similar cell types in vitro; and (3) CMV possesses genes that are capable of increasing the expression of the HIV genome by transactivation.[31,32]

A wide range of disease symptoms of active viral infection can result from iatrogenic transmission of CMV by transfusion or transplantation. The exact illness depends, at least in part, on the host's previous experience with CMV. One well-described CMV syndrome is a self-limiting infectious mononucleosis that is EBV-negative.[33,34] CMV can infect almost any organ, but clinical manifestations most commonly recognized are hepatitis, pneumonitis, malaise, arthralgia, retinitis, central nervous system disease, gastrointestinal disease, and hematologic involvement including leukopenia, thrombocytopenia, and anemia.

In addition to syndromes of viral infection, CMV has been etiologically linked with conditions traditionally classified as neoplastic and degenerative, including several malignant neoplasms and atherosclerosis. Possible association of CMV with endothelial cell damage preceding atherosclerosis has been suggested by work demonstrating CMV antigens and nucleic acid sequences in smooth muscle cells cultured from aortic punch biopsy specimens and plaque samples, and from cell cultures of human arterial tissue.[35,36] A recent report of elevated CMV antibody levels in male patients undergoing vascular surgery for atherosclerosis lends support to this suggestion.[37]

A possible etiologic role for CMV in the development of neoplastic disease has long been postulated. Human CMV laboratory strain AD169 contains a specific DNA fragment within its genome that upon in vitro transfection into mouse cells transformed these cells sufficiently so that they caused tumors when implanted into mice.[38] Other reports demonstrating successful transformation using several regions of the CMV genome have been published.[39,40] Additional evidence for CMV oncogenic potential is suggested by the presence of CMV antigen or nucleic acid in tissues of several human malignancies: neuroblastoma, Wilms' tumor, adenocarcinoma of the colon, and prostatic cancer.[41-44] CMV has also been associated with Kaposi's sarcoma;[45] however, other reports have failed to demonstrate a clear association with this tumor.[46,47] A direct relationship of CMV with some of these diseases will be difficult to establish because of the high prevalence of CMV and its ability to exist in latent form in multiple cell types.

Diagnosis

Two types of laboratory approaches have been developed to diagnose CMV infections: (1) detection of CMV-specific antibody in serum, and (2) detection of virus in body secretions or tissues. Both approaches can provide useful information about the CMV status of the individual being tested if certain characteristics of the host and the viral infection are carefully considered. Serologic assays can establish previous exposure, which is useful for blood donor screening, prenatal testing, or pretransplant assessment. They are not useful, however, in assessing reactivation or reinfection in a CMV-seropositive individual, or in establishing whether a clinical viral illness is caused by CMV. Furthermore, use of CMV serologic assays to follow a patient's clinical course could be confounded by transfusion therapy, particularly by administration of intravenous immunoglobulin. On the other hand, viral cultures for CMV are critical for diagnosis in patients with viral syndromes and not at all helpful in healthy individuals. When a symptomatic patient has active CMV infection, the virus can be readily cultured from multiple body sites, but is almost never recoverable from an asymptomatic, seropositive individual.

An outline of the typical course of a CMV infection from the laboratory viewpoint may be useful to illustrate why appropriate selection of a CMV assay is necessary to determine the current status of a patient's CMV infection. A primary infection is characterized by a period of viruria, viremia, and detectable serum levels of antibody to CMV. CMV infection in both normal and immunocompromised persons induces the production of specific IgG, IgM, and IgA to the three major types of viral antigens: IE, E and L. Generally, CMV seropositivity is defined as the presence of IgG to L antigens that develops soon after infection and persists for life. Although prospective studies of transfusion recipients clearly suggest that the virus is present in blood, isolation of CMV from blood of healthy individuals who are beyond the initial stages of the infection has been extremely difficult. After an acute primary infection, the virus enters a period of latency, during which antibody titers persist and are readily detectable. Later, at sporadic, unpredictable times, the virus can be reactivated from the latent state with recurrence of viral shedding. During such reactivation, viruria is frequently detectable, but there is at best only a minimal increase in the CMV-specific IgM level. Sometimes CMV-specific IgG levels become elevated, showing the typical anamnestic response. The cells that maintain viral latency and the mechanism of reactivation are not known. Reinfection with a second strain of CMV with viral shedding and increased IgG levels is possible because the infection provides only partial immunity.[48] Reactivation and reinfection are not clinically distinguishable. In short, CMV infection exists in a lifelong dynamic balance between the virus and the host.

Detection of CMV-specific antibody is easily accomplished with several readily available assays. Currently, ELISA, latex agglutination, and immunofluorescence (both conventional and solid-phase) are the assays most widely used. In contrast, complement fixation and hemagglutination inhibition assays, which were used widely before the early 1980s, are no longer routinely used. Comparative studies of current assays have reported excellent concordance among assays, uniform ability to use plasma or serum samples for testing, and ability to determine an antibody titer if desired.[49-51] Therefore, selection of a CMV screening method can be made on the basis of ease of performance, cost, availability of equipment, compatibility with laboratory staff, and time requirements for testing.

Since detection of CMV antibody indicates previous exposure but not current active infection, serologic study alone is not adequate for detection of CMV infection in patients at risk for severe disease. Rather, detection of replicating virus by culture is more useful. Options currently available include conventional and rapid viral culture. Traditionally, CMV laboratory diagnosis has been based on the development of typical cytopathic effects produced by the virus in cell cultures. These procedures are slow because CMV cytopathic effects can take as long as 6 weeks after inoculation of the specimen to become evident. The speed of conventional CMV culture has been greatly increased by the technique of shell vial centrifugation cultures, which includes confirmation by a monoclonal antibody to IE viral antigens. Results using this rapid method are available in 24 to 48 hours. Briefly, human fibroblasts are seeded onto coverslips contained in 1-dram shell vials. The clinical specimen is inoculated onto the cells, centrifuged at low speed, overlaid with culture medium, and incubated overnight. Then, the coverslips are washed, fixed, stained with the IE antibody, and examined by fluorescence microscopy. In addition to being significantly faster, several studies have shown that centrifugation cultures have equal or greater sensitivity than conventional cell cultures.[52,53] Components necessary to perform centrifugation cultures are readily available commercially and are adaptable to a variety of clinical specimens.

An alternative to demonstrating viral replication in culture that may allow rapid diagnosis of CMV infections is a direct examination of patient's samples for viral antigens and nucleic acids. Direct detection of CMV antigens in tissue using fluorescein-labeled monoclonal antibodies has been reported to be useful for the rapid immunodiagnosis of CMV pneumonia.[54] Specimens used for these studies have included frozen sections from open lung biopsy or cell suspensions and cytocentrifugation preparations of cells obtained from bronchoalveolar lavage. The sensitivity of CMV detection by immunofluorescence was equal to viral culture in these studies.

The CMV genome can be detected in clinical specimens using nucleic acid hybridization techniques. DNA hybridization has been successful for rapid detection of CMV genome in urine and peripheral blood leukocyte preparations.[55,56] Hybridization techniques allow quantitation of viral DNA that could be useful for correlating the quantity of virus with clinical findings.[57] In situ hybridization has been performed using commercially available DNA probes to detect CMV nucleic acids from both formalin-fixed, embedded tissue sections and bronchoalveolar washings.[58,59] Newer techniques, such as gene amplification procedures for the detection of viral nucleic acid sequences,[60,61] offer considerable promise for studying certain aspects of infection with CMV and may be well suited to the diagnosis of viral diseases such as CMV, in which culture is difficult, expensive, and time consuming, and serologic analysis is complex.

Prevention

Prevention of CMV transmission to all transfusion recipients is not medically indicated since most CMV infections are subclinical. This relative absence of disease, together with the virus' high prevalence, explain why measures to block natural routes of CMV transmission have not been attempted. However, efforts have been made to prevent CMV infections in distinct groups of transfusion recipients at high risk for severe CMV disease: premature neonates, CMV-seronegative pregnant women, and bone marrow transplant recipients. Many premature neonates and bone marrow transplant recipients are so severely immunosuppressed that CMV infection can develop into devastating disease. Likewise, prevention of congenital CMV infection by avoiding transmission to CMV-seronegative pregnant transfusion recipients is important. For these patients, selective prevention strategies have been developed. Transfusion recommendations were formalized in 1984 by the Committee on Transfusion Transmitted Diseases of the AABB[62] to provide CMV-seronegative blood products to seronegative neonates weighing less than 1250 g, seronegative pregnant women, and bone marrow transplant patients receiving prophylactic granulocyte transfusions. The recommendations for neonates were modified in 1987 to allow blood banks to implement either CMV serologic screening or preparation procedures such as freezing for providing cellular blood products with reduced risk of CMV transmission.[63]

Two basic approaches are being explored for the prevention of CMV transmission to transfusion recipients at risk for serious disease: serologic screening and special processing of blood products. Transfusion-associated CMV infection can indeed be reduced by transfusing only CMV-seronegative blood products.[7,8] However, the supply of seronegative blood is limited because of the high seroprevalence in donor populations. While there is widespread agreement (from transfusion studies) that only a small subset of CMV-seropositive donors is infectious, there is no method for distinguishing an infectious seropositive unit of blood from a noninfectious seropositive one. IgM to CMV has been suggested as a marker for this infectious subset of donors.[64] However, an attempt to exclude infectious seropositive donors by interdicting CMV-specific IgM positive blood products from transfusion reduced, but did not completely eliminate, CMV transmission.[65] Therefore, a working assumption prevails that all CMV-seropositive blood is potentially infectious for the transfusion recipient.

Provision of CMV-seronegative blood products for the transfusion needs of small numbers of patients, such as in a neonatal intensive care unit, is usually not a supply problem for blood banks. However, blood bank support for a bone marrow transplantation program that may require large quantities of CMV-seronegative platelet and red blood cell products is a real and growing problem.

The development of effective alternatives to serologic screening is imperative; such techniques include those that render blood products noninfectious by leukocyte-depletion or viral inactivation. Attempts to wash red blood cells in saline solution to deplete leukocytes and prevent CMV transmission were successful in one study[66] and unsuccessful in another.[67] Use of freezing and deglycerolization procedures for red blood cell products effectively prevented transfusion-associated CMV in neonates.[68-70] However, procedures to produce these products are costly, and many patients require blood products such as platelets, which cannot be readily frozen. Attempts to reduce transfusion-associated CMV by attaching leukocyte trapping filters to red blood cells and platelets could be predicted to efficiently remove a highly cell-associated virus like CMV, but filtration is also expensive and studies to evaluate efficacy for CMV removal are currently being performed. Gilbert et al[71] were the first to demonstrate that transfusion-acquired CMV infection in neonates was preventable by using blood that was leukocyte-depleted by filtration. Preliminary results from an ongoing study have reported that depletion of leukocytes from platelets reduces the transmission of CMV to marrow transplant recipients.[72] Additional results from prospective transfusion studies of this type will be forthcoming and will help define alternatives for providing blood products of low CMV infectivity to patient populations in the quantities needed.

Photosensitive chemicals or radiation treatment of blood products are being studied for their utility in viral inactivation as an alternative to viral removal. Demonstration of the effectiveness of these approaches to reduction of CMV infectivity will not be possible by routine viral culture of blood since, with only one exception, multiple attempts to culture CMV from the blood of healthy blood donors have been unsuccessful.[73] Therefore, prospective clinical evaluations will be required to assess the efficacy of measures to prevent transfusion-transmitted CMV. Such studies will require the detailed follow-up of large numbers of transfusion recipients in view of the extremely low incidence of transfusion-associated CMV infection and the high prevalence of CMV seropositivity in the recipient population. Furthermore, ethical considerations prevent the possibility of studying transmission in patient groups at risk for clinically significant CMV disease since transmission can be prevented by interdicting CMV-seropositive blood products. Molecular biologic approaches to the detection of CMV nucleic acids may eventually offer a means to detect effective depletion of the virus from cellular blood products.

Transfusion needs for CMV-noninfectious blood products are currently being met because the number of patients requiring seronegative blood products is small. However, an increasing awareness of transfusion-transmitted infections has heightened safety concerns in transfusion medicine that could promote more requests for CMV-seronegative blood products. For example, immunosuppressed CMV-seronegative patients such as those with hematologic malignancies, or HIV infection, or patients undergoing solid organ transplantation could be at increased risk for severe CMV disease. Specific prevention measures for these patients are currently managed on an individual basis. If transfusion to all recipients in these categories with CMV-seronegative blood becomes necessary, supplies might be inadequate. Therefore, the feasibility of implementing viral depletion or viral inactivation processing to produce CMV-noninfectious blood products will be eagerly anticipated.

References

1. Salahuddin SZ, Ablashi DV, Markham PD, et al: Isolation of a new virus, HBLV, in patients with lymphoproliferative disorders. *Science* 234:596–601, 1986.
2. Josephs SF, Salahuddin SZ, Ablashi DV, et al: Genomic analysis of the human B-lymphotropic virus (HBLV). *Science* 234:601–603, 1986.
3. Frenkel N, Schirmer EC, Wyatt LS, et al: Isolation of a new herpesvirus from human CD4+ T cells. *Proc Natl Acad Sci USA* 87:748–752, 1990.
4. Lopez C, Pellett P, Stewart J, et al: Characteristics of human herpesvirus-6. *J Infect Dis* 157:1271–1273, 1988.

5. Henle W, Henle G: Epstein-Barr virus and blood transfusions, in Dodd RY, Barker LF (eds): *Infection, Immunity, and Blood Transfusion.* New York, Alan R Liss, 1985, pp 201–209.

6. Pass RF, Hutton C, Ricks R, et al: Increased rate of cytomegalovirus infection among parents of children attending day-care centers. *N Engl J Med* 314:1414–1418, 1986.

7. Adler SP: Transfusion-associated cytomegalovirus infections. *Rev Infect Dis* 5:977–993, 1983.

8. Tegtmeier GE: Cytomegalovirus infection as a complication of blood transfusion. *Semin Liver Dis* 6:82–95, 1986.

9. Glenn J: Cytomegalovirus infections following renal transplantation. *Rev Infect Dis* 3:1151–1178, 1981.

10. Onorato IM, Morens DM, Martone WJ, et al: Epidemiology of cytomegaloviral infections: Recommendations for prevention and control. *Rev Infect Dis* 7:479–497, 1985.

11. Ribbert D: Uber protozoanartigen zellen in der niere eines Syphilitischen Neugeborenen und in der parotis van kindern. *Zentralbl Allg Pathol* 15:945–948, 1904.

12. Goodpasture E, Talbot F: Concerning the nature of 'protozoan-like' cells in certain lesions of infancy. *AJDC* 21:415–425, 1921.

13. Smith M: Propagation in tissue cultures of a cytopathogenic virus from human salivary gland virus (SGV) disease. *Proc Soc Exp Biol Med* 92:424–430, 1956.

14. Alford CA Jr, Britt WJ. Cytomegalovirus, in Fields BN (ed): *Virology.* New York, Raven Press, 1985, pp 629–659.

15. Zerbini M, Musiani M, LaPlaca ML: Effects of heat shock on Epstein-Barr virus and cytomegalovirus expression. *J Gen Virol* 66:633–636, 1989.

16. Wathen MW, Stinski MF: Temporal patterns of human cytomegalovirus transcription: Mapping the viral RNAs synthesized at immediate early, early, and late times after infection. *J Virol* 41:462–477, 1982.

17. DeMarchi JM: Post-transcriptional control of human cytomegalovirus gene expression. *Virology* 124:390–402, 1983.

18. Smith JD, deHarven E: Herpes simplex virus and human cytomegalovirus replication in WI-38 cells. *J Virol* 12:919–930, 1973.

19. Stinski MF: The proteins of human cytomegalovirus. *Birth Defects* 20:49–62, 1984.

20. Somogyi T, Colimon R, Michelson S: An illustrated guide to the structure of the human cytomegalovirus genome and a review of transcription data. *Prog Med Virol* 33:99–113, 1986.

21. Kilpatrick BA, Huang ES: Human cytomegalovirus genome: Partial denaturation map and organization of genome sequences. *J Virol* 24:261–276, 1977.

22. Chou S: Acquisition of donor strains of cytomegalovirus by renal transplant recipients. *N Engl J Med* 314:1418–1423, 1986.

23. Collier A, Chandler SH, Handsfield H, et al: Identification of multiple strains of cytomegalovirus in homosexual men. *J Infect Dis* 159:123–126, 1989.

24. Adler SP: Molecular epidemiology of cytomegalovirus: Viral transmission among children attending a day care center, their parents, and caretakers. *J Pediatr* 112:366–372, 1988.

25. Schrier RD, Rice GPA, Oldstone M: Suppression of natural killer cell activity and T cell proliferation by fresh isolates of human cytomegalovirus. *J Infect Dis* 153:1084–1091, 1986.

26. Hirsch MS, Schooley RT: Resistance to antiviral drugs: The end of innocence. *N Engl J Med* 320:313–314, 1989.

27. Weller TH: The cytomegaloviruses: Ubiquitous agents with protean clinical manifestations. *N Engl J Med* 285:203–214, 1971.

28. Stagno S, Pass RF, Dworsky ME, et al: Congenital cytomegalovirus infection: The relative importance of primary and recurrent maternal infection. *N Engl J Med* 306:945–949, 1982.

29. Adler SP: Neonatal cytomegalovirus infections due to blood. *CRC Crit Rev Clin Lab Sci* 23:1–14, 1986.

30. Yeager AS, Palumbo PE, Malachowski N, et al: Sequelae of maternally derived cytomegalovirus infections on premature infants. *J Pediatr* 102:918–922, 1983.

31. Rice GPA, Schrier RD, Oldstone MBA: Cytomegalovirus infects human lymphocytes and monocytes: Virus expression is restricted to immediate-early gene products. *Proc Natl Acad Sci USA* 81:6134–6138, 1984.

32. Rando RF, Pellett PA, Luciw PA, et al: Transactivation of human immunodeficiency virus by herpes virus. *Oncogene* 1:13–18, 1987.

33. Smith DR: A syndrome resembling infectious mononucleosis after open-heart surgery. *Br Med J* 1:945, 1964.

34. Kaariainen L, Klemola E, Paloheimo J: Rise of cytomegalovirus antibodies in an infectious mononucleosis-like syndrome after transfusion. *Br Med J* 1:1270–1272, 1966.

35. Melnick JL, Dreesman GR, McCollum CH, et al: Cytomegalovirus antigen within human arterial smooth muscle cells. *Lancet* 2:644–647, 1983.

36. Petrie BL, Melnick JL, Adam E, et al: Nucleic acid sequences of cytomegalovirus in cells cultured from human arterial tissue. *J Infect Dis* 155:158–159, 1987.

37. Adam E, Probtsfield JL, Burek J, et al: High levels of cytomegalovirus antibody in patients requiring vascular surgery for atherosclerosis. *Lancet* 2:291–293, 1987.

38. Nelson JA, Fleckenstein B, Galloway DA, et al: Transformation of NIH 3T3 cells with cloned fragments of human cytomegalovirus strain AD169. *J Virol* 43:83–91, 1982.

39. Clanton DJ, Jariwalla RJ, Kress C, et al: Neoplastic transformation by a cloned human cytomegalovirus DNA fragment uniquely homologous to one of the transforming regions of herpes simplex virus type 2. *Proc Natl Acad Sci USA* 80:3826–3830, 1983.

40. El-Beik E, Razzaque A, Jariwalla R, et al: Multiple transforming regions of human cytomegalovirus DNA. *J Virol* 60:645–652, 1986.

41. Wertheim P, Voute PA: Neuroblastoma, Wilms' tumor and cytomegalovirus. *JNCI* 57:701–703, 1976.

42. Huang ES, Mar EC, Boldogh I, et al: The oncogenicity of human cytomegalovirus. *Birth Defects* 20:193–211, 1984.

43. Rapp F, Geder L, Murasko D, et al: Long term persistence of cytomegalovirus genome in cultured human cells of prostatic origin. *J Virol* 16:982–990, 1975.

44. Spector DH, Spector SA: The oncogenic potential of human cytomegalovirus. *Prog Med Virol* 29:45–89, 1984.

45. Boldogh I, Beth E, Huang ES, et al: Kaposi's sarcoma detection of CMV DNA, CMV RNA and tumor biopsies. *Int J Cancer* 28:469–474, 1981.

46. Ambinder RF, Newman C, Hayward GS, et al: Lack of association of cytomegalovirus with endemic African Kaposi's sarcoma. *J Infect Dis* 156:193–197, 1987.

47. Civantos F, Penneys NS, Ziegels-Weissman J: Kaposi's sarcoma: Absence of cytomegalovirus antigens. *Invest Dermatol* 79:79–80, 1982.

48. Chou S: Neutralizing antibody responses to reinfecting strains of cytomegalovirus in transplant recipients. *J Infect Dis* 160:16–21, 1989.

49. Beckwith DG, Halstead DC, Alpaugh K, et al: Comparison of a latex agglutination test with five other methods for determining the presence of antibody against cytomegalovirus. *J Clin Microbiol* 21:328–331, 1985.

50. Fend CS, Williams IB, Gohd RS, et al: A comparison of four commercial test kits for detection of cytomegalovirus antibodies in blood donors. *Transfusion* 26:203–204, 1986.

51. Lentz EB, Dock NL, McMahon CA, et al: Detection of antibody to cytomegalovirus induced early antigens and comparison with four serologic assays and presence of viruria in blood donors. *J Clin Microbiol* 26:133–135, 1988.

52. Gleaves CA, Smith TF, Shuster EA, et al: Comparison of standard tube and shell vial cell culture techniques for the detection of cytomegalovirus in clinical specimens. *J Clin Microbiol* 21:217–221, 1985.

53. Forbes BA, Bartholoma NY: Detection of cytomegalovirus in clinical specimens using shell vial centrifugation and conventional cell culture. *Diagn Microbiol Infect Dis* 10:121–124, 1988.

54. Volpi A, Whitley, R, Ceballos R, et al: Rapid diagnosis of pneumonia due to cytomegalovirus with specific monoclonal antibodies. *J Infect Dis* 147:1119–1120, 1983.

55. Chou S, Merigan TC: Rapid detection and quantitation of human cytomegalovirus in urine through DNA hybridization. *N Engl J Med* 308:921–925, 1983.

56. Spector SA, Rua JA, Spector DH, et al: Detection of human cytomegalovirus in clinical specimens by DNA-DNA hybridization. *J Infect Dis* 150:121–126, 1984.

57. Churchill MA, Zaia JA, Forman SJ, et al: Quantitation of human cytomegalovirus DNA in lungs from bone marrow transplant recipients with interstitial pneumonia. *J Infect Dis* 155:501–509, 1987.

58. Hilborne LH, Nieberg RK, Cheng L, et al: Direct in situ hybridization for rapid detection of cytomegalovirus in bronchoalveolar lavage. *Am J Clin Pathol* 87:766–769, 1986.

59. Seto E, Yen TSB: Detection of cytomegalovirus by means of DNA isolated from paraffin-embedded tissues and dot hybridization. *Am J Pathol* 127:409–413, 1987.

60. Shibata D, Martin WJ, Appleman MD, et al: Detection of cytomegalovirus DNA in peripheral blood of patients infected with human immunodeficiency virus. *J Infect Dis* 158:1185–1192, 1988.

61. Demmler GJ, Buffone GH, Schimbor CM, et al: Detection of cytomegalovirus in urine from newborns by using polymerase chain reaction DNA amplification. *J Infect Dis* 158:1177–1184, 1988.

62. Committee on Transfusion Transmitted Diseases of the American Association of Blood Banks: Cytomegalovirus infection and blood transfusion. *Am Assoc Blood Banks News Briefs* 7:1–2, 1984.

63. Committee on Standards American Association of Blood Banks: Special problems of the neonatal (under 4 months) recipient, in *Standards for Blood Banks and Transfusion Services*, ed 12. Arlington, VA, American Association of Blood Banks, 1987, pp 30–31.

64. Beneke JS, Tegtmeier GE, Alter HJ, et al: Relation of titers of antibodies to CMV in blood donors to the transmission of cytomegalovirus infection. *J Infect Dis* 150:883–888, 1984.

65. Lamberson HV, McMillan JA, Weiner LB, et al: Prevention of transfusion associated cytomegalovirus (CMV) infection in neonates by screening blood donors for IgM to CMV. *J Infect Dis* 157:820–823, 1988.

66. Luban NLC, Williams AE, MacDonald MG, et al: Low incidence of acquired cytomegalovirus infection in neonates transfused with washed red blood cells. *AJDC* 141:416–419, 1987.

67. Demmler GJ, Brady MT, Bijou H, et al: Posttransfusion cytomegalovirus infection in neonates: Role of saline-washed red blood cells. *J Pediatr* 108:762–765, 1986.

68. Adler SP, Lawrence LT, Biro BV, et al: Prevention of transfusion-associated CMV infections in very low-birth weight infants using frozen blood and donors seronegative for cytomegalovirus. *Transfusion* 24:333–335, 1984.

69. Taylor BJ, Jacobs RF, Baker RL, et al: Frozen deglycerolyzed blood prevents transfusion-acquired cytomegalovirus infections in neonates. *Pediatr Infect Dis* 5:188–191, 1986.

70. Brady MT, Milam JD, Anderson DC, et al: Use of deglycerolized red blood cells to prevent posttransfusion infection with cytomegalovirus in neonates. *J Infect Dis* 150:334–339, 1984.

71. Gilbert GL, Hayes K, Hudson IL, et al: Prevention of transfusion-acquired cytomegalovirus infection in infants by blood filtration to remove leucocytes. *Lancet* 1:1228–1231, 1989.

72. Bowden RA, Sayers M, Cays M, et al: The role of blood product filtration in the prevention of transfusion associated cytomegalovirus (CMV) infection after bone marrow transplant. *Transfusion* 29(Suppl):57S, 1989.

73. Diosi P, Moldovan E, Tomescu N: Latent cytomegalovirus infection in blood donors. *Br Med J* 4:660–662, 1969.

8
Other Viruses Transmitted by Blood Transfusion

Robert Westphal, MD

The 1980s have been a difficult decade for those in blood banking and transfusion medicine. The discovery of HIV and its relatives, the implementation of surrogate tests for non-A, non-B hepatitis, and the introduction of still another new test for HTLV-I have occurred with great rapidity. We have seen the addition of a specific test for the hepatitis C virus, and there is speculation about the addition of more tests for retroviruses such as HIV-2, HTLV-II, and HTLV-V. There has never been such concern about the transmission of infectious diseases by blood transfusion; at times it defies rational thought. For these reasons, it is probably appropriate to look at some of the viruses that, however unlikely, may be transmitted by transfusion.

'Slow' Viruses

Although in some cases it may be a misnomer, the term "slow virus" is descriptive in that the diseases associated with it are transmissible to animal models from cell-free filtrates of blood or infected tissue and have long incubation times, on the order of years. HTLV-I (see Chapter 5) is perhaps the "slowest" of these, although it appears to require leukocytes for transmission. There are three recognized degenerative neurologic diseases in humans that can be transmitted in the laboratory to animals: Creutzfeldt-Jakob disease, kuru, and the Gerstmann-Straussler syndrome, which is a cerebellar syndrome characterized by ataxia and tremor. Gerstmann-Straussler syndrome occurs primarily in Europe, with vertical family clustering, and it has an apparent autosomal-dominant inherited predisposition to disease. Dementia occurs quite late in its course. The plaques seen in biopsy or autopsy material are different from those seen in Alzheimer's disease and in Creutzfeldt-Jakob disease. The late development of dementia is also true of kuru, another cerebellar syndrome discovered in certain tribes in New Guinea and thought to be spread by ritualistic cannibalism. The disease is believed to have died out, perhaps because of cessation of the practice.[1]

Creutzfeldt-Jakob disease, on the other hand, presents as a progressive dementia with memory loss and poor judgment and intellectual function, although in some cases tremor and ataxia may be the earliest signs. In addition, Creutzfeldt-Jakob disease has been documented to occur after corneal transplantation[2] and dura mater transplantation[3] from affected donors; recently, several cases have been reported in humans receiving human pituitary-derived growth hormone.[4] Because of the long incubation period and its transmissibility by human tissue, the FDA now requires the screening out of blood or tissue donors who received human-derived growth hormone before its removal from the market, despite the fact that transmission by transfusion has not been demonstrated.

Concerns have been raised that other degenerative diseases may be due to biologic agents with long incubation times that have not yet been identified and that could perhaps be transmissible by blood transfusion. Speculations have included Alzheimer's disease, multiple sclerosis, and progressive multifocal leukoencephalopathy (PML). JC virus, a papovavirus isolated from a patient with the initials J.C. (JC does not stand for Jakob-Creutzfeldt), has recently been isolated from bone marrow and splenic mononuclear cells from a patient with AIDS and PML and from marrow B lymphocytes in another patient with PML.[5] There is evidence that immunosuppressed patients shed JC virus in their urine[6]; however, there is no evidence that it is present in healthy persons or that it can be transmitted by blood transfusion.

Perhaps it is best not to speculate idly in a climate already fraught with hysteria, but it is worth examining Creutzfeldt-Jakob disease in more depth since the biology of the presumed transmissible agent is so fascinating and mysterious.

Epidemiology

Creutzfeldt-Jakob disease is a worldwide disorder with an incidence of about one death per million population per year. It was first described by Creutzfeldt in 1920 in a young woman, but the next four cases were reported by Jakob in older patients in the following year. The age at onset is usually in the sixth decade. Curiously, its incidence among Libyan Jews is 30-fold higher than average and a clustering of cases has occurred in the Slovakian Soviet Socialist Republic.[7] 10% of cases are familial but only two instances in which husband and wife were affected have been reported, suggesting that familial clustering is related more to genetic susceptibility than to transmissibility. Although human-to-human spread has been documented, it is not known whether subclinical infections occur. Greenlee[7] points out that it is unlikely that such a uniformly fatal disease with such a low incidence could maintain itself without spread through subclinical cases or some other, perhaps nonhuman, reservoir.

Creutzfeldt-Jakob disease seems to be related to other encephalopathies, including kuru, which derives its name from the tremors and shaking associated with cerebellar degeneration, and scrapie, a fatal infectious encephalopathy of sheep. Visna, another form of degenerative encephalopathy in sheep, has been shown to be caused by a "true" slow virus, a retrovirus similar to that of HIV.[8] In both Creutzfeldt-Jakob disease and kuru, incubation periods of 30 years have been noted.

The Infectious Agent

The neuropathology and electron microscopy of the agent causing CJD and scrapie are remarkably similar and the major efforts of Prusiner[8,9] have focused on both. The transmissible agents are called prions—"small proteinaceous infectious particles which resist inactivation by procedures that modify nucleic acids."[8] Prions are infectious but do not invoke an immune response. Prions contain little or no nucleic acid and the prion protein (PrP) is encoded by a cellular gene, whereas viruses contain a nucleic acid genome that encodes its progeny with most or all of the proteins in their envelopes.

Creutzfeldt-Jakob disease has been experimentally transmitted to animals by inoculation with blood or urine from an affected human.[10] It seems to defy biologic logic, but inoculation with either scrapie PrP or Creutzfeldt-Jakob disease PrP can reproduce the infection in cultured neuroblastoma cells or in susceptible animals. Prion proteins are found in the brain tissue of patients dying of Creutzfeldt-Jakob disease and rod-shaped amyloids have been found in fractions purified from such tissues, suggesting that the amyloid plaques in the brains of patients with Creutzfeldt-Jakob disease are composed of crystals of PrP similar to those seen in scrapie. This is also true of kuru and the Gerstmann-Straussler syndrome, both of which can also be transmitted to animals by inoculation. Human PrP have epitopes distinct from those of mice, but after transmission of human PrP into mice the resulting PrP have no human specific epitopes. This suggests that prions in some way turn on the production of more PrP by host cells, not that they themselves reproduce.

There are apparently host genes in experimental scrapie and Creutzfeldt-Jakob disease that influence the incubation times for prions, suggesting that perhaps some people are more susceptible than others. This complex interaction involves host susceptibility, infectious proteins that do not appear to contain genetic material, biologic response modifiers and, undoubtedly, other, interrelated factors. The reader is referred to Prusiner's article[8] for more detail.

Not everyone agrees with the prion story, which, on its face, is quite curious, to say the least. Others[11] have argued that the transmissible agents of scrapie and Creutzfeldt-Jakob disease are really RNA viruses that have escaped detection for a variety of reasons.

Relationships to Other Neurologic Disorders

The cellular origin of prions and their replication into macromolecules that appear to be causing disease opens a whole new avenue of investigation.

Abnormal proteins that accumulate as amyloids are seen in both Alzheimer's disease and in Parkinson's disease; however, neither have been transmitted to laboratory animals. These amyloids may only represent the accumulation of pathologic products from some other source, though this seems clearly not to be the case in Creutzfeldt-Jakob disease. As Prusiner states, these studies suggest that infectious, environmental, and genetic events may sometimes come together to convert normal proteins into lethal macromolecules and they may improve our understanding of some systemic degenerative diseases.

Finding transmissible agents for kuru, Creutzfeldt-Jakob disease, PML, and subacute sclerosing panencephalitis (measles virus) has led to attempts to identify similar agents for Parkinson's disease, amyotrophic lateral sclerosis, Alzheimer's disease, and multiple sclerosis. All have been unsuccessful, despite the fact that epidemiologic studies have suggested that multiple sclerosis seems to be associated with exposure to some agent or factor during childhood. Whether further work related to HTLV-I and tropical spastic paraparesis (see Chapter 5) will lead to information about multiple sclerosis remains to be seen.

Prevention of Creutzfeldt-Jakob Disease From Transfusion or Transplantation

The initial guidelines designed to screen out donors who had received human pituitary-derived growth hormone deferred those who received it between 1963 and 1985. The FDA's informational statement now indicates that anyone who has ever received the human product should be permanently deferred. Recombinant DNA–produced growth hormone is now available from several manufacturers and is the product of choice. Pituitary-derived hormone is no longer available. These same standards will undoubtedly be promulgated for sperm donors as well as for donors of other tissues and organs, and such a standard has already been adopted by the AABB, the American Red Cross, and other blood- and tissue-banking organizations.

Tropical Viruses

The potential for blood-borne transmission of tropical viruses in the United States is probably very, very small. On the other hand, the world is much smaller, functionally, than even a decade ago. All over the developing world, rural populations are migrating to urban areas for economic, agricultural, and political reasons. This has become a very important consideration regarding Chagas' disease (see Chapter 11). According to Tabor,[12] in an earlier work on infections and transfusion, it was recommended in 1958 that travelers to tropical regions be excluded as blood donors for 4 weeks after returning. Current exclusions of 6 months for travelers to areas endemic for malaria clearly also exclude donors likely to have been infected by arboviruses, those infections that are transmitted by mosquitoes. Because professionals working in blood banks and transfusion services often are asked questions by patients and prospective travelers, as well as donor room personnel, it is worth discussing a few of these viral diseases since it is clear that they *can* be bloodborne. Though transmission by transfusion of healthy donor blood is remote, the changing demographic characteristics of our population, plus the fact that many of us might work at some time in an endemic area, suggest that some knowledge of these illnesses is useful. Tabor[12] and Warren and Mahmoud[13] provide further information on this subject.

Diseases Transmitted by Arboviruses

There are over 350 candidates, of which two families, togaviruses and bunyaviruses, are responsible for most of the human disease that we associate with these arthropod-borne viruses. In all cases, the mosquito is the vector between an animal reservoir and humans. Some better known examples of these viruses include the various American and Asian encephalitis viruses, yellow fever, and dengue. A brief discussion of some of the tropical arboviruses of more specific concern follows.

Rift Valley fever.   The Rift Valley is a large area of land in western Kenya, just northeast of Lake Victoria in east central Africa. Many important archeological finds have occurred there. The virus causing Rift Valley Fever is endemic in goats, sheep, cattle, and undoubtedly, some wild species. It is not confined to the Rift Valley, but is present in many parts of Africa. A new outbreak in Mauritania, in western Africa, occurred in the fall of 1987, leaving 28 people dead of the 245 hospitalized. This was the first outbreak of this disease in West Africa, and the Pasteur Institute of Dakar estimates that there were 1264 cases with 224 deaths.[14]

The virus of Rift Valley fever is a single-stranded RNA bunyavirus of the same family as the California and La Crosse encephalitis viruses. Most commonly, it produces an influenza-like illness but occasionally causes severe hepatic necrosis, meningoencephalitis, and death. During infection the virus may be isolated from serum, making it at least theoretically possible to transmit the illness by blood transfusion. It can also be transmitted by direct contact with infected blood in aerosol form. In some locations antibody prevalence is as high as 10%, and in southern Mauritanian shepherds it is 13%, suggesting that some asymptomatic infections have occurred. It is not known if there is a chronic carrier state in apparently uninfected humans that would make the virus a major concern for blood bankers.

Yellow fever.   Yellow fever is not of great importance currently in the western hemisphere but played a major role in the history of its development. For decades it was a serious deterrent for immigration into both western Africa and the Caribbean and foiled the attempts of the French to build the first Panama Canal. Benjamin Rush, the only physician to sign the Declaration of Independence, is also remembered for his prescriptions for bloodletting as a therapy during the yellow fever outbreak in Philadelphia at the end of the 18th century. The last yellow fever epidemic in the United States occurred in New Orleans in 1905.[13]

The yellow fever virus, an RNA virus, is prevalent among certain non-human primates in the jungles of Central Africa, South America, and parts of Central America. As was convincingly demonstrated by Dr Walter Reed, working in Cuba with the US Army in 1910 and 1911, it is transmitted to man by infected mosquitoes. Originally, Reed thought it had to be transmitted from one infected human to another; it is now known that it can also be transmitted to humans from infected animal reservoirs in nonurban settings. Several species of mosquitoes can transmit the infection, but *Aedes aegypti* is most commonly involved in outbreaks in more settled areas. Although that species of mosquito exists in Asia and the Far East, there is no yellow fever seen there.

In 1986 there was an epidemic of yellow fever in eastern Nigeria, which was followed by an urban epidemic in western Nigeria in early 1987. This was the first urban epidemic in 40 years and probably resulted from the migration of viremic individuals into an urban area with abundant *A aegypti*. In 1988 and 1989, yellow fever was cultured from some mosquito isolates in Trinidad, but no human cases were identified.

Clinically, yellow fever presents as an acute febrile illness of sudden onset with nausea, vomiting, myalgia, and headache, following a usual incubation period of 3 to 6 days. Although there are some asymptomatic cases, other patients go on to develop a severe illness with jaundice, soft palate hemorrhages, hematemesis, and hepatorenal syndrome. The majority of cases, however, are of the mild, symptomatic variety. The mortality rate is reportedly 2% to 5% in endemic areas, but in some epidemics has been as high as 60%. As with dengue, a relative bradycardia may develop and shock may occur if cardiac involvement is extensive. Antibodies are present in about two thirds of the population in endemic areas.

The diagnosis should be suspected in anyone presenting with fever, vomiting, and myalgia and a positive geographic history. Although usually the incubation period is 3 to 6 days, in some cases it has been as long as 2 weeks.[13] If the patient has received the vaccine in the past 10 years, the diagnosis is very unlikely, since the vaccine is quite effective. Immunity is likely to be lifelong after vaccination. The virus can be found in the blood during the first few days of infection, but is unlikely to be transmitted by transfusion in developed countries since exposure to mosquitoes is required and the overlap with malaria in endemic areas is very close, leading to donor deferral. In endemic countries, however, especially in areas where specific standards concerning blood transfusion are not delineated or not known, it is possible that transmission by transfusion has occurred, although there are no reports of it.

Therapy for yellow fever is simply supportive and symptomatic, with special attention paid to fluid balance and renal function in severe cases. The vaccine is safe and effective and is required for entrance into some countries. Specific information about endemic areas and requirements for travel can be found in the *Handbook of Information for International Travelers*, published by the CDC.

Dengue fever and dengue hemorrhagic fever. Compared with yellow fever, dengue is a disease of much greater worldwide importance. An estimated 100 million cases occur yearly, worldwide, and there is almost universal distribution of the virus between 30° north latitude and 20° south latitude,[15] which includes parts of Florida, Louisiana, and Texas. It is found in some monkey species which may serve as a reservoir for isolated cases in the bush, but in urban settings it is transmitted from infected humans by *A aegypti*, the yellow fever vector.

An Asian strain of Aedes, *A albopticus*, which is reportedly more voracious than *A aegypti*, has arrived in this hemisphere in the stagnant water inside imported tires. This stagnant, "rubberized" water is a favorite breeding place for this species, and they have now been found in 17 states in the continental United States.[16] Current surveillance data suggest that the pattern of dengue infection in the Americas is evolving in a manner similar to what happened in Asia in the 1960s, where it is now a leading cause of hospitalization and death among children. Dengue hemorrhagic fever has now been documented in Brazil, Puerto Rico, Nicaragua, the Dominican Republic, and St Lucia.

Although most cases in children are mild, there is a severe syndrome of shock and hemorrhagic fever seen primarily in Southeast Asian children, but which was recently identified in an outbreak among children in Puerto Rico in 1986.[17] At least 1.5 million children have been hospitalized and 33,000 have died of this syndrome since it was first reported in the 1950s.[15] It occurs in children who have been previously infected by one strain of dengue, have an antibody to it, and then are infected with another strain. The viruses replicate in monocytes, and subneutralizing concentrations of antibody to one strain seem to enhance the rapid proliferation of virus of a second serotype.[15]

There are four distinct serotypes of this RNA virus, and often more than one at a time is involved in a specific outbreak. The mosquito can acquire the virus from patients 6 to 18 hours before or anytime after the outbreak of fever. The mosquito remains infected throughout its lifespan. Young infants born to immune mothers or older children previously infected are at risk for the development of the hemorrhagic syndrome. Since tropical Asia is the region of highest dengue endemicity, this probably explains why the severe childhood form has primarily been seen there.

After an incubation period of 2 to 7 days, dengue presents clinically with a high fever associated with chills, headache, backache, and muscle and joint pain, leading to its common name of "bone-break fever." A transient macular rash may appear on the first day, and there is a characteristic "dengue facies" of puffy eyelids, facial flushing, and conjunctival erythema, often with retro-orbital pain. During the next several days nausea and vomiting, lymphade-nopathy, anorexia, and constipation occur. Often there is a temporary re-mission of fever on the third day, giving rise to another name, "saddleback fever." Some patients feel depressed out of proportion to their clinical status; others express feelings of anxiety. As the fever declines after 6 or 7 days, a generalized, slightly grainy rash develops that spares the palms and soles. A striking bradycardia, which may persist for several weeks, is common.

Although mild hemorrhagic symptoms may occur in adults, the severe hemorrhagic syndrome is almost entirely confined to young children. There is a marked increase in vascular permeability with severe physiologic consequences, including hypovolemia and abnormal hemostasis characterized by decreased platelet and fibrinogen levels, elevated fibrin degradation product levels, and a reduction in the complement level. Circulating immune complexes are found and are probably the cause of this consumptive coagulopathy.

Virus can be isolated from the blood in 100% of patients with their first infection and about half of those with their second.[12] Although there are four distinct serologic subtypes, the signs and symptoms of the illnesses are the same. Since vaccination with one strain, or three of the four, would leave the recipient susceptible to the development of dengue hemorrhagic fever, it is believed that vaccine should be administered only for all four subtypes. There currently is no available vaccine, however, and prevention must focus on the eradication of mosquitoes from urbanized endemic areas and avoidance of mosquito bites by the wearing of appropriate clothing and the use of insect repellents.

Although the potential for transmission of dengue by blood transfusion exists, it is unlikely to occur since the viremia occurs during the time that the donor/patient is quite ill. There does not seem to be a carrier state despite the fact that asymptomatic infections do occur. Given the migrations of both vectors and humans from endemic areas in the United States, one cannot help but believe we will hear more of this disease. Cases of "imported" dengue reported to the CDC numbered 94 in 1987 and 124 in 1988, but only about 20% were subsequently confirmed.

Hemorrhagic Fevers Transmitted by Arena and Marburg/Ebola Viruses

The arena viruses derive their name from the Latin "arenaceus," meaning sandy, because of their grainy appearance on electron microscopy. The group includes the virus that causes lymphocytic choriomeningitis. Only the lymphocytic choriomeningitis virus, the Lassa virus, and the two subgroup viruses that cause Argentine hemorrhagic fever and Bolivian hemorrhagic fever are pathogenic in man. These are single-stranded RNA viruses.

These viruses are found in the rodent populations in endemic areas and are transmitted to humans by contact with excreta, including aerosolization of urine or bites. Person-to-person transmission of the Lassa virus occurs by similar mechanisms. All are rural diseases, Lassa fever is found primarily in West and Central Africa. Case fatality ratios in untreated patients with Argentine hemorrhagic fever and Bolivian hemorrhagic fever are on the order of 15% to 20%.

Lassa fever.   Lassa fever was first described in 1969 and laboratory-acquired needle-stick transmission has also been documented.[18] Persons of all ages are affected, but pregnant women seem to be especially prone to severe disease. Following an incubation period of 3 to 16 days, there is a gradual development of fever and malaise, often accompanied by persistent headache and myalgia. Diarrhea, cough, nausea, and vomiting occur in about 50% of cases. Severe pharyngitis with a white patchy exudate is seen in about 80% of patients, along with hypotension and lymphadenopathy. Hearing loss is common, and in some cases is permanent. A macular rash and conjunctival erythema often occur. In severe cases there is abnormal bleeding and thrombocytopenia. In fatal cases the disease progresses with an altered mental state, pulmonary infiltrates and edema, pleural effusions, ascites, and hypovolemic shock, which are believed to be due to an alteration in capillary permeability. Myocarditis may occur.

The diagnosis is suggested in a patient with high fever, prostration, erosive or exudative pharyngitis, and severe myalgias, particularly lumbar, who has just returned from sylvan areas of West Africa. Definitive diagnosis can be made by isolation of the virus from blood or body fluids, including urine. However, great caution should be exercised in handling these patients and their fluids since the illness is highly contagious. Patients should be kept in strict isolation. Treatment is simply supportive and symptomatic. Immune plasma has been used in some severe cases, but the data are anecdotal.

Marburg and Ebola viruses. Marburg and Ebola viruses are African viruses first isolated in 1967 and 1976, respectively. They are very long, single-stranded RNA viruses present in central and south-central Africa. The initial isolation of the Marburg virus occurred in Germany, where it was traced to infected green monkeys imported from Uganda.[13] These monkeys also carry the HIV virus but do not seem to be clinically affected by it.

Transmission in all outbreaks has been from person to person. Both agents cause an acute hemorrhagic fever with a very high mortality rate. There have been several outbreaks of Marburg or Ebola disease. In every instance the index case was fatal, and person-to-person spread, often in a hospital setting, was the cause of dissemination to the community. How the disease spreads from monkeys to humans is uncertain but may relate to the use of monkeys as food or ritual use of their blood. The virus is found in the blood of infected monkeys and humans.

After an incubation period of 6 to 8 days, there is an abrupt onset of fever, rash, myalgias, nausea and vomiting, abdominal pain and diarrhea, often bloody. A severe hemorrhagic diathesis may develop and mortality rates are between 25% and 80% in both Marburg and Ebola virus disease. The management of such cases is simply supportive and even in a modern hospital setting is difficult.

The titer of Marburg virus in blood is highest just after the onset of symptoms and is found to be higher in whole blood than in serum, suggesting that the virus associates with cells.[19] Transmission by transfusion has not been reported and is probably extremely unlikely, given the short viremic period and the severity of the illnesses. Certainly it is not likely to occur outside of the endemic areas.

Management of Patients with Suspected Viral Hemorrhagic Fever

The CDC have recently released a supplement to the *Morbidity and Mortality Weekly Report*[20] with recommendations concerning patients with suspected viral hemorrhagic fever, specifically addressing Lassa, Marburg, Ebola, and Crimean-Congo hemorrhagic fevers. The other viral diseases noted above are less likely to be hemorrhagic and are generally less severe. A geographic or travel history is of utmost importance; specifically, if the patient has visited only urban areas, viral hemorrhagic fever is improbable. An interval of 3 weeks or more between exposure and the onset of symptoms excludes the diagnosis.

Initial symptoms, as we have seen, may be quite nonspecific and include fever, sore throat, headache, myalgia, abdominal pain, and diarrhea. Symptoms and signs more specific for viral hemorrhagic fever in general are pharyngitis and conjunctivitis, a skin rash (particularly Marburg and Ebola), and, later, hemorrhage and shock. Blood cultures and a smear for malaria should be obtained immediately from any suspect patient. If viral hemorrhagic fever is a likely diagnosis, the patient should be immediately isolated and the CDC and local health departments should be notified. Strict barrier techniques and body fluid precautions should be put in place. Specific diagnosis can only be established by viral cultures and should only be attempted in a biosafety level 4 facility, such as the CDC.

Therapy is largely supportive; ie, fluids, blood replacement, and airway maintenance. Heparin and steroids are not effective and probably are contraindicated. Patients with Lassa fever do respond to ribavirin, but this drug does not have in vitro effects against Marburg or Ebola viruses. It may be helpful for Crimean-Congo infection. Analogues of prostacyclin are being evaluated, and convalescent plasma may be therapeutic in all but Lassa fever, although there have not been useful clinical trials in this area.

Conclusion

Needle-stick transmission has occurred, either in the field or in the laboratory with all of these arboviruses discussed above. Thus, it is *possible* that transmission could occur by blood transfusion. The likelihood of this occurring in the United States is small. The likelihood of it occurring in a remote part of a developing country is also small, but probably greater. These viruses have a short incubation period with symptoms beginning at the time, or very shortly after, viremia occurs. Theoretically, a person could become infected, depart by jet 2 days later, and offer themselves for blood donation on day 4 or 5. Since blood bank standards include requisite delays for travelers from malaria-endemic countries (see Chapter 10), such a scenario is *extremely* unlikely, but should probably never be absolutely ruled out. More than one half of cases of transfusion-transmitted malaria reported in the United States from 1972 to 1981 resulted from failure of donors or blood banks to adhere to appropriate standards.

Transmission of Creutzfeldt-Jakob disease from tissue transplantation and by injection of processed human pituitary glands has been documented in humans and animals have been infected by inoculation with blood from infected humans. The virus, or prion, may not always be present in blood but is persistent in neural tissue. It is not known if the vertical spread of kuru was facilitated only by eating brain tissue of infected persons or if any tissue could be implicated. Given the long incubation period, the nature of the proposed infectious agent and our lack of knowledge about it, and the current regulatory climate in blood banking, the recent restrictions with regard to recipients of human pituitary-derived growth hormone are probably reasonable.

Parvovirus

The B19 parvovirus is neither "slow" nor "tropical," but is worth mentioning since it has been associated with aplastic crises in chronic hemolytic syndromes,[21,22] acute lymphocytic leukemia,[23] and hydrops fetalis,[24] occurs in patients with congenital or acquired immunodeficiency syndromes,[25] and is thought to be the cause of a case of red cell aplasia of 10 years' duration in one patient.[26] It is transmitted by blood component transfusion, including plasma and cryoprecipitate, and has also been identified in concentrates used to treat hemophilia and in hemophilic patients.[27] It is the cause of a common childhood exanthem called erythema infectiosum, or fifth disease.

The illness has been transmitted to health care workers by patients with sickle cell anemia who are having an acute attack of parvovirus infection[28] and it can cause erythroblastopenia in persons with iron deficiency and in others without underlying hemolysis.[29] Transient reticulocytopenia occurs in all those infected but actual anemia, severe enough to be recognized, is manifest only when the demand for red blood cell production is high (hemolysis) or another underlying condition (immunosuppression) precludes antibody formation and rapid clearing of the infection.

B19 parvovirus is a single-stranded DNA virus discovered in 1975 in the serum of normal blood donors.[30,31] Infected adults are more likely to present with a polyarthralgia syndrome than with a skin rash. The virus infects and is propagated within the marrow's erythroid progenitor compartment, resulting in the reticulocytopenia noted above. Neutropenia and thrombocytopenia may occur,[32] although in vitro myeloid suppression is much less marked than in erythroid cultures.

In most serosurveys, approximately 50% of adults show evidence of past infection. The incubation period may vary from 6 to 16 days. Illness begins with fever, malaise, and the development of an erythematous rash on the face and a reddish, reticulated rash on the trunk and extremities. The rash may recur for several weeks, although most patients appear otherwise healthy. A moderately severe, but relatively brief, polyarthropathy also may occur and in adults is very common, occurring in 100% of contacts in one nosocomial outbreak.[28] In healthy persons, neutralizing antibodies develop in about 1 week and the infection is fairly rapidly cleared. It is believed that in most healthy persons (not immunocompromised) the virus does not persist in the circulation. However, the fact that it has been identified in unpasteurized coagulation factor concentrates and was first isolated from the serum of asymptomatic blood donors suggests a chronic carrier state. Since as many as 20% of those infected in several studies remained asymptomatic, it seems more likely these individuals may be the source of spread by blood transfusion.

Recommendations with regard to blood transfusion seem fairly obvious. First, testing is available at only a few research sites and through the CDC, and the presence of antibody, as opposed to virus, is not indicative of infectivity. Second, at least half of the persons old enough to donate have been infected and have the antibody. Thus, widespread donor testing is clearly not indicated.

In patients with anemia and reticulocytopenia who are receiving immunosuppressive therapy, who have chronic hemolysis, or who have reduced immunocompetence for any of a variety of reasons (congenital or acquired immunodeficiency, lymphoproliferative disorders, cancer therapy) the illness should be suspected and arrangements made for appropriate testing. Since the disease is easily spread to health care workers and to other patients,[28] young patients with, for example, chronic hemolysis and an acute febrile illness, should probably be placed in contact isolation, as should immunocompromised patients with documented or suspected chronic B19 infection. Most patients with parvovirus infection, however, are past the period of infectivity and do not pose a risk to others. Isolation of most patients is not warranted.[25]

Treatment of most patients is unnecessary; however, in those with severe aplastic crisis or documented chronic infection, a course of intravenous immunoglobulin at a dosage of 400 mg/K for several days seems warranted, based on current information.[23,26]

References

1. Gajdusek DC: Unconventional viruses and the origin and disappearance of kuru. *Science* 197:943–960, 1977.

2. Duffy P, Wolf J, Collins G, et al: *N Engl J Med* 290:692–693, 1974.

3. Morbidity and Mortality Weekly Report, 4 February, 1987.

4. NIDDK Fact Sheet: *Human Growth Hormone and Creutzfeldt-Jakob Disease.* Bethesda, Md, National Institutes of Health, Publication No. 86–2793, May, 1986.

5. Houff SA, Major EO, Katz DA, et al: Involvement of JC virus-infected mononuclear cells from the bone marrow and spleen in the pathogenesis of progressive multifocal leukoencephalopathy. *N Engl J Med* 318:301–305, 1988.

6. Gardner SD, MacKenzie EFD, Smith C, Porter AA: Prospective study of the human polyoma viruses BK and JC and cytomegalovirus in renal transplant recipients. *J Clin Pathol* 37:578–586, 1984.

7. Greenlee JE: Slow Virus Infections, in Stein JH (ed): *Internal Medicine*. Boston, Little Brown & Co, 1983.

8. Prusiner SB: Prions and neurodegenerative diseases. *N Engl J Med* 317:1571–1581, 1987.

9. Prusiner SB: Novel proteinaceous infectious particles cause scrapie. *Science* 216:136–144, 1982.

10. Tateishi J: Transmission of Creutzfeldt-Jakob disease from human blood and urine into mice. *Lancet* 2:897–898, 1985.

11. Clawson GA: Antiheretical speculations on the prion protein and scrapie. *Persp Biol Med* 31:212–223, 1988.

12. Tabor E: *Infectious Complications of Blood Transfusion*. New York, Academic Press, 1982.

13. Warren KE, Mahmoud AAF: *Geographic Medicine for the Practitioner*. New York, Springer-Verlag, 1985.

14. Walsh, J: Rift Valley fever rears its head. *Science* 240:1397–1399, 1988.

15. Halstead SB: Pathogenesis of dengue: challenges to molecular biology. *Science* 239:476–480, 1988.

16. Dengue and dengue hemorrhagic fever in the Americas, 1986. *MMWR* 37:129–131, 1988.

17. Dengue in the Americas, 1985. *MMWR* 35:732–733, 1986.

18. International Notes: Lassa Fever–Sierra Leone. *MMWR* 21:386–387, 1972.

19. Wulff H, Slenczka W, Gear JHS. *Bull WHO* 56:633–639, 1978.

20. Management of patients with suspected viral hemorrhagic fever. *MMWR* 37 (suppl)3:1–13, 1988.

21. Pattison JR, Jones SE, Hodgson J, et al: Parvovirus infections and hypoplastic crises in sickle-cell anaemia. *Lancet* 1:664–665, 1981.

22. Young N: Hematologic and hematopoietic consequences of B19 parvovirus infection. *Semin Hematol* 25:159–172, 1988.

23. Kurtzman GJ, Cohen B, Myers P, et al: Persistent B19 parvovirus infection as a cause of severe chronic anemia in children with acute lymphocytic leukemia. *Lancet* 2:1159–1162, 1988.

24. Anderson LJ, Hurwitz ES: Human parvovirus B19 and pregnancy. *Clin Perinatol* 15:273–286, 1988.

25. Risks associated with human parvovirus B19 infection. *MMWR* 38:81–97, 1989.

26. Kurtzman G, Frickhofen N, Kimball J, et al: Pure red cell aplasia of ten years' duration due to persistent parvovirus B19 infection and its cure with immuno-globulin therapy. *N Engl J Med* 321:519–523, 1989.

27. Mortimer PP, Luban NLC, Kelleher JF, Cohen BJ: Transmission of serum parvovirus-like virus by clotting factor concentrates. *Lancet* 2:482–484, 1983.

28. LaFrere JJ, Burgeois H: Human parvovirus associated with erythroblastopenia in iron deficiency anemia. *J Clin Pathol* 39:1277–1278, 1986.

29. Van Horn DK, Mortimer PP, Young N, Hason GR: Human parvovirus-associated red cell aplasia in the absence of underlying hemolytic anemia. *Am J Pediatr Hematol Oncol* 8:235–239, 1986.

30. Cossart YE, Field AM, Cant B, Widdows D: Parvovirus-like particles in human sera. *Lancet* 1:72–73, 1975.

31. Bachman PA, Hoggan MD, Melnick JL, et al: Parvoviridae. *Intervirology* 5:83–92, 1975.

32. Kurtzman GJ, Ozawa K, Cohen B, et al: Chronic bone marrow failure due to persistent B19 parvovirus infection. *N Engl J Med* 317:287–294, 1987.

9
Transfusion-Transmitted Treponemal Infections

Asa Barnes, MD

All donors of blood must have a negative serologic test for syphilis (STS) because it is required by the FDA in the Code of Federal Regulations (No. 640.5a). This test is an ancient but recently controversial requirement.[1] The AABB also has required an STS on all blood donors in their *Standards for Blood Banks and Transfusion Services* beginning with the first edition, until publication of the ninth edition in 1978, when the requirement was discontinued. Recently, the Presidential Commission on the AIDS Epidemic issued recommendations. Recommendations No. 6-24 in Section IV, entitled "Safety of The Blood Supply and Donated Tissue," states that "surrogate tests, such as serology for syphilis, should be required" to be performed on all blood donors. Why is there such a variation of opinion about the need for, and utility of, the serologic test for syphilis?

Epidemiology

Before the era of antibiotics, syphilis occupied an exalted position among medical diseases. "To know syphilis is to know medicine," a quotation attributed to Osler, referred to the diversity of manifestations of the disease. Public Health and Syphilology was a recognized, board-certified medical specialty. In 1943 penicillin changed all that. Adequate treatment with penicillin of patients with early syphilis produces an absolute, or biologic, cure with complete healing of lesions and reversal of serologic test results and spinal fluid findings. Treated patients become entirely well, are not infectious, and do not develop any of the late manifestations of the disease.

Syphilis is usually transmitted by direct and intimate contact with moist infectious lesions of the skin and mucus membranes. Sexual contact is the commonest means of infection but transfer of the disease by kissing or biting may occur. Infection is transmitted to the fetus through the placenta. It also can be transmitted by inoculation of infected blood. Indirect transmission by contaminated objects is rare since *Treponema pallidum* quickly dies if allowed to dry.

Since the late 1950s syphilis has been considered an infectious disease that was brought under control. The availability of an effective antibiotic, an intensive national campaign, laws requiring premarital and prenatal screening, and mandatory reporting of all new cases to the local health department made such control possible. Until 1986, the national rate of infectious syphilis was low, holding steady at approximately ten cases per 100,000 population. Since that time the number of cases has increased geometrically. In 1987 the rate increased by 31%, to 14.7 cases per 100,000. Rates in California, New York, and Florida have consistently been higher than the national average, reaching 55.6 per 100,000 in Los Angeles County, a 60% increase.[2] One of the factors deemed responsible for the growing incidence of syphilis is the spreading use of drugs. Both men and women have admitted exchanging sexual favors for drugs. A random review of 50 syphilis patients from sexually transmitted diseases clinics showed that 16% of the cases were drug-related and 26% were prostitution-related. Some of the prostitution cases may also be drug-related, because men and women often turn to prostitution to support their drug habits. These findings may have implications in the spread of AIDS, because ulcerative lesions of the genitalia, like syphilis chancres, may promote transmission of HIV.[3]

Agents

T pallidum is a slender spirochete with regular, evenly spaced spirals. It varies in length from 5 to 20 μm. The organism does not stain well with ordinary dyes but can be demonstrated in fixed tissues by silver impregnation methods. For clinical purposes it can be demonstrated by dark-field microscopy of material from primary or secondary syphilitic lesions. When viewed with the dark-field microscope, *T pallidum* shows characteristic motility, rotating on its long axis and moving slowly backward and forward. The spirals usually keep their uniform size and shape, although the body of the organism may bend in the middle.

T pallidum does not survive in blood stored at 4 °C beyond 72 hours.[4] However, it can be frozen and remain viable for many years. Thus, red blood cells stored longer than 3 days cannot transmit syphilis, but conceivably it could be transmitted by platelets stored at room temperature or fresh-frozen plasma. When direct vein-to-vein transfusions were given, before the development of modern blood storage technology, transmission of syphilis by transfusion was a real danger. Hence, the requirement in the first AABB "Standards" mandating the STS. However, since that time only one possible instance of transfusion-induced syphilis has been recorded in the American medical literature.[5] The patient was a 28-year-old man with lymphoma who received 6 units of stored red blood cells and 25 units of platelet concentrate stored at room temperature. All of the platelet donors had a nonreactive Venereal Disease Research Laboratory (VDRL) test, and upon repeated testing, 22 of these donors had a nonreactive STS and three donors were unavailable for follow-up. Eight weeks after transfusion the patient developed the rash of secondary syphilis, which persisted for 6 weeks. The VDRL test became reactive at a dilution of 1:128, whereas it had been nonreactive before transfusion. The fluorescent treponemal antibody tests were also positive. The patient had received whole-body radiation therapy, so he was immunosuppressed.

Disease

T pallidum can penetrate small abrasions in the epithelium or normal mucosal membranes. In the primary stage, a lesion called a *chancre* appears at the portal of entry after an incubation period of 10 to 90 days (usually around 21 days). Initially this is a painless papule, surrounded by an inflammatory cuff, that breaks and forms an ulcer. The chancre may persist for 2 to 6 weeks and heals spontaneously. This sequence represents the primary stage of syphilis and is infectious. The STS is negative during this period. In the secondary stage, the infected individual may develop low-grade fever, headache, malaise, lymphadenopathy, and a generalized skin eruption that may be papular or maculopapular, but not vesicular. It often involves the palms, soles, and face in addition to the trunk and extremities. Also, the mucous membranes of the mouth and genitalia are commonly involved in secondary syphilis. Syphilid lesions of the mouth appear as painless, superficial erosions covered with a thin gray exudate known as *mucous patches*. They contain a large number of spirochetes but may be very inconspicuous. Syphilitic mucosal lesions of the genitalia or perianal regions may become hypertrophic and are called *condylomata lata*. The lesions of secondary syphilis are very infectious and spirochetemia occurs early. However, during this time the STS is sometimes negative. After 2 to 6 weeks the rash heals, symptoms disappear spontaneously, and the serologic test results become positive. Anytime thereafter the tertiary stage of syphilis may develop, taking one of three forms: neurosyphilis, cardiovascular syphilis, or a form that involves skin, bones, and viscera. Between healing of the secondary form of syphilis and development of the tertiary, a latent period may intervene when the infected individual is asymptomatic. Routine serologic testing is the only way to obtain a diagnosis in the majority of patients with latent syphilis.

Serologic Diagnosis

Serologic tests for the diagnosis of syphilis may be divided into nontreponemal, or cardiolipin, and treponemal tests. The first serologic test for syphilis used complement fixation methodology and human fetal liver from a case of congenital syphilis as a source of antigen because it was heavily infected with *T pallidum*. (To this day the organism has never been grown in artificial media.) Soon it was discovered that extracts of normal liver served equally well as antigen. Later the optimal antigen was found to be an alcoholic extract of beef heart combined with lecithin and cholesterol. This cardiolipin antigen is employed in current flocculation tests for syphilis, such as the VDRL and RPR (rapid plasma reagent). These nontreponemal tests have a high degree of sensitivity but are not specific for syphilis. Thus they are appropriate for screening large populations but require a specific treponemial test for confirmation. The most commonly used of these specific tests is the FTA-ABS (fluorescent treponemal antibody absorption), which measures antibodies that react with killed *T pallidum* after absorption with the patient's serum. When the screening tests are positive but the confirmatory test is negative, it is termed a biologic false-positive (BFP) reaction. Acute febrile illnesses and collagen-vascular diseases, such as systemic lupus erythematosus, commonly produce BFP reactions. In volunteer blood donors BFP reactions may account for 80% to 90% of positive nontreponemal tests.[6]

Another spirochetal disease, yaws, which is not transmitted by transfusion, may produce seropositivity with both nontreponemal and treponemal tests. Yaws is caused by *Treponema peretenue*, an organism closely related to *T pallidum*, but it is not a venereal disease. It occurs only in tropical, moist lowland countries, being epidemic in Samoa, Cambodia, and Vietnam.[7] Recent immigrants from these countries may have false-positive STS results on the basis of past yaws.

The Controversy

The presence of a negative cardiolipin reaction does not always exclude syphilis, nor is a positive reaction always proof of the existence of the disease.[8] The STS is negative in the incubation phase of syphilis and during much of the primary stage, even when spirochetemia is occurring. It is also negative during many of the late manifestations, such as cardiovascular symptoms and neurosyphilis. Conversely, most persons whose serum is STS-reactive do not have circulating spirochetes. Thus, *T pallidum* is more likely to be present in the blood during the seronegative phase of syphilis and absent during the seropositive phase. Obviously then, the routine STS does not insure protection against transfusion-transmitted syphilis. This is why the AABB in their ninth edition of *Standards for Blood Banks and Transfusion Services* (1978) dropped the requirement that an STS be performed on all blood donors. The FDA has not yet followed the AABB's example and changed their requirement as stated in the Code of Federal Regulations.

Recently the FDA received reinforcement of their requirement for performing an STS on all blood donors. The Presidential Commission on the Human Immunodeficiency Virus Epidemic made the following recommendation: "The Food and Drug Administration, in collaboration with the Blood Products Advisory Committee, should identify principles on which to base the introduction of new testing requirements and actively assess additional direct or surrogate tests in order to consider their introduction. Surrogate tests, such as serology for syphilis, should be required" (recommendation No. 6–24).

What timing! Just as the STS seemed to be breathing its last as a commonly performed blood donor screening procedure, the fear of transmission of another sexually transmitted disease, AIDS, restores an element of legitimacy and probably prolongs indefinitely the use of the STS as a test for screening blood donors.

Is the recommendation of the President's Commission justified? Utility as a surrogate test for AIDS should be based on frequent coexistence of a positive STS and infection with HIV. In a study of patients attending clinics for sexually transmitted diseases, a history of syphilis or a positive STS was significantly associated with HIV seropositivity in men.[9] But these clinic patients are a totally different population from volunteer blood donors, and the risk of transmitting HIV by transfusion of blood from donors who are seronegative for HIV antibody is minimal.[10,11] Also, the test for antibody to hepatitis B core antigen, which is now required as a surrogate test for non-A non-B hepatitis, was utilized as a surrogate test for HIV infection by several blood centers in areas where there was a high incidence of AIDS during the early days of the epidemic.[12] One direct test (HIV antibody) and one surrogate test (hepatitis B core antibody) would seem to provide sufficient protection against transmission of HIV. Finally, the population being tested must be considered to evaluate the utility of a surrogate test. When screening volunteer blood donors, as opposed to patients at a sexually transmitted disease clinic, the known high incidence of biologic false-positive reactions, which would also be false-positive for infection by HIV, would make the STS a dubious surrogate test to detect carriers of the AIDS virus.

References

1. International Forum: Does it make sense for blood transfusion services to continue the time-honored syphilis screening with cardiolipin antigen? *Vox Sang* 41:183–192, 1981.

2. Cohen DA: Shadow across Los Angeles: The county's syphilis epidemic. *LACMA Physician* 118:28–34, 1988.

3. Potterat JJ: Does syphilis facilitate sexual acquisition of HIV? *JAMA* 258:473–474, 1987.

4. Turner TB, Diseker TH: Duration of infectivity of *Treponema pallidum* in citrated blood stored under conditions obtaining in blood banks. *Bull Johns Hopkins Hosp* 68:269–279, 1941.

5. Chambers RW, Foley HT, Schmidt PJ: Transmission of syphilis by fresh blood components. *Transfusion* 9:32–34, 1969.

6. Barker LF: Viral hepatitis and other infections transmitted by transfusion, in Petz LD, Swisher SN (eds): *Clinical Practice of Blood Transfusion*. New York, Churchill Livingstone, 1981, pp 757–782.

7. Davis GE: Yaws and bejel, in Swartzwelder JC, Hunter GW, Frye WW (eds): *Manual of Tropical Medicine*. Philadelphia, WB Saunders, 1960, pp 119–126.

8. Walker RH: Bacteria and spirochetes, in Greenwalt TJ, Jamieson GA (eds): *Transmissable Disease and Blood Transfusion*. New York, Grune & Stratton, 1974, pp 221–240.

9. Quinn TC, Glasser D, Cannon RD, et al: Human immunodeficiency virus infection among patients attending clinics for sexually transmitted diseases. *N Engl J Med* 318:197–203, 1988.

10. Bove JR: Transfusion-associated hepatitis and AIDS: What is the risk? *N Engl J Med* 317:242–245, 1987.

11. Peterman TA, Lui K-J, Lawerence DN, Allen JR: Estimating the risks of transfusion-asssociated acquired immune deficiency syndrome and human immunodeficiency virus infection. *Transfusion* 27:371–374, 1987.

12. Perkins HA: Transfusion-associated AIDS. *Am J. Hematol* 19:307–313, 1985.

10
Transfusion-Transmitted Malarial Infections

Robert Westphal, MD

In medical school in the early 1960s, very little time was spent learning about malaria; it was a disease of the tropics, soon to be eradicated even in such places as Haiti, thanks to the widespread use of DDT. Seventeen years later, while working in Haiti, I saw my second and 20th cases of malaria on the same day in clinic. The first case, seen 2 years before going to Haiti, occurred in a man in the midwest who received approximately 20 units of blood for esophageal varices, splenectomy, and a splenorenal shunt. He died of blackwater fever.

From 1972 to 1981 there were 26 cases of transfusion-transmitted malaria reported to the CDC[1] and probably more that were not. In 1982, nine cases were reported to the CDC, the most since 1971.[2] Data compiled by Dr Bernard Nahlen of the CDC (now with the Los Angeles County Division of the California Health Department) (personal communication, Aug 22, 1988) included only an additional 11 cases of transfusion-transmitted malaria from 1983 to 1986.

From 1978 to 1982, 5,204 cases of malaria were imported into the United States, of which 26% occurred in US citizens, 33% occurred in refugees from Southeast Asia, and 41% occurred in other foreigners, primarily from India, Haiti, and Latin America.[3] In addition, an outbreak involving 26 cases of vivax malaria occurred in San Diego county, California, in 1986, that primarily was due to infection by local mosquitoes.[4] There has clearly been a worldwide resurgence of malaria, and a resurgence of basic research, including vaccine development, as a result of the failure of the eradication program begun by the WHO in the late 1950s.

Before World War II, approximately two thirds of the world's population was at risk of contracting malaria. The eradication program worked in most temperate climates, but by 1983 the potential for transmission appeared to have returned to near its original level, with approximately 300 million cases occurring annually and more than 1 million malaria-related deaths occurring annually in tropical Africa alone.[5] The eradication program has failed for a variety of complex reasons, including agricultural irrigation, large-scale population migrations, political upheaval, economic recession, resistance to DDT, and the development of many strains of *P falciparum* resistant to chloroquine and other antimalarial drugs. The situation in Europe is similar to that in the United States, with imported malaria becoming more common. There was even an outbreak in France and Switzerland in persons living near an international airport who became infected by mosquitoes imported on flights from Africa, thus making jet aircraft into a new type of "vector."

Life Cycle and Epidemiology

There are over 100 species of *plasmodia* that infect reptiles, birds and mammals, but only four of these, *Plasmodium falciparum*, *Plasmodium malariae*, *Plasmodium ovale*, and *Plasmodium vivax*, infect humans. They are transmitted by infected female *Anopheles* mosquitoes, which require a blood meal for maturation of their eggs. Humans are the primary, if not the sole, reservoir for such infections, although many monkey species are infected with *Plasmodium knowlesi*, a close relative of *P vivax*. In addition, some nonhuman primates are susceptible to *P falciparum*, and chimpanzees can be rendered so by splenectomy.

Plasmodia have a complex life cycle, consisting of a sexual stage occurring in the mosquito vector and an asexual stage, called schizogony, that occurs in humans. After feeding on an infected human, it takes about 2 weeks for the sporozoites to develop, which then may be inoculated into another human at a subsequent blood meal. These sporozoites circulate only briefly, 1 hour or less, before entering hepatic cells. This pre-erythrocytic phase lasts from 5 to 16 days, depending on the species of plasmodia. At this point the parasites, now called merozoites, rupture the hepatic cells, enter the circulation, penetrate circulating red blood cells and initiate the erythrocytic phase of infection.

It appears that there may be species-specific receptors that allow for attachment and penetration of the merozoites since En(a−) erythrocytes that lack glycophorin A are much more resistant to invasion by *P falciparum*[6] and glycophorin antibodies or high concentrations of glycophorin A added to cultures of En(a+) red blood cells have similar effects.[7] Similarly, the antigens of the Duffy group seem to confer a susceptibility to invasion by *P vivax*, explaining the natural resistance to vivax seen in Duffy-negative black populations. This has been experimentally confirmed with *P knowlesi* but not yet with *P vivax* since continuous in vitro cultivation of the latter organism has yet to be realized.[5]

Once inside a red blood cell, the parasites replicate asexually by a process called *schizogony*, using hemoglobin as a substrate for growth. Hemoglobin S is poorly metabolized by *P falciparum*, and parasite growth is also inhibited in cells with large amounts of hemoglobin F.[8] The assumption that G6PD deficiency and the various forms of thalassemia also confer some protection against malarial infection has not been borne out in the laboratory. As the merozoites mature into larger, more ameboid forms, they are called trophozoites. After 48 hours, red blood cells containing *P falciparum, P ovale*, and *P vivax* rupture, and red blood cells containing *P malariae* rupture after 72 hours, causing clinical symptoms and releasing schizonts that contain 16 to 32 merozoites that can then invade additional red blood cells. Some merozoites develop into male or female gametocytes after a few of these cycles, which can be taken up by the mosquito during the next meal. In the mosquito, the female gametocytes are fertilized, forming a zygote that replicates in cysts in the stomach wall of the insect. When these cysts eventually rupture, approximately 2 weeks later, sporozoites are released and migrate to the salivary glands of the now infective mosquito, thus completing the life cycle.

Merozoites from *P vivax* and *P ovale* may exist in the hepatic phase for long periods, causing both of these organisms to be associated with relapsing episodes of clinical illness. *P falciparum* and *P malariae* do not have a chronic exoerythrocytic phase; however, very low levels of parasitemia with *P malariae* may persist for years. In malaria induced by sharing of dirty needles or by transfusion, parasite-containing red blood cells enter the circulation directly, bypassing the hepatic stage. Because of this no relapses occur in transfusion-transmitted malaria.[9]

The malarial organisms have a world-wide distribution and are endemic in areas with *Anopheles* mosquitoes and a human reservoir. Malaria has essentially been eradicated from most of Europe, the United States, Australia, and Japan. It has not been naturally transmitted in climates such as exist in Canada, the Nordic countries, and the northern Soviet Union. Countries where some or all of the population is at risk are listed in Table 10–1.

The risk for developing malaria is shared by all ages, sexes and races, except as noted above. The risk is directly proportional to the density of the human reservoir, the density of the vector population, and the resulting amount of exposure. In general, even in endemic countries, there is little risk at altitudes above 1500 to 1800 m of elevation (5000 feet), and less in more temperate climates. Urban areas are generally safer than rural ones and the use of protective clothing and netting is helpful. Specific information on a country-by-country basis is available from the CDC.[10]

Chloroquine-resistant *P falciparum* malaria has been reported from many countries in the northern half of South America, some countries in central Africa, and most countries of Southeast Asia, the Indian subcontinent, and the island nations of the archipelago extending from the South China Sea across to the north of Australia.

Pathology of Malaria

For a complete discussion of the pathologic changes related to malarial infection, the reader is referred to other texts, such as *Manson's Tropical Dis-*

Table 10–1   Countries Reporting Malaria Transmission[10]

Afghanistan, Algeria, Angola, Argentina

Bangladesh, Belize, Bhutan, Benin, Botswana, Bolivia, Brazil, Burma, Burundi

Cameroon, Cape Verde, Central African Republic, Chad, China, Colombia, Comoros, Congo, Costa Rica, Cambodia (Kampuchea)

Djibouti, Dominican Republic

Ecuador, Egypt, El Salvador, Equatorial Guinea, Ethiopia

French Guiana

Gabon, Gambia, Ghana, Guatemala, Guinea, Guinea-Bissau, Guyana

Haiti, Honduras

India, Indonesia, Iran, Iraq, Ivory Coast

Kenya

Laos, Liberia, Libya

Madagascar, Malawi, Malaysia, Maldives, Mali, Mauritania, Mexico, Morocco, Mauritius, Mozambique

Namibia, Nepal, Nicaragua, Niger, Nigeria

Oman

Pakistan, Panama, Papua New Guinea, Paraguay, Peru, Phillipines

Ruanda

Sao Tome and Principe, Saudi Arabia, Senegal, Sierra Leone, Solomon Islands, Somalia, South Africa, Sri Lanka, Sudan, Surinam, Swaziland, Syria

Tanzania, Thailand, Togo, Tunisia, Turkey

Uganda, USSR, United Arab Emirates, Upper Volta

Vanuatu (New Hebrides), Venezuela, Viet Nam

Yemen, Democratic Yemen (North and South Yemen)

Zaire, Zambia, Zimbabwe

eases.[11] Invasion of red cells by parasites occurs in all four forms of malaria and immunopathologic mechanisms are responsible for some aspects of the anemia, bone marrow suppression, and, in *P malariae*, the nephrosis associated with malaria.

In nonfalciparum malaria, the infected red cells are sequestered and hemolyzed in the spleen and reticuloendothelial system. In falciparum malaria, with high rates of parasitemia, the red cells develop knoblike projections that make them less deformable and more adherent to the vascular endothelium. These knobs have been shown to react with antibodies raised to whole cultures of malarial organisms, suggesting that they contain fragments of malarial antigens. Such rigidity leads to vascular occlusion and tissue hypoxia, the principal pathologic lesion in falciparum malaria. Intravascular hemolysis occurs, leading to severe hemoglobinemia, hemoglobinuria, and renal failure (blackwater fever). In cerebral malaria, there is diffuse hypoperfusion of the brain with severe sludging and stasis seen in the cerebral vasculature. Disseminated intravascular coagulation may occur. In falciparum infestations hypoglycemia, lactic acidosis, and hyperkalemia may develop if hemolysis is severe. Hepatic dysfunction with elevations of bilirubin and liver enzyme levels occurs as a result of red cell stasis, not because of initial infection of the liver with the parasite.

Clinical Characteristics of the 4 Types of Malaria

Malaria may be associated with a number of nonspecific symptoms, such as cough, myalgias, abdominal pain, nausea, and vomiting. Since liver dysfunction is common the diagnosis may be confused with a variety of viral or bacterial infections, including hepatitis. Typically, a patient who becomes infected with malaria will describe a rigorous shaking chill, followed by high fever, headache, malaise, and myalgia. The patient's temperature may be as high as 40 to 41 °C. The chill, or cold stage, may last for 15 to 60 minutes, followed by the hot stage, which lasts for 2 to 6 hours. This is followed by a drenching sweat and defervescence lasting 2 to 4 hours, after which the patient often falls asleep and awakens feeling tired but well.

During early stages of the infection a milder fever may occur daily; however, within 2 weeks the typical pattern develops of alternate day chills and fever (tertian malaria) or symptoms occurring every third day (quartan malaria), the latter seen only with *P malariae* infection. In addition to the fever, there may be enlargement of the spleen over a few weeks, particularly in vivax and ovale malaria. In those patients who are partially immune, the signs and symptoms may be blunted and splenomegaly is almost always found. In *P falciparum* infection the pulse is often quite slow in the presence of fever, but rises during a rigor.

P falciparum Infection

A very high degree of parasitism characterizes falciparum infection, making it the most dangerous of the malarial infections. In the nonimmune patient a primary attack may rapidly become fatal, but in the immune resident of an endemic area reinfection may not be accompanied by any symptoms. In the absence of new infections, falciparum dies out in the host after approximately 2 years, since there is no exoerythrocytic phase after the first infestation. Although the fever tends to be tertian, the parasite broods do not become as synchronized as in other forms of malaria, so that the fever is not always regular. The spleen does not always enlarge, although the liver usually does, so the absence of splenomegaly should not be used to rule out the diagnosis, especially in a newly suspected case.

Anemia is due to intravascular and extravascular hemolysis and may become severe by the fifth or sixth day. In addition, as with other forms of malaria, there is suppression of myelopoiesis aggravating the anemia and also causing leukopenia. Thrombocytopenia, which may be profound in the presence of disseminated intravascular coagulation, is due primarily to a shortened platelet lifespan. Malarial organisms do not usually cause eosinophilia, though it may be present for other reasons. A moderate monocytosis is common. In tropical countries a left-shifted mild neutrophilia may be observed, but moderate neutropenia is more common.

In falciparum infection there is usually parasitization of more than 2% to 3% of the red cells, often as high as 10% to 30% or more, and there may be more than one parasite in a cell. Falciparum is almost always seen as small ring forms; in cases where there is absolutely overwhelming infection with falciparum, schizonts may be seen in the peripheral blood. This is called algid malaria. There is circulatory collapse and shock; the patient is cold and clammy, the pulse is rapid and weak, the blood pressure is low, and the temperature is subnormal. Death is usually imminent.

Severe falciparum infection can lead to cerebral malaria, the hepatorenal syndrome, disseminated intravascular coagulation, pulmonary edema, and a profuse, watery diarrhea with cramps and dehydration. This severe diarrhea is called the *choleraic* form of malaria. The dark brown urine of blackwater fever is due to the oxidation of hemoglobin during intravascular hemolysis to methemoglobin and methemalbumin, both of which are brown or black in acidic urine.

P vivax Infection

Malaria caused by *P vivax* is often called *benign tertian malaria*, to differentiate it from the "malignant" tertian malaria of *P falciparum*. If untreated, it becomes a chronic, relapsing infection, which gives it, along with *P ovale*, its other name of relapsing malaria. There are different strains of the parasite but not much variety in the severity of the infection, which is not fatal. Unlike *P falciparum* and *P malariae* infections, there is not much of an immune antibody response.

The initial symptoms are somewhat nondescript, and include headache, myalgia and arthralgia, nausea, and general malaise. The fever is somewhat irregular for a few days before becoming intermittent. Symptoms tend to occur in the afternoon and occasionally on a daily basis if a concomitant infection with *P falciparum* has occurred. There may be mild cerebral symptoms, such as drowsiness or giddiness, but serious cerebral malaria or other severe complications such as described above for falciparum infection do not occur. Splenic enlargement is quite common and characteristic, again in contrast to falciparum, and, much as in infectious mononucleosis, the spleen is more vulnerable to traumatic rupture. The hemolysis is primarily extravascular and jaundice and hepatomegaly are unlikely.

P vivax seems to have a predilection for reticulocytes and cannot penetrate older red cells, making one wonder if the loss or development of some specific antigen on the red cell membrane is responsible for this specificity. Because of this, the rate of parasitization is low, rarely more than 1%. Ring forms, trophozoites, and schizonts are all commonly seen by the time tertian periodicity is established, differentiating it again from falciparum, which has mostly only ring forms and a higher percentage of affected red cells. In vivax infection, the red cells that are infected tend to appear larger, perhaps because they are younger. Gametocytes may be seen in the peripheral blood a week after the primary attack and there is often stippling of the affected red cells.

Because vivax merozoites do reinvade the liver, an untreated attack can be followed by relapses up to 2 or 3 years later. A single untreated attack lasts approximately 1 week, and in approximately two thirds of the cases relapse occurs. The relapse pattern varies between the three known strains of vivax and also varies geographically in that tropical strains have more frequent relapses and a shorter latency period.

P ovale Infection

Infection with *P ovale* resembles that of *P vivax* very closely, except that relapse is less frequent and spontaneous recovery within a few weeks to months is usual. The ovale parasites tend to cause the formation of ovalocytes in the cells they infect, thus the appellation.

P malariae Infection

P malariae causes *quartan malaria*, so named because of the periodicity of 72 hours associated with the attacks of fever. Infection is mild and the parasitization rate is less than 1%. There is no exoerythrocytic stage, but chronic low levels of parasitemia may persist without symptoms for years, leading to apparent relapses as many as 50 years later.[11]

The primary attack resembles that of *P vivax*, but the rigors may be more severe. Splenomegaly is a common feature, but hepatomegaly and jaundice seldom occur. The anemia is less severe than in vivax or other forms of malaria. Although perhaps the most benign of these three forms of "benign" malaria, it has the propensity for persistence noted above with recurrent attacks of malaise, fever, headaches, and sweats. In chronically infected persons, a nephrotic syndrome probably due to circulating immune complexes may develop.

In *P malariae* infections, the red cells are not smaller, as is often seen in falciparum infection, ovoid, as in ovale infections, nor larger than uninfected cells, as in vivax infections. Ring forms (merozoites), trophozoites (slightly ameboid forms), and schizonts are present in the peripheral blood smear.

The principal distinction among the four types of infection is that "malignant" malaria, infection with *P falciparum*, is different from the other three types as manifested by a greater than 1% parasitization rate of red cells, usually on the order of 10% or more when developed, and the presence of primarily ring forms (merozoites, some trophoizoites) that often occur at a rate of more than one per parasitized red cell. The presence of schizonts or gametocytes is common in the "benign" forms of malaria but is seen only in severely ill patients with *P falciparum* infection. Preparation of thick-film blood smears allows more rapid identification of the illness in question as malaria; however, careful examination of thin films is required to arrive at a reasonable suspicion of the implicated species. Table 10–2 provides a summary of the clinical and

Table 10–2   Differential Diagnosis of Human Malarial Infection

	Plasmodium falciparum	*Plasmodium vivax*	*Plasmodium ovale*	*Plasmodium malariae*
Splenomegaly	Unlikely	Common	Common	Common
Jaundice	Common	Uncommon	Uncommon	Uncommon
Anemia	May be severe	Mild-Moderate	Mild-Moderate	Mild
Exoerythrocytic phase	No	Yes	Yes	No
Relapses	No	Yes	Yes	Yes
Immunity	Slight	Yes	Yes	Yes
Parasitemia	High	1% or less	1% or less	1%
Morphology	Ring forms	Ring forms	Ring forms	Ring forms
	Often 1/RBC	Trophozoites	Trophozoites	Trophozoites
	Rarely other forms	Schizonts	Schizonts	Schizonts
Infected RBCs	Small	Large	Ovalocytes	"Normal"
Incubation time	8-20 days	12-15 days	16-18 days	22-24 days

microscopic differentiation between the various species of human malarial infections.

Transfusion-Transmitted Malarial Infection

Imported malaria will continue to be a problem in the United States and other countries with a temperate climate but little or no reservoir of infection. Reduced travel times mean that the incubation period may not even be complete by the time an infected traveler returns home (Table 10–2). Immunity and prophylactic drugs lengthen this time, or may even submerge overt infection, thus allowing unsuspecting persons to be basically free of symptoms even though infected. This poses obvious problems for transfusion services and led to the adoption of revised standards by the AABB in 1981, which currently state that: 1. travelers may donate blood 6 months after returning from endemic areas if they have been free of symptoms and have not taken antimalarial drugs; 2. persons who have had malaria or who had been taking chemoprophylaxis shall be deferred from donating blood for 3 years after either becoming asymptomatic or stopping therapy or chemoprophylaxis.

Because partially suppressed malaria may present no symptoms, or none specific enough to suggest the diagnosis, transfusion-transmitted cases will continue to occur. Many travelers forget to continue their chemoprophylaxis for the recommended 6 weeks after returning from an endemic area. In 1983, Guerrero and colleagues[1] estimated that 0.25 cases of transfusion malaria would occur for every 1 million units of blood collected. This was based on their review of the reported 26 cases from 1972 to 1981 and is undoubtedly a low estimate. They suggested that donor guidelines be amended to include the country of birth of blood donors with subsequent verbal questioning to ascertain the last visit to an endemic area and that anyone with an unexplained febrile illness occurring within 1 year of travel to an endemic area be deferred and investigated.

Although cell-free blood components are believed to be exempt from transmission of malaria, transmission has been reported from cryoprecipitate as well as from red cells, platelet, and leukocyte concentrates.[12] Plasmodia even survive for years in frozen red cells, although it seems unlikely that the thawing and washing of such units would permit survival of such infected red blood cells, as was reported in a case in Nashville in 1976.[13]

In 1982 the CDC reviewed the indications for which serologic testing for malaria is indicated. Because an indirect fluorescent antibody response is usually associated with current or prior malarial infection, serologic testing may be a useful adjunct in identifying donors potentially responsible for transfusion-transmitted malaria. The CDC review noted that the diagnosis is best made by thorough and proper preparation and examination of blood smears, but that indirect fluorescent antibody testing may be useful in identifying a donor in a transfusion-related case or to assist in diagnosis of a clinically suspected case in a patient with persistently negative blood smears, two cases of which occurred in 1982.[14]

Whether or not current donor screening criteria should be augmented or changed is problematical. Standards must strike a reasonable balance between the need to prevent disease transmission, the need to maintain adequate numbers of donors, and the costs of additional screening or testing. The current standards work well, although not perfectly. In fact, approximately one half the cases in the 1972 to 1981 study occurred because either the blood bank or the donor did not adhere to the proper standards.[1] Transmission of malaria by transfusion will continue to occur, for a variety of reasons. Physicians need to be educated to consider the diagnosis in patients with fever who have recently received a transfusion.

Transfusion-transmitted malaria can be lethal, particularly falciparum malaria, which may also be confused with babesia infection on the peripheral smear. In the case noted in the introduction, the splenectomized patient was suspected of having babesiosis *or* malaria initially and died of severe intravascular hemolysis and acute renal failure within 24 hours of the diagnosis being established. Other severe cases have been successfully treated with chemotherapy and a massive exchange transfusion, either manual[15,16] or automated.[17]

Chloroquine and quinine remain mainstays of chemotherapy for malaria, but the emergence of chloroquine-resistant strains of *P falciparum* complicates the problem. The other strains of malaria have remained sensitive to chloroquine. Prophylaxis with Fansidar™ (Hoffman-La Roche), a combination of sulfadoxine and pyrimethamine, has been recommended for travelers to areas of chloroquine-resistant malaria and the drug has been useful in the treatment of *P falciparum* infection. However, adverse reactions, particularly the occurrence of a severe form of the Stevens-Johnson syndrome, have led to changes in the CDC's recommendations for travelers to such areas. Ineffectiveness of Fansidar™ has been identified as well in a few scattered regions such as the Thai-Kampuchean border, Papua New Guinea, and parts of Brazil.[5] Travelers and their physicians should refer to the most recent CDC recommendations for advice about chemoprophylaxis.[18] An excellent review of malarial prophylaxis and advice on immunizations and specific health information for international travelers has been published by the *Annals of Internal Medicine.*[19]

Specific details on the chemotherapeutic treatment of malaria are similarly complicated by the problem of drug resistance in *P falciparum*. Few alternative drugs are available and various combinations of quinine, tetracyclines, sulfonamides, and folate antagonists have been used with some success. A new drug, mefloquine, appears promising for the treatment of chloroquine-resistant strains of falciparum, and the active ingredient of an ancient Chinese herbal medicine used to treat malaria, qinghaosu, has also been shown to have some unique properties.[5] If a chloroquine-resistant strain of *P falciparum* is suspected, therapy with mefloquine should be instituted and the Malaria Branch of the CDC should be contacted at once.

Immunity and Vaccination

Given the immense morbidity and mortality associated with malaria, one would think it would be a prime target for the development of a vaccine.

Malaria is far and away the biggest public health scourge in the world. Not only is malaria itself a big problem, but the anemia that it causes, particularly among African children, leads to blood transfusion, which is one of the major factors in the exposure of children in Kinshasa, Zaire, to HIV infection.[20] Estimates are that up to 1 billion potential recipients for a malarial vaccine would exist in the few years following its introduction,[21] but who in the third world will be able to afford it? The cost of recombinant vaccine for hepatitis B approaches $150 per person, for example, about one half the annual per capita income of a native Haitian.

Though the market is huge, it will take more than the usual market relationships to deliver an effective vaccine. It is quite clear that the only hope for gaining any semblance of control over this major health problem of the world lies in the appropriate application of vaccination for prevention. The project deserves a major effort, and major expenditures on the part of the developed countries for the ultimate benefit of not just the underdeveloped, emerging countries, but for mankind.

Infection with malarial parasites does provoke an immune response in humans, as well as in animals, but it does not always have a protective effect, especially in falciparum malaria. Protective immunity to *P falciparum* develops slowly, is often only partial, and may be rapidly lost. Resistance to malarial rechallenge can be transferred by immunoglobulin infusion, particularly with vivax, and appears to be due to the infused IgG fraction.[5] Antibody can agglutinate merozoites in vitro and block their entrance into red cells, but the presence of such in vitro activity does not always predict similar effects in vivo. It has also been noted that in residents of endemic areas protective immunity develops slowly, confirming clinically the experimental observations that infection with malaria tends to be immunosuppressive. These and other factors have posed significant obstacles to vaccine development.

In malarial infection the spleen becomes enlarged in 70% to 80% of patients,[8] with marked proliferation of splenic macrophages. These macrophages ingest normal as well as infected red cells during a malarial attack, and in many studies complement (C3D) can be found on normal as well as infected red cells, producing a positive Coombs test. Specific red cell antibodies are lacking, however, suggesting that circulating immune complexes are involved in the anemia and thrombocytopenia of malarial infection, and perhaps in the glomerular lesion seen in *P malariae* infection. High levels of circulating immune complexes are indeed found in humans suffering from malarial infection, but their specific role in the pathophysiology of the illness has not been fully elaborated.

Some patients living in endemic areas develop massive, persistent splenomegaly with high levels (polyclonal) of IgM, increased levels of malarial antibody, and loss of these signs following prolonged malarial prophylaxis. This tropical splenomegaly syndrome has been identified in approximately one third of adult patients with splenomegaly in parts of Africa.[8] The IgM levels in patients with tropical splenomegaly syndrome are as much as ten times normal, but only a small portion of the IgM reacts with malarial antigens, the remainder reflecting a broad repertoire of B-cell activity, including heterophile antibodies and autoantibodies. High levels of cryoglobulins and circulating immune complexes also occur in tropical splenomegaly syndrome.

In the 1940s, the principal that malaria could be prevented by vaccination was established in animals.[22] The difficulties of human vaccine development have been well stated by Wyler[5]: "The challenges are formidable and include the isolation, purification and mass production of defined parasite antigens; the development of safe adjuvants; the selection of appropriate populations to be vaccinated; the monitoring of the efficacy and duration of protection; and the establishment of an appropriate health care infrastructure to carry out a mass vaccination campaign."

Despite many setbacks, much work continues toward the development of a vaccine, with the main focus on falciparum, since it is lethal and has developed resistance to drug therapy. There have been successful vaccines against falciparum in owl monkeys, but the vaccine required the use of an adjuvant unsuitable for use in humans.[23] Three basic types of vaccine have been under development: sporozoite vaccines, to block hepatic invasion; merozoite vaccines, to block red cell invasion; and transmission-blocking vaccines to prevent fertilization of female gametes of the parasite in the mosquito gut, or to somehow interfere with the growth of the oocyst if fertilization takes place.[24]

Work on the sporozoite vaccine has progressed to the point of field trials. Sporozoite vaccines utilize circumsporozoite proteins, which are found on the surface of the sporozoites located in the salivary glands of the mosquito. These circumsporozoite proteins are structurally important and contribute significantly to the antigenicity of the organism. On contact with specific circumsporozoite antibodies, sporozoites shed these circumsporozoite proteins. Circumsporozoite proteins of all malarial parasites have some similar antigenic properties[24] and their structure has been clarified by the cloning of circumsporozoite genes. The circumsporozoite protein for *P falciparum* has a large central domain of 412 amino acids, which constitute almost one half of the polypeptide chain. These protein segments are composed of 37 tetrapeptides with the sequence asparagine–aspartic acid–asparagine-proline interspersed with four tetrapeptides with a slightly modified sequence that includes valine. This repeating sequence is found in all strains of falciparum investigated and the monoclonal antibody that binds it neutralizes infectivity. Mice and rabbits produce high antibody titers when immunized with a recombinant-DNA–produced synthetic peptide coupled with tetanus toxoid as a carrier and adsorbed onto aluminum hydroxide. This work has been ongoing at New York University.[25]

A second circumsporozoite vaccine has been developed by workers at the Walter Reed Army and US Navy Medical Research Institutes and at the NIH. The vaccine is based on a recombinant *P falciparum* circumsporozoite protein expressed in *E coli*. The initial results of trials in 15 humans were presented at a conference convened by the US Agency for International Development in December 1986 (which has been a prime sponsor of malaria vaccine research). Fairly low antibody titers developed in the volunteers, lower than those in immune patients in endemic areas, but there were no significant side effects.[24] Meanwhile, studies have also been underway at the University of Maryland using the vaccine developed at New York University, and the US Agency for International Development had been laying the groundwork for phase III trials to be done in the field in Asia, Africa, and Latin America in 1987.[25] In July 1988, it was reported in *Science*[26] that trials with both vaccines in 1987 were disappointing. Only about one in three subjects developed immunity, which was of short duration, suggesting that more work on fundamentals must precede further development efforts.

Despite all this activity, literally years of fieldwork will be necessary to bring these projects to fruition. In the meantime, malaria must still be considered a potentially lethal, transfusion-transmitted infectious disease. Appropriate precautions must be taken to prevent it and to teach our colleagues to consider it as a real problem, especially as US demographic characteristics change.

Unlike in the United States, in countries where malaria is endemic it is not possible to accept as donors only those persons who have not had malaria or in whom 3 years have elapsed since antimalarial therapy or prophylaxis has been taken. A recent report from India,[27] in which a monoclonal antibody against malarial antigens was used to determine infectivity, found that donors who tested positive and were treated with chloroquine and primaquine could safely donate 3 months after therapy when the malarial antigens could no longer be detected in the blood. When this antibody becomes more available, and less costly, further studies along such lines might demonstrate an effective strategy to reduce transfusion-transmitted malarial infections in endemic areas of the world.

References

1. Guerrero IC, Weniger BC, Schultz MG: Transfusion malaria in the United States, 1972–1981. *Ann Intern Med* 99:221–226, 1983.

2. Transfusion Malaria: Serologic identification of infected donors—Pennsylvania, Georgia. *MMWR* 32:222–229, 1983

3. Lobel HO, Campbell CC: Trends in imported malaria, United States. *MMWR* 32(suppl):15–18ss, 1983.

4. *Plasmodium Vivax* Malaria—San Diego County, California, 1986 *MMWR* 35:679–681, 1986.

5. Wyler DJ: Malaria: Resurgence, resistance and research. *N Engl J Med* 308:875–878, 934–940, 1983.

6. Miller LH, Haynes JD, McAuliffe FM, et al: Evidence for differences in erythrocyte surface receptors for the malarial parasites *P falciparum* and *P knowlesi. J Exp Med* 146:277–281, 1977.

7. Perkins M: Inhibitory effects of erythrocyte membrane proteins on the in vitro invasion of the human malarial parasite (*P falciparum*) into its host cell. *J Cell Biol* 90:563–567, 1981.

8. Perrin LH, Mackey LJ, Miescher PA: The hematology of malaria in man. *Semin Hematol* 19:70–82, 1982

9. Warren KS, Mahmoud AAF: *Geographic Medicine for the Practitioner*. New York, Springer-Verlag, 1985, p 87.

10. Health Information for International Travel, 1984. Atlanta, Centers for Disease Control, HHS Publication No. (CDC) 84–8280.

11. Manson-Bahr PEC, Bell DR: *Manson's Tropical Diseases*, ed 19. Philadelphia, Balliere Tindall, 1987.

12. Wells L, Ala FA: Malaria and blood transfusion. *Lancet* 1:1317–1318, 1985.

13. Najem GR, Sulzer AJ: Transfusion-induced malaria from an asymptomatic carrier. *Transfusion* 16:473–476, 1976.

14. Transfusion Malaria: Serologic Identification of Infected Donors—Pennsylvania, Georgia. *MMWR* 32:222–229, 1983.

15. Yarrish RL, Janos JS, Nosanchuk JL, et al: Transfusion malaria: Treatment with exchange transfusion after delayed diagnosis. *Arch Intern Med* 142:187–188, 1982.

16. Kramer SL, Campbell CC, Moncrieff RE: Fulminant *Plasmodium falciparum* infection treated with exchange blood transfusion. *JAMA* 249:244–245, 1983.

17. Files JC, Case CJ, Morrison FS: Automated erythrocyte exchange in fulminant falciparum malaria. *Ann Intern Med* 100:396–397, 1984.

18. Recommendation for the Prevention of Malaria Among Travelers. *MMWR* 39:1–10, No. RR-3.

19. Hill DR, Pearson RD: Health advice for international travel. *Ann Intern Med* 108:839–852, 1988.

20. Greenberg AE, Nguyen-Dinh P, Mann JM, et al: The associations between malaria, blood transfusion and HIV seropositivity in a pediatric population in Kinshasa, Zaire. *JAMA* 259:545–549, 1988.

21. Graff, G: A Billion Potential Customers At Risk for Malaria. *New York Times*. May 15, 1988:15.

22. Freund J, Thomson KJ, Sommer HE, et al: Immunization of monkeys against malaria by means of killed parasites with adjuvants. *Am J Trop Med* 28:1–22, 1948.

23. Mitchell GH, Richards WHG, Butcher GA, Cohen S: Merozoite vaccination of douroucouli monkeys against falciparum malaria. *Lancet* 1:335–338, 1977.

24. Bruce-Chwatt LJ: The challenge of malaria vaccine: Trials and tribulations. *Lancet* 1:371–372, 1987.

25. Walsh J: Human trials begin for malaria vaccine. *Science* 235:1319–1320, 1987.

26. Marshall E: Crisis in AID malaria network. *Science* 241:521–523, 1988.

27. Choudhury N, Jolly JG, Mahajan RC, et al: Selection of blood donors in malaria-endemic countries. *Lancet* 2:972, 1988.

11
Other Parasitic Organisms Transmitted by Transfusion

Robert Westphal, MD

There are four classes of nonmalarial parasites that infect man and that can be transmitted by blood transfusion. Diseases in the group that causes filariasis are rarely transmitted this way, at least in North America. The transmission of babesiosis is uncommon but has occurred in Europe and North America. Toxoplasmosis, because it is so often a mild or unrecognized illness, is not widely reported but probably occurs much more frequently than we recognize and may become of greater importance as more immunocompromised recipients patients receive transfusions. The fourth parasite to be discussed causes American trypanosomiasis, or Chagas' disease, named for the Brazilian physician, Dr Carlos Chagas, who described it in 1909. Chagas' disease has assumed major importance in blood transfusion in parts of South and Central America and may become more important in North America, given the current changes in the US population.

Chagas' Disease

Chagas' disease, or *Trypanosomiasis cruzi*, occurs only in the Western hemisphere and should not be confused with the two African forms of trypanosomiasis, one of which causes "sleeping sickness." It is prevalent in Brazil, Argentina, Uruguay, Paraguay, Peru, Bolivia, Chile, and Venezuela and has also been found in Colombia, Costa Rica, Ecuador, El Salvador, Guatemala, Honduras, and Mexico.[1] Table 11–1, adapted from several tables in Schmunis'[1] article, provides information on seropositivity in blood donors from some of the areas mentioned. Note that a seroprevalence of 63% was found in Santa Cruz, Bolivia.

Jesus Linares, MD, director of the municipal blood bank of Caracas, Venezuela, estimates that approximately 90 million people are at risk, 16 to

Table 11–1   Prevalence of *T. cruzi* Seropositivity in Selected Donor Populations*

Location	Number of samples	Percent positive
Metropolitan Santiago	311	7.3
Buenos Aires (suburbs)	97,308	6.05
Catamarca province, Argentina	156	17.0
Brasilia	2,413	14.6
Rio de Janeiro	1,191	1.8
Santa Cruz, Bolivia	268	63.0
San Jose, Costa Rica	221	7.6
San Salvador	537	8.7
Guatemala	1,132	7.8
Caracas	98,620	5.1

*Adapted from a series of tables in Schmunis.[1]

18 million are infected, and there is an annual incidence of infection of about 200,000 persons. Trypanosomiasis is a disease of the countryside, but the vast destruction of forested lands in Latin American and other economic pressures are driving hundreds of thousands of rural people into the urban areas of their own or other countries. In search of work and money, many of these people sell their blood in order to feed themselves or their families. Another colleague from Brazil (Augusto Gonzaga, MD, Personal Communication, 1987) has reported he is seeing more cases of transfusion-transmitted trypanosomiasis. There have been reports of Chagas' disease in Latin American immigrants to the United States,[3] and the third reported case of indigenous (to the United States) Chagas' disease occurred in California in 1984.[4] The first two indigenous cases were found in 1955 in two infants from Texas.[5]

Although humans serve as a reservoir for *T cruzi* in some locales, the parasite can be found in many kinds of wild and domestic animals. The most important reservoirs in the United States are opossums and raccoons, with infection rates of 17% and 2%, respectively.[6] It is transmitted to humans from infected animals (or humans) by a variety of bedbugs called reduvids, including species such as *Triatoma* and *Rhodnius*. These bloodsucking insects deposit their contaminated feces as they feed. The organism can penetrate unbroken skin but most commonly it is inoculated when the bite is scratched. It can also be transmitted by a needle stick. The bedbugs are associated with poverty conditions, particularly rural poverty, favoring cracked or decaying wood or adobe housing. Crowded homes, often with many domestic animals sharing the living space, are common in much of Latin America and the bedbugs are not particular about what they feed on. Tabor[7] reports that analysis of reduvid stomach contents has shown evidence of blood from humans, dogs, cats, mice, rats, chickens, cows, toads, opossums, snakes, and rabbits.

T cruzi is a 15- to 20-μm protozoa propelled by a flagellum. Human infection has an acute parasitemic phase, during which the organism may be seen in peripheral blood smears, that lasts for a few weeks, and a chronic phase that is lifelong. An inflammatory lesion appears at the site of insect inoculation (chagoma), but these lesions may not be noted in some environments. The organism may fall directly in bedbug feces onto mucous membranes. The classic Romaña sign, unilateral conjunctivitis and periorbital edema, is not always seen, but it lasts for weeks, differentiating it from other allergic responses to insect bites. After a 10- to 14-day incubation period the patient manifests fever, lymphadenopathy, and hepatosplenomegaly. In endemic areas this illness in younger children may pass undetected. A tachycardia reflects early cardiac involvement, and the presence of arrhythmia, cardiomegaly, or congestive failure are bad prognostic signs. Infections in young children may carry a mortality rate of 10%[7] in some areas. Older patients are more likely to develop a chronic illness with no obvious signs of infection, and two thirds of infected persons have no initial symptoms.

The parasite has a predilection for myocardial cells and for smooth muscle cells of the esophagus and colon. An intense inflammatory reaction occurs, with eventual damage to the muscle tissue itself, leading to cardiomyopathy or to the "megasyndromes" of the colon, esophagus, or, rarely, stomach, gallbladder, or urinary bladder, as a result of the degeneration of autonomic ganglia in those smooth muscles. This classic form of Chagas' disease usually occurs decades after infection; however, exceptions are well documented, particularly of cardiac disease occurring in the subacute phase.[8]

There are three ways to establish the diagnosis: by seeing the parasite in blood films or stained serum samples during the acute phase of the "mononucleosis-like" syndrome, by xenodiagnosis (feeding uninfected triatomids on the patient and examining their stools 25 to 33 days later), or by a variety of serologic tests. The first two tests are useful only about 50% of the time. Serologic study is the usual method of diagnosis, even in endemic areas. Although indirect hemagglutination, immunofluorescence, and an ELISA test are available, a complement fixation test using *T cruzi* antigens is most commonly used, according to Strickland.[8] Schmunis,[1] however, states that the indirect hemagglutination assay and the indirect immunofluorescent test are the most widely used and available methods. Seropositivity varies with the method, but the test is almost always positive a few months after infection. Some patients with leishmaniasis may have false-positive reactions; however, a positive serologic test typically implies active, ongoing infection since there are no curative drugs that can be employed once the parasites are embedded in the target tissues.

In the acute phase, nifurtimox or benzonidazol may abolish the parasitemia and effect a cure in more than 50% of the patients, but these drugs do not always eradicate the disease. They are of no value in the chronic phase of the illness.[8] Symptomatic treatment of the cardiac disease or surgical removal of dilated esophagus or colon are effective but not curative. Heart failure appears between 20 and 50 years of age and, once it is established, the patient may live only a few more months to years. Control of the vector reduvid bugs is the best means of prevention, but is difficult in remote areas.

It is certain that infection with *T cruzi* can occur through the transfusion of blood from an infected individual. Given the data on seroprevalence in Table 11–1, it is also certain that this is a major public health problem in some parts of the Western Hemisphere. Blood transfusion is the second most important mechanism of transmission of *T cruzi*. Risks of becoming infected after receiving blood or plasma from a seropositive donor vary from 12% to 50%.[1] Hemophiliacs, being at the high end of the recipient scale, are at the greatest risk in developing countries, where they are likely to be treated with whole blood, depending of course on the seropositivity status of the particular blood supply they are dependent on.

To prevent transmission by transfusion, blood donors with a positive serologic test should be permanently deferred and, in endemic areas or countries with a high seroprevalence, such testing often is, or should be, mandatory. Similarly, even in nonendemic countries those donors who come from endemic parts of the hemisphere should probably be tested. The parasites survive for at least 10 days in refrigerated, citrated blood and have been recovered from frozen plasma.

Gentian violet or crystal violet (250 mg/L), if added to the blood and allowed to sit for 24 hours before transfusion, prevents infection. There are some side effects (principally, patients become "stained" for a period), and there may be some mutagenic effects in pregnant women. Amphotericin B has been shown to be effective in eradicating organisms under laboratory conditions, as have nystatin and some tetracyclines, but they have not yet been evaluated in actual clinical situations.

It should be clear that transmission of *T cruzi* by transfusion is a very real problem in Latin America and will grow in importance in the United States as our Hispanic population increases rapidly. Until recently, there has been virtually no information available on the seroprevalence of the disease in the United States, in blood donors in general, or in specific immigrant populations. However, a presentation at the October 1988 meeting of the AABB reported a serosurvey of 988 volunteer donors at a major Los Angeles hospital in which 1.8% to 2.4% of the donors, depending on the test used, had positive titers for antibodies to *T cruzi*.[9] Positive donors were 3.6 times more likely to come from Central America and 11.8 times more likely to have a history of malaria.

Two recent reports on transfusion-transmitted Chagas' disease underscore these concerns. The first involved a young girl with Hodgkin's disease who had never been to an endemic area. She received platelets from a Bolivian immigrant who had serologic evidence of Chagas' infection.[10] The second involved a young Canadian woman with leukemia who received blood products from over 100 donors, several of whom had modest antibody titers for *T cruzi*. One donor, from rural Paraguay, was asymptomatic but had a titer greater than 1:2000.[11] In both of these immunosuppressed patients, blood transfusion appears to have transmitted Chagas' disease.

Filariasis

In its various forms, filariasis affects more than 300 million persons world-wide.[12] Of the eight varieties of filariae found in humans only six are pathogens,[7] and five of the eight can be found in human blood and have the potential to be transmitted by transfusion.[6] *Mansonella perstans* and *Mansonella ozzardi* are remarkably well tolerated by humans, with even massive infestations apparently causing no clinical illness. *Mansonella streptocerca, Brugia timori*, and *Onchocerca volvulus*, which are responsible for serious clinical illnesses, have not been observed to be transmitted by blood. This leaves *Brugia malayi* in Southeast Asia, *Loa loa* in Africa and *Wuchereria bancrofti* in tropical Africa, Asia, and Latin America as organisms of potential concern for blood transfusion.

B malayi and *W bancrofti* cause elephantiasis and other lymphopathic problems, and *Loa loa* produces Calabar swelling and other allergic manifestations. (Calabar swellings are recurrent subcutaneous swellings commonly seen on the extremities after trauma. They represent a hypersensitivity response to antigenic material released by a migrating worm.) Because of its worldwide distribution, and to avoid confusion and redundancy, we will discuss only *W bancrofti* and bancroftian filariasis, which also may serve as a model for the other blood-transmissible filarial infections as it is the principal cause of elephantiasis around the tropical world.

Generally, the organism is found between the Tropic of Cancer and the Tropic of Capricorn (30° north and south latitudes, respectively), although in Southeast Asia it is found as far north as the 40th parallel. Most affected people live in south Asia or tropical Africa, but bancroftian filariasis came to the western hemisphere from Africa when slaves were imported in the 18th and 19th centuries. It became endemic in most of the major Caribbean islands south of the Bahamas and the eastern coastal plains of South and Central America, and an apparently indigenous case was reported early in this century from Charleston, SC.[6] The disease has been greatly reduced in the Americas and now is an isolated and generally uncommon public health problem in Haiti, the Dominican Republic, the Guianas, and some coastal areas of Brazil. It appears that there are no animal reservoirs; it is transmitted from humans to humans.

Adult filarial worms are white and threadlike and vary from 5 to 10 cm in length, with females being the larger. Adult females give birth to microfilariae which, though convoluted like the adults, are 200 to 300 μm long. Microfilariae develop into infective larvae after penetrating the intestinal tract of the various species of mosquitoes that serve as vectors, from whence they migrate to the thoracic muscles of the mosquito, where they mature and become infective in about 2 weeks.

Thus, an individual bitten by a mosquito who has recently fed on another human with microfilariae in his or her blood cannot become infected unless the microfilariae have developed into the infective larval stage within the mosquito. When the infective larvae are inoculated into humans, they mature to the third stage, the adult worm, and (in the case of *W bancrofti*) invade the lymphatics, giving birth to more microfilariae. Microfilariae first appear in the peripheral blood after 6 months and may persist for years, even in the absence of reinfection.

An amazing and curious relationship between the mosquito vectors and the organism has developed. The parasites peak in their swarming in the bloodstream in coincidence with the peak feeding times of the mosquitoes that are their secondary hosts. In Southeast Asia, swarms and feeding times are greatest around midnight, the vector being strains of *Anopheles*. In the Pacific islands, the parasite has adapted to the day-biting *Aedes*. The density of the microfilarialemia at the right time for vector ingestion is critical to the maintenance of the organism. Some other filariae, such as *Loa loa*, are transmitted by flies or midges. Over 48 species of mosquitoes transmit *W bancrofti*.[6]

Microfilarial infections generally cause only mild symptoms, even at high levels of parasitemia. Fever, headache, and rash may occur in reaction to dead microfilariae transmitted by blood transfusion or primary infection. Tropical pulmonary eosinophilia is believed to result from the immune response to the presence of microfilariae in the lungs. Infection with the adult larvae, however, can cause severe illness, including elephantiasis.

The adult worms of *W bancrofti* take up residence in the lymphatics, most often within the dilated lymph vessels of inguinal, epitrochlear, and axillary nodes. They are also found in retroperitoneal nodes and seem to have a special predilection for the lymphatics of the testis, epididymis, and spermatic cord. Perhaps for this reason, men seem to be more affected than women in the same endemic area. The most severe inflammatory response seems to surround dead or dying worms, which are probably releasing more antigenic material. Fibrosis and lymphatic abscesses develop at these sites, producing the characteristic swelling and lymphedema of elephantiasis of legs, scrotum, arms, and breasts. Rupture of abdominal lymphatics can cause chylous ascites.

The diagnosis is established by identifying microfilariae in a blood smear. It is important to obtain the blood sample when the organism is swarming, which may be a diurnal or nocturnal pattern.

The paucity of symptoms following transmission of microfilariae suggests that routine donor screening is not warranted. On the other hand, increased international travel means that the possibility of such a microfilarial infection occurring is increasing, even though it may not lead to serious consequences. Weller et al[13] reported just such an occurrence in a blood recipient whose donor had briefly visited the Caribbean.

Toxoplasmosis

Seropositivity for *Toxoplasma gondii* is common in the United States and the organism may be present in the blood for months in some individuals.[6] Seropositivity in the United States varies from 20% to 70%[5] and congenital toxoplasmosis is estimated to occur in 0.5 to five cases per 1000 live births. In addition to causing lymphadenopathy, it may cause a lethal infection in the immunocompromised host, and considerable morbidity and mortality have been noted in such patients, including those with AIDS.

T gondii is found throughout the world in many species of animals, both wild and domestic, including humans. In Paris, up to 90% of adults have chronic (latent) infection and up to 50% of adults in the United States are similarly affected.[14] In most cases, both the acute and chronic phases are asymptomatic and, although never recognized or treated, cause no problems. However, millions of dollars are spent each year to care for the approximately 3000 infants born with congenital toxoplasmosis and subsequent blindness and mental retardation. Immunodeficient patients may contract severe systemic toxoplasmosis, encephalitis, or both. McCabe and Remington[14] state that approximately 30% of toxoplasma antibody–positive patients with AIDS will develop toxoplasmosis encephalitis because of reactivation of their latent infection. Thus, approximately 25% of European AIDS victims and 5% to 10% of those in the United States may be so affected.[14]

The toxoplasma protozoa exists in three forms: trophozoite, cyst, and oocyst. The trophozoite is the invasive form that is responsible for the acute infectious symptoms. The cyst is found in many organs and represents the latent form of the disease. The oocyst is found exclusively in the cat, the only animal that hosts the complete lifecycle. Oocysts from cats are one of the common modes of infection of humans, but otherwise the oocyst plays no role in the pathology seen in humans. After formation in the cat intestine, and excretion in the feces, the oocyst undergoes a period of maturation of 1 to 21 days and is then infective.[15]

Primary infection in humans occurs after ingestion of the cyst or oocyst from inadequately cooked meat or soil contaminated with cat feces. The disrupted organisms invade the epithelium of the intestine and spread hematogenously to virtually all organs. They multiply intracellularly and form cysts, particularly in brain and muscle tissue. Ingestion, parasitemia, organ invasion, and chronic infection may all occur with no clinical evidence of disease, or disease may occur at any time after or during parasitemia. During the short-lived parasitemia, the crescent-shaped trophozoites, or tachyzoites, which measure 2 to 7 μm, may be seen in the blood smear. In 1969, Miller et al[16] reported isolation of toxoplasmosis parasites from a donor's blood 14 months after the acute infection. They also cited references in the Brazilian literature in which parasites were found in the blood of a donor and a Uruguayan study demonstrating survival of the parasite in blood stored at refrigerator temperatures for up to 50 days. Leukocyte donors have been shown to transmit fatal infections to immunocompromised recipients,[17] suggesting that chronic carriers are probably not uncommon among blood donors.

They most common clinical manifestation of toxoplasmosis in the adult is local or generalized lymphadenopathy, usually cervical. Although fever, malaise, and occasionally a rash may occur, suggesting a mononucleosis-like syndrome, asymptomatic localized adenopathy is the most common clinical symptom in the adult. Although there may be some fluctuation in symptoms or nodes, spontaneous resolution in weeks to months is the rule. Rarely does more serious disease occur. Congenital toxoplasmosis occurs only in infants whose mothers acquire the primary infection during pregnancy, and the earlier it occurs during gestation, the more likely are serious sequelae.

In the immunocompromised host the story is much different, and the infection is often fatal, particularly in patients with leukemia, lymphoma, or AIDS. The infection may be acquired through blood transfusion or organ transplantation, or, more commonly, the immune mechanisms responsible for containing the organism in a latent state from a previous infection break down. More than one half of such patients will present with neurologic symptoms, and in fatal cases more than 90% have encephalitis.[15] Myocarditis and pneumonitis may also occur.

Treatment, when needed, consists of the combination of sulfadiazine and pyrimethamine, the latter therapy requiring supplemental folinic acid. Prevention is more important and, in children and pregnant women, consists of avoiding the eating of raw or undercooked meat and hand washing after handling raw meat, cats, or soil contaminated with cat feces. Since most adults are already infected and since most cases of severe illness (not congenital) are due to reactivation of the infection in an immunocompromised host, it does not seem that testing of donated blood or other tissues is warranted. The prevention of congenital toxoplasmosis may be a more important issue and has recently been reviewed.[15]

Babesiosis

Babesiosis is an uncommon intraerythrocytic parasitemia that has been reported with increasing frequency, particularly in splenectomized patients and, more recently, in a patient with AIDS.[18] The first case was reported in Yugoslavia in 1957[19] and, as in most following reports, occurred in a splenectomized man. There are now reports involving residents of Massachusetts, New York, Georgia, New Hampshire, Wisconsin, California, Ireland, France, Scotland, Mexico, and Yugoslavia.

There are at least 40 recognized species of Babesia,[6] of which only two have been reported in humans, *Babesia divergens* (*Babesia bovis*) from Europe and *Babesia microti* from the United States. Transmission by blood transfusion has only been reported in the United States. Tick vectors in Europe include a *Dermacentor* species and *Ixodes ricinus*; in the United States the principal tick vector has been *Ixodes dammini*, the northern deer tick. Although *B bovis* used to infect plains cattle in the western United States, the species and its *Dermacentor* host have been virtually eliminated. Animal hosts for the parasite in New England include deer mice and the white-tailed deer, but *Babesia* organisms have been found in other rodents and in cattle in Europe.

Babesia does not have a nonerythrocytic life cycle in humans. The tick that transmits the parasite spends its larval and nymphal life in deer mice and its adult life on deer. The tick is also responsible for transmission of the spirochete that causes Lyme disease. The first reported case of babesiosis in

Wisconsin occurred in an asplenic man whose wife had one of 117 cases of an outbreak of Lyme disease occurring in Wisconsin and Minnesota between 1980 and 1983. She had serologic evidence of *Babesia* infection, but none of the other 116 patients was found to have *Babesia* antibodies.[20] At the same time, however, Benach et al[20] reported on a serological survey of patients with Lyme disease in regions endemic for babesiosis and found that 60% of them had *Babesia* antibodies.

Before 1979, there were no reports of transfusion-transmitted *Babesia* infection, although the possibility of its occurrence was raised in 1977[22] and a suspected but unproven case was reported in 1976 from Georgia.[23] Most reported cases up to that time were that of a prolonged illness with fever, chills, sweats, myalgias, and variable degrees of hemolytic anemia. A serologic study of patients admitted to the Nantucket (MA) Hospital in 1977 showed that 11 of 577 patients had significant antibody titers to *B microti* and that, of patients with a history of tick bite or fever of 3 days' or more duration in the past 6 months, ten of 133 had titers greater than 1:64.[22] The authors concluded that *Babesia* infection may have a wide range of expression, including asymptomatic infection, in the normal host.

The splenectomized host offers an ideal setting for severe parasitemia and hemolysis, and such a case was seen at the Massachusetts General Hospital, Boston, in 1979 and documented to have been transfusion-acquired.[24] An elderly man with idiopathic thrombocytopenic purpura was treated with prednisone and 20 units of platelet concentrate, though his platelet count was 10,000 and he did not have life-threatening bleeding. One month later his spleen was removed, and 1 month after that procedure he was found to have a severe hemolytic anemia and *Babesia* parasites in up to 40% of his red blood cells. Chloroquine therapy failed and the patient underwent an exchange transfusion of red blood cells and plasma as well as pentamidine therapy. He relapsed approximately 6 weeks later with more hemolysis and again underwent exchange transfusion, remaining well subsequently. The suspected donor was a summer resident of Nantucket who had not recently been ill and who had no parasites demonstrable in his blood, but who did have an antibody titer of 1:256. The patient had never been in a recognized endemic area. If the proper indications for platelet transfusion had been followed, the patient would probably not have become infected.

Babesiosis has an incubation period of approximately 1 month and a maximum period of parasitemia of 4 to 6 months. Most cases probably go unrecognized, but the diagnosis should be suspected in patients with hemolytic anemia who have recently visited an endemic area, or who reside in one. In any case of anemia, thorough examination of the blood smear by the clinician is imperative; in fact, most reported cases were at first thought to be due to malaria. Like falciparum malaria, *Babesia* can infect red blood cells of any age, leading to a high degree of red blood cell parasitemia being noted in blood smears and severe hemolysis of the "blackwater fever" type. The other three varieties of human malaria infect primarily reticulocytes and rarely have infestation rates of more than 1% to 2%, whereas babesiosis and falciparum may be seen in greater than 10% of the red blood cells.

Unlike falciparum, *Babesia* organisms in red blood cells are smaller and more ameboid, and have a clear area within the ring. Rod forms or dividing forms may be seen and some cells may contain tetrads of organisms with filamentous connections, resembling a Maltese cross. A geographic history is important in the differential diagnosis, although a history of blood transfusion may not be helpful in discriminating between the two possibilities. Definitive diagnosis is obtained by injecting hamsters, which are quite susceptible, with the patient's blood or by an indirect immunofluorescence test for antibody, which can be arranged through most state health department laboratories or the CDC in Atlanta. Titers of antibody begin to decrease after a few months. If the patient is asplenic or severely immunocompromised and parasitemia is noted but there has been no exposure to malaria, rapid identification and therapy are critical.

Appropriate therapy is still evolving, and even such heroic measures as exchange transfusion may need to be considered. Pentamidine is useful in controlling the infection but is painful, may cause abscesses, and does not eradicate the parasite from the bloodstream, especially in the splenectomized patient.[25] Neither chloroquine, chloroquine plus pyrimethamine, quinine plus cotrimoxazole, or other combinations have been totally effective. The combination of pentamidine with cotrimoxazole was reported to be successful in a French patient with *B divergens*.[26] Work in hamsters[27] suggested that the use of clindamycin, with or without oral quinine, was safe and effective and was recommended by the CDC in 1983.[28] However, Smith et al[29] reported on a transfusion-acquired case in 1986 that did not respond to this combination. This unsplenectomized elderly man continued to show parasitemia of approximately 1%, dying of a noninfectious cause a few weeks later. Thus, therapy is not only difficult, it may not be effective, particularly in the splenectomized host.

Babesia infections in European cattle have led to work to develop an animal vaccine, since in heavily infested areas stock losses due to "redwater," the blackwater fever equivalent in cattle, can be very high. Commercial development of such a vaccine for cattle was discussed in 1988 at a European conference on babesiosis and malaria,[30] but it is not likely that a vaccine in humans would be useful.

Although prevention is of prime importance as it applies to transfusion-transmitted babesiosis, it is simply not practical to screen out donors from endemic areas, nor is it feasible to examine smears or perform antibody tests on such units of blood. Even the logistics of providing *Babesia*-free blood from donors in endemic areas to immunocompromised recipients would be a formidable task. A recent serologic survey of blood donors, 779 from Cape Cod and 148 from metropolitan Boston, showed no difference in seropositivity to *B microti*.[31] 3.7% of the Cape Cod donors and 4.7% of the Boston donors had clinically significant antibody titers, though no travel histories were obtained from either group. Thus, simply being from, or even having been to, an endemic area is not a useful criterion for donor exclusion.

Lyme Disease

Although the causative agent is a spirochete, not a parasite, it seems appropriate to briefly mention Lyme disease, or borreliosis, since it is also spread by the same ticks (and other species on the West coast) responsible for human infection with *Babesia* species.

It is an interesting paradox to note that migration of the rural poor into urban areas of Latin America has increased the spread of Chagas' disease, while the migration of the urban affluent into the countryside is clearly responsible for the increase in cases of Lyme borreliosis in the United States. Sylvatic reservoirs of the disease have been invaded by suburban and rural development, particularly in the northeastern United States. Cases have been reported from 41 states.[32] In Connecticut, the index community that gave its name to the illness, twice as many cases were reported in 1988 compared with 1987.[33] It is now the most common tick-transmitted infection in the United States.[34]

The classic localized skin rash, erythema chronicum migrans (now called simply erythema migrans), with which Lyme disease often (but not always) presents was first described in Europe in 1909.[35] The presentation is usually associated with malaise, fever, and fatigue, with or without headache and nuchal rigidity. Not all patients give a history of tick bite. Patients with untreated or unrecognized cases go on to develop a protean illness with arthritic, neurologic, or cardiac manifestations.

The spirochete involved, *Borrelia burgdorferi*, was cultured from the deer tick, *Ixodes dammini*, in 1982 and from patients with Lyme disease in 1983.[34] However, routine blood cultures from patients with suspected disease are not usually positive; a special medium is required. Antibody testing is routinely unreliable, as well.[36] The organism can be found in the blood as late as 14 days after the onset of symptoms.[37] Most workers agree that the spirochetemia phase is short, but there are no data about whether it can be recurrent.

Unlike *Treponema pallidum*, the spirochete of Lyme disease survives storage in blood components quite well. After inoculation of red blood cells, plasma to be frozen, and platelet concentrates, the spirochete was found to survive for 45 days in red blood cells stored at 4 °C and in plasma frozen at −18 °C, and it was, of course, found in platelet concentrates stored at room temperature for 6 days.[38]

Although no cases of transfusion-transmitted Lyme disease have been found, transmission by transfusion is at the least theoretically possible. As pointed out by Aoki and Holland,[34] large-scale testing of healthy donor blood is not indicated since we have no evidence of transmission by this method and do not yet have a reliable test. However, the increasing incidence of the disease has led to the following recommendations from the American Red Cross and the AABB:

1. Since donors with acute Lyme borreliosis are symptomatic, additional questions for the purpose of deferring donors to prevent transmission by transfusion are not necessary.

2. Although tests for Lyme borreliosis are under development, implementation of these tests, even in endemic areas, is not recommended.
3. Health care workers should be encouraged to be alert in making the diagnosis and, once made, to determine whether the patient had previously been a blood donor or recipient. In either event, the appropriate collection or transfusion facility should be notified so that the potential risk, if any, for transfusion transmission can be evaluated.
4. Individuals with a history of Lyme borreliosis may donate blood after they have completed a course of antibiotics and are totally asymptomatic.

References

1. Schmuñis GA: Chagas' disease and blood transfusion, in Dodd RY (ed): *Infection, Immunity and Blood Transfusion*. New York, Alan R Liss Inc, 1985, pp 127–145.
2. Linares J: Malaria and Chagas' Disease: Role in Transfusion and Prospects for Testing. VIIth Interamerican Red Cross Seminar on Blood Transfusion; San Juan, Puerto Rico, November 1–5, 1987.
3. Kirchoff LV, Neva FA: Chagas' disease in Latin American immigrants. *JAMA* 254:3058–3060, 1985.
4. Schiffler RJ, Mansur GP, Navin TR, Limpakarnajanarat K: Indigenous Chagas' disease in California. *JAMA* 251:2983–2984, 1984.
5. Greer DA: Found: Two cases of Chagas' disease. *Texas Health Bull* 9:11–13, 1955.
6. Warren KS, Mahmoud AAF: *Geographic Medicine for the Practitioner*. New York, Springer-Verlag, 1985.
7. Tabor E: *Infectious Complications of Blood Transfusion*. New York, Academic Press, 1982.
8. Strickland GT: *Hunter's Tropical Medicine*, ed 6. Philadelphia, WB Saunders, 1984.
9. Kerndt P, Waskin H, Shulman I, et al: *Trypanosoma cruzi* antibody among blood donors in Los Angeles, California. *Transfusion* 28(suppl):31S, 1988.
10. Grant IH, Gold JWM, Wittner M, et al: Transfusion-associated acute Chagas' disease acquired in the United States. *Ann Intern Med* 111:849–851, 1989.
11. Nickerson P, Orr P, Schroeder ML, et al: Transfusion-associated *Trypanosoma cruzi* infection in a non-endemic area. *Ann Intern Med* 11:851–853, 1989.
12. Schultz MG: Current concepts in parasitology. *N Engl J Med* 297:1259–1261, 1977.
13. Weller PF, Simon HB, Parkhurst BH, Medrek TF: Tourism-acquired *Mansonella ozzardi* microfilaremia in a regular blood donor. *JAMA* 240:858–859, 1978.
14. McCabe R, Remington JS: Toxoplasmosis: The time has come (editorial). *N Engl J Med* 318:313–315, 1988.
15. Krick JA, Remington JS: Toxoplasmosis in the adult: An overview. *N Engl J Med* 298:550–553, 1978.
16. Miller MJ, Aronson WJ, Remington JS: Late parasitemia in asymptomatic acquired toxoplasmosis. *Ann Intern Med* 71:139–145, 1969.
17. Siegel SE, Lunde MN, Gelderman AH, et al: Transmission of toxoplasmosis by leukocyte transfusion. *Blood* 37:388–394, 1971.

18. Benezra D, Brown AE, Polsky B, et al: Babebiosis and infection with human immunodeficiency virus (letter). *Ann Intern Med.* 107:944, 1987.

19. Skrabalo Z, Deanovic Z: Piroplasmosis in man. *Doc Med Geograph Trop* 9:11–16, 1957.

20. Steketee RW, Eckman MR, Burgess EC, et al: Babesiosis in Wisconsin: a new focus of disease transmission. *JAMA* 253:2675–2678, 1985.

21. Benach JL, Coleman JL, Habicht JS: Serological evidence for simultaneous occurrences of Lyme disease and babesiosis. *J Infect Dis* 152:473–477, 1985.

22. Ruebush TK, Juranek DD, Chisholm ES, et al: Human babesiosis on Nantucket Island: Evidence for self-limited and subclinical infections. *N Engl J Med* 297:825–827, 1977.

23. Healy GR, Walzer PD, Sulzer AJ: A case of asymptomatic babesiosis in Georgia. *Am J Trop Med Hyg* 25:376–378, 1978.

24. Jacoby GA, Hunt JV, Kosinski KS, et al: Treatment of transfusion-transmitted babesiosis by exchange transfusion. *N Engl J Med* 303:1098–1100, 1980.

25. Francioli PB, Keithly JS, Jones TC, et al: Response of babesiosis to pentamidine therapy. *Ann Intern Med* 94:326–330, 1981.

26. Racult D, Soulayrol L, Toga B, et al: Babesiosis, pentamidine and cotrimoxazole (letter). *Ann Intern Med* 107:944, 1987.

27. Rowen KS, Tanowitz HB, Wittner M: Therapy of experimental babesiosis. *Ann Intern Med* 97:556–558, 1982.

28. *MMWR* 32:65–72, 1983.

29. Smith RP, Evans AT, Popovsky MA, et al: Transfusion-acquired babesiosis and failure of antibiotic treatment. *JAMA* 256:2726–2727, 1986.

30. Vaccines against malaria and babesiosis (editorial). *Lancet* 2:1232–1233, 1983.

31. Popovsky MA, Lindberg LE, Syrek AL, Page PL: Prevalence of *Babesia* antibody in a selected blood donor population. *Transfusion* 28:59–61, 1988.

32. Lyme disease: United States. *MMWR* 38:668–672, 1989.

33. Carter ML, Mshar P, Hadler JL: The epidemiology of Lyme disease in Connecticut. *Conn Med* 53:320–323, 1989.

34. Aoki SK, Holland PL: Lyme disease: Another transfusion risk? *Transfusion* 29:646–650, 1989.

35. Afzelius A: Erythema chronicum migrans. *Acta Derm Venereol* 2:120–125, 1921.

36. Schwartz BS, Goldstein MD, Ribeiro JMC, et al: Antibody testing in Lyme disease, a comparison of results in four laboratories. *JAMA* 262:3431–3434, 1989.

37. Nadelman RB, Pavia CS, Magnarelli LA, Wormser GP: Isolation of *Borrelia burgdorferi* from the blood of seven patients with Lyme disease. *Am J Med* 88:21–26, 1990.

38. Badon SJ, Fister RD, Cable RG: Survival of *Borrelia burgdorferi* in blood products. *Transfusion* 29:581–583, 1989.

12
Transfusion of Blood Components Contaminated With Bacteria

Charles H. Wallas, MD

Fatal reactions due to transfusion of blood contaminated with bacteria have been noted since the 1930s, when the use of blood became a common form of therapy.[1] Most cases involving whole blood and red blood cells have been caused by bacteria that were introduced at the time of collection or processing[2] and that grew preferentially at cold temperatures (psychrophilic organisms). With improved refrigeration and the substitution of disposable plastic bags, needles, and tubes for reusable glass bottles, rubber tubing, and needles, the incidence of sepsis associated with red blood cell transfusion decreased from 5% to 25% in the 1930s and 1940s and 2.2% to 4.5% in the 1950s to 0.1% in the 1970s. Nonetheless, cases continued to be reported in the 1980s.[3-5] More recently, it has become recognized that sepsis can also be caused by platelet transfusion, apparently augmented by the fact that platelets are now routinely stored at 20 to 24 °C. This chapter will review those factors producing or promoting transfusion-associated sepsis as well as the clinical diagnosis and prevention of this potentially catastrophic complication.

Mechanisms for Contamination of Blood

Bacteria can enter blood at the time of collection because of infection in the donor. Two reports of fatal salmonella infections in recipients of platelet transfusions occurred because of sepsis in the donor. In one case salmonella osteomyelitis in a platelet pheresis donor produced sepsis in seven recipients, one of whom died.[6] In a second report, salmonella gastroenteritis associated with sepsis produced a fatal outcome in the recipient of donated platelets.[7]

Small numbers of bacteria can also be introduced at the time of collection because of mechanical problems. Early reports stressed the techniques that must be used to prevent contamination,[8-10] and Novak[11] even suggested that sulfanilamide be added prophylactically to collected blood to inhibit bacterial growth. Thus, use of contaminated disinfectants or inadequate cleansing of the venipuncture site[2] may allow entrance of contaminants into the unit of blood either directly or through a small plug of contaminated skin that may be excised by the needle and carried into the bag. In addition, bacteria may gain entrance through cracks in glass bottles or pinholes in plastic bags or from intravenous solutions used in conjunction with transfusion therapy.[12-14] In this regard, there is a report of a donor who developed gram-negative sepsis during a leukapheresis procedure because of infusion of contaminated hydroxyethyl starch.[15] Finally, the anticoagulant solution in a pilot tube contaminated with microorganisms is capable of entering the bag of blood if the tube is filled with blood from the bag and the tubing is then stripped toward the bag. In one report, one of two patients died who received platelet concentrates prepared from blood contaminated with *Serratia marcescens* present in the EDTA solution in the pilot tube[16]; in another report, febrile reactions occurred in two patients who were given transfusions of blood with contaminated acid citrate dextrose (ACD) in the pilot tube.[17] This problem is similar to that noted by Katz et al[18] and McLeish et al,[19] who reported *S marcescens* sepsis in patients from whom blood samples were collected using contaminated vacuum tubes.

With the introduction of a closed collection system using plastic bags and tubing in the 1950s, contamination of blood components during processing became an uncommon event although, theoretically, inadequate skin cleansing or the use of contaminated equipment (eg, scissors, heat sealers, or water baths) could lead to introduction of bacteria into individual components. In this regard, it was recognized that cryoprecipitate can transmit organisms contaminating the transfusion ports of the bag at the time the product is thawed.[20] Rhame et al[20] found that *Pseudomonas cepacia* was present in the water of the thawing bath at a concentration of 2×10^8 organisms per milliliter, even though the incubator was cleaned with povidone-iodine and the water was changed daily. Rhame et al[20] demonstrated that as little as 0.025 mL of water, when placed between the unopened tabs covering the transfusion ports, may contaminate the port when the tabs are pulled apart before pooling. Sepsis was produced in two patients and a mediastinal wound infection developed in a third patient. Although not reported, similar problems could occur when thawing frozen plasma or red blood cells. Use of a plastic overwrap has been recommended to prevent contamination of transfusion ports from a contaminated waterbath.[21]

Studies of Whole Blood and Red Blood Cells

The prevalence of contaminated units of blood varies widely depending on whether open or closed collection systems were used, how long the blood was stored before sampling, and the temperature of incubation of the cultured material.[22] Braude et al[23] found that 2.2% of 1697 units of blood stored at

4 °C for 24 hours and cultured at 37 °C were contaminated primarily with staphylococci. Presumably, most of these contaminants would not have survived longer storage at 4 °C nor would this high a frequency have been seen if contaminants only growing at 25 to 30 °C were sought. Thus, when blood was cultured at 20 to 25 °C, the ideal temperature to identify the cold-growing (psychrophilic) bacteria implicated in reports of fatal reactions to infected blood,[24] James and Stokes[25] detected 1 contaminated unit among 406 tested and Chaplin et al[26] noted none among 200 outdated units tested. The psychrophilic bacteria implicated in cases of fatal sepsis following transfusion of contaminated blood are mainly gram-negative, endotoxin-producing organisms. These organisms are found in soil, water, and feces and grow slowly at 4 to 8 °C, rapidly at 25 to 30 °C, and often not at all at 37 °C. Occasionally, gram-positive organisms are implicated.[23,25,27,28] Most organisms isolated are capable of using citrate as the carbon source. Organisms probably enter the unit of blood in small numbers at the time of collection and multiply readily at 1 to 6 °C beginning after the third to fourth day of storage, with dangerous levels achieved after 2 weeks of storage.[29-31] For example, Braude et al[32,33] noted that many gram-negative strains isolated grew rapidly in blood after only 1 to 2 weeks of cold storage, reaching concentrations of 10^8 to 10^{10} bacteria per milliliter. A recent study implicated *Yersinia enterocolita* in stored blood as causing sepsis and death of one of two patients given transfusions of contaminated blood.[3]

Since most organisms contaminating whole blood and red blood cells are not hemolytic, even blood heavily contaminated may appear normal, although with 10^9 organisms per milliliter of blood, a permanganate color may be seen.[31] Examination of a Gram's stained preparation to exclude bacterial contamination is usually unsatisfactory because debris is often present that is difficult to distinguish from bacteria. In addition, Walter et al[28] noted that upon adding serial dilutions of bacteria to blood, a concentration of 2.4×10^6 organisms could be easily detected, while a concentration of 2.4×10^5 was difficult to detect since only one organism was seen in every 100 fields examined. Conversely, when only 24 organisms per milliliter were present, a culture could demonstrate bacteria after 24 hours.

There are several special circumstances in which sterility of red blood cells has been a concern, but studies have not documented that a problem with contamination exists. Thus, transfusion of placental blood to the newborn has not been associated with sepsis if the blood is taken aseptically from the umbilical vein into a heparinized syringe and used within 24 hours of collection.[34] Similarly, blood taken in syringes from blood bags and stored for up to 24 hours for replacement of blood lost in the neonatal period has not become septic.[35] Finally, two studies have shown that there was a 2-log decrease in the concentration of bacteria intentionally inoculated into red blood cells before glycerolization and freezing as a result of dilution by glycerol and post-thaw washing with 3000 mL of glucose and saline solution.[36,37] Furthermore, there was no increase in bacterial counts in these units when they were stored for up to 10 days at 4 °C.[37] Although results of these studies suggested that post-thaw (4 °C) storage could be extended for up to 72 hours since contamination of blood during glycerolization or during postfreeze washing did not lead to significant levels of bacterial contamination, psychrophilic organisms were not utilized, making it uncertain if post-thaw storage could be prolonged past the currently mandated 24 hours.

Studies of Platelets

Although the occurrence of sepsis following transfusion of whole blood and red blood cells has been decreasing during the past 30 years, the incidence of sepsis from platelet transfusions has been increasing. Thus, from 1976 to 1978, one of 64 evaluable fatalities resulting from transfusion reported to the FDA was due to sepsis from a psychrophilic pseudomonas organism transfused in red blood cells.[38] With an estimated 27 million units of blood given during that time, it appears that such occurrences are now exceedingly rare events. There was also one death described in this same report as a consequence of transfusion of platelets contaminated with gram-positive cocci. In another report encompassing a similar period that evaluated 113 fatalities reported to the FDA, an additional report involved the death of a recipient due to transfusion of cryoprecipitate contaminated with gram-negative organisms.[39] However, between 1980 and 1983 there were six more deaths attributable to infusion of contaminated platelets, four of which occurred in 1983.[40]

There are numerous reports in the literature indicating that platelet concentrates are usually sterile. Katz and Tilton,[41] Mallin et al,[42] and Silver et al[43] cultured 100, 110, and 40 concentrates, respectively, none of which demonstrated bacterial growth. Conversely, Buchholz et al[44] cultured pools prepared from 2188 units of platelets and calculated that 2.4% of them were contaminated, yielding predominately diptheroids and *Staphylococcus epidermidis*. Recovery of bacteria was noted to increase as a function of storage time.[45] Cunningham and Cash[46] demonstrated that 6.3% of 1000 platelet concentrates cultured were contaminated immediately after preparation, although with exceedingly few bacteria (<10 organisms per milliliter in 78% of the cultures), predominately *S epidermidis*. However, these workers could not demonstrate postinfusion sepsis in 175 patients receiving 1800 units of platelets; these findings are similar to those of Wrenn and Speicher,[47] who cultured 400 concentrates and evaluated patients receiving 10,024 concentrates. Goddard et al[48] also noted that 350 platelet concentrates were sterile at the time of preparation, although they suggested that, once stored, concentrates should not be issued until a negative culture is obtained.

In view of a report by Kahn et al,[49] it is possible that those studies showing that platelet concentrates are regularly contaminated may have reached this conclusion as a result of contamination of the platelets during the culturing process. Kahn et al,[49] using intentionally contaminated platelets, showed that, to isolate one to ten per milliliter of concentrate immediately after preparation (the level found by Cunningham and Cash[46]) it was necessary to inoculate the original whole blood unit with 42 to 125 bacteria per milliliter, given the dilutional effect of dividing the original unit into three components as well as the sedimentation characteristics of bacteria relative to the platelets. Since it is unlikely that approximately 5% of whole blood units contain this level of bacterial contamination because of the low frequency of sepsis following red blood cell infusion, it is more likely that the high rate of platelet contamination reported was an artifact. Furthermore, Myhre et al[50] also demonstrated by intentionally contaminating platelets with *P aeruginosa* or *Staphylococcus aureus* or *epidermidis* that unless $>10^3$ organisms per milliliter were introduced into the concentrate, no growth was seen after 48-hour storage at 22 °C, suggesting that platelets have bacterostatic properties. This observation also further supports the hypothesis that the reported high incidence of contamination of platelet concentrates may be an artifact.

Before 1980, reports of a 2.4% to 6.3% contamination rate in a product stored for 3 days at temperatures noninhibitory to bacterial growth (20 to 24 °C), suggested that platelet transfusion might cause sepsis. Only three isolated reports of sepsis following the receipt of platelets actually appeared. One case stemmed from a platelet pheresis donor who had salmonella osteomyelitis[6] and the other from contaminated EDTA solution in the pilot tubes that was backwashed into the unit of blood.[16] The third report involved two patients who developed fever due to transfusion of platelets contaminated with *Enterbacter cloacae*; both recovered.[44]

In 1983, the outdating period of platelets was extended to 5 days with the introduction of gas-permeable storage bags; in 1984 it was extended to 7 days. In 1986 Braine et al[51] reported four nonfatal cases of sepsis associated with platelet transfusion, three due to *S epidermidis* and one due to *S viridans*; all patients had received platelet pools in which at least one concentrate had been stored for more than 5 days. While three of four patients on antibiotic therapy developed transient fever, the fourth patient not on antibiotics developed fever and transient hypotension as well. To evaluate the ability of platelets to support bacteria growth, concentrates were intentionally inoculated. If only one organism of *S epidermidis* was introduced, there was a 24- to 48-hour lag phase followed by a log growth that yielded 10^7 to 10^8 organisms per 0.1 mL in 7 days; if greater numbers of bacteria were introduced, similar levels were seen in as few as 3 days. Because of these findings, the hospital involved in this study reduced the storage time for platelets from 7 to 5 days. Heal et al[40] similarly noted that inoculation of platelets with *Salmonella typhi* at concentrations of 10^1 to 10^5 organisms per milliliter yielded $\geq 10^8$ organisms per milliliter in 10 of 18 concentrates, usually after 3 to 7 days of storage at 20 to 24 °C. No growth occurred in six of 18 concentrates inoculated with 10^1 to 10^2 organisms per milliliter. These workers concluded that bacterial contamination of platelets not clinically significant at 3 days of storage might become so if platelets are stored for 7 days. Interestingly, no visible evidence of bacterial contamination was evident until there were $>10^8$ organisms per milliliter, at which point irregular white aggregates and strands of material were noted.

Anderson et al[2] similarly reported on the occurrence of sepsis due to the presence of gram-positive cocci in four patients. They concluded that the organisms entered the blood collection bag because the anticubital fossa had been inadequately sterilized due to scarring at the venipuncture site. The cocci had then multiplied during prolonged storage at room temperature.

Finally, after the appearance of a nonfatal case of *E coli* sepsis from platelets, Arnow et al[52] noted that 36 of 500 platelet concentrates retrospectively cultured contained microorganisms. In 35 of 36 concentrates, there were <20 organisms per milliliter and no symptoms were seen in the recipients. In one concentrate, there were 1000 organisms per milliliter and a transient febrile reaction was seen. In none of these concentrates were the segments culture-positive, probably because initial contamination occurred with only a few bacteria that were not distributed into the small volume in the tubing.

Clinical Presentation

In general, the symptoms and ultimate clinical outcome in patients receiving contaminated blood are dependent on the number of organisms infused, the immune status of the patient, and whether or not the patient is receiving antibiotics.

Sepsis is produced by whole blood or red blood cells when such units are contaminated with psychrophilic organisms. These bacteria are usually introduced at the time of collection. Seven to 14 days of storage are required before the bacterial content can cause a sequence of signs and symptoms at transfusion. These signs and symptoms are caused by infusion of bacterial endotoxin as well as release of endogenous pyrogens. Typical presentation has been summarized by Stevens et al[53] as follows: from 0 to 30 minutes after initiation of transfusion, the patient complains of headache, restlessness and chilliness; 30 to 60 minutes later, violent chills and high fever occur, 60 minutes later, flushing, vomiting, and diarrhea ensue. From 1 to 6 hours later, shock and disseminated intravascular coagulation occur. Death, which occurs in 60% of patients in some series, can occur after transfusion of as little as 25 mL of blood and may happen within 3 hours after transfusion, with 65% of patients dying within the first 24 hours. Apparently, a concentration of approximately 10^8 bacteria per milliliter can be associated with fatal reactions. Before the introduction of plastic storage bags, contamination of whole blood and red blood cells was not infrequent; currently this is a rare event.

When contaminated platelets are transfused, most patients develop fever; rarely hypotension is seen, usually in patients not taking antibiotics for preexisting infections. Among 18 cases reported in the United States since 1971, two patients died, both secondary to salmonella sepsis. All cases were due to the presence of gram-negative organisms, except for three cases due to *S epidermidis* and one to *S viridans*. During the 1980s, increased use of platelets and prolonging of shelf life from 3 to 7 days (recently reduced to 5 days), have been associated with an increase in the number of cases of sepsis produced by platelet transfusion.

Diagnosis

Since the transfusion of blood products contaminated with bacteria is a rare event, a critical element in diagnosing this condition is to consider it in the differential diagnosis. Since the signs and symptoms are nearly identical to those seen in an ABO hemolytic transfusion reaction, it is crucial to differentiate between these two conditions. Hemolytic reactions, in addition to producing fever, shock, and disseminated intravascular coagulation, usually are associated with hemoglobinuria, which is not typically seen when contaminated blood is transfused since most of the psychrophilic organisms do not hemolyze red blood cells during blood storage. In addition, a hemolytic reaction usually results from a clerical error and is associated with hemoglobinemia, a positive direct Coombs test, and evidence of an ABO mismatch, also not seen with a septic reaction.

Ultimately, however, the confirmation of a septic transfusion reaction depends on identifying the responsible organism. As indicated above, Gram stain evaluation of the contents of the blood product is usually not productive. There must be at least 10^5 to 10^6 organisms per milliliter present to be visible on a smear and often it is difficult to differentiate bacteria from debris in the blood product. Moreover, visual examination of the bag is also nonproductive since it appears to require 10^9 organisms per milliliter to produce a permanganate color in whole blood or red blood cells and 10^8 organisms per milliliter to produce aggregates and strands of whitish material in platelets. When the transfusion of a contaminated unit is suspected, a sample taken from the blood product (not the segment) and from the patient should be cultured using a technique capable of detecting as few as 1 to 2×10^2 organisms per milliliter. Even if the diagnosis of a septic reaction is not immediately considered and the blood product has been left for up to 24 hours at room temperature, it is still usually productive to culture it since such blood is usually sterile or only minimally contaminated.[25] When whole blood or red blood cells are involved, the blood product should be cultured at 25 to 30 °C as well as at 1 to 6 °C and 37 °C to detect the presence of psychrophilic bacteria. When platelets are involved, the contents of the bag should be cultured at 25 to 30 °C, as well as 37 °C. Cultures should be held at these temperatures for at least as long as the blood has been stored before transfusion. In addition, efforts should be made to locate, quarantine, and evaluate other blood products obtained from the same donor as the implicated components. While a negative culture virtually excludes the possibility that the blood product was significantly contaminated with bacteria at the time of transfusion, a positive culture does not indicate with certainty that the blood was contaminated before transfusion; it is possible that the unit became contaminated between the time of transfusion and bacterial evaluation. The type of organisms isolated from the implicated blood component (usually gram-negative pseudomonas and enterobacter species), the level of contamination on culture, and identity between the organism cultured from the blood product and the patient must all be considered in determining if a patient's signs and symptoms are a result of receiving contaminated blood.

Treatment

Patients who become infected from transfusion of blood components contaminated with bacteria often are septic. Accordingly, clinical manifestations include hemodynamic instability, hyperventilation, metabolic acidosis, and fever. Immediate therapy must be aimed at correction of abnormal hemodynamic parameters, metabolic acidosis, and fluid and electrolyte disorders as well as the initiation of effective antibiotic therapy. Since a patient's outcome from a septic episode is critically dependent on the correct antibiotic selection, a drug or combination of drugs that is active against all potential pathogens is desirable. A review of microorganisms that have been reported to cause infection following transmission by whole blood and red blood cells and by platelet concentrates reveals a wide spectrum of both gram-positive and gram-negative pathogens. Standard empiric therapy for sepsis has traditionally included a β-lactam antibiotic and an aminoglycoside. This approach, using an extended-spectrum antipseudomonal β-lactam agent such as ticarcillin–clavulanic acid (Timentin) combined with an aminoglycoside,[54,55] would be appropriate. A newer β-lactam agent such as imipenem (Primaxin) could be used alone.[56,57] The final choice of antibiotic would be dictated by the results of cultures and sensitivities.

Prevention

The use of closed blood collection systems, made possible by the introduction of disposable plastic equipment, has resulted in a significant reduction in the incidence of bacterial contamination of blood. Nonetheless, reports of transfusion of bacterial contaminated blood continues; therefore, blood banks and transfusion services must adhere to strict protocols to limit introduction of bacteria into blood products by careful donor processing, by limiting the potential for bacterial growth through proper storage and shipping, and by appropriately limiting the storage period.

Regarding blood collection, it appears extremely unlikely that a blood donor will unknowingly present with sepsis. Even in individuals undergoing a variety of procedures in which transient bacteremia occurs, such as oral surgery, genitourinary tract manipulations, and upper gastrointestinal tract endoscopy, it is unlikely that bacteria will be present in the blood even 24 hours later. For example, a group of 128 patients were studied who underwent dental extractions performed under local or general anesthesia with or without penicillin therapy.[58] In those patients not receiving penicillin, positive blood cultures were detected 5 minutes after completion of the procedure in 77% of patients receiving a general anesthetic and in 59% of those receiving a local anesthetic, while 42% of those receiving penicillin therapy had bacteremia 5 minutes after surgery. This incidence of bacteremia fell sharply 25 minutes later to 52%, 27%, and 13%, respectively. Streptococci were recovered most frequently in patients not receiving penicillin while bacteroides species were seen in those given penicillin. Since neither of these organisms grows well at either 1 to 6°C or 20 to 24 °C and since an individual is unlikely to donate blood immediately after dental surgery, the previous requirement that prohibits blood donation for 72 hours after dental surgery was deleted from the 10th edition of AABB standards published in 1981. Conversely, although it is unlikely that bacteria will be introduced into a collected unit of blood by virtue of sepsis in the donor, bacteria present on the donor's skin can be introduced into the blood if careful scrub techniques are not utilized.

During the first 8 to 12 hours after blood collection, maintenance of the collected blood at 20 to 24 °C does not lead to bacterial multiplication because of the presence of viable phagocytes.[53] Therefore, it is essential to store blood continuously at 1 to 6 °C within 8 hours of collection and to ship blood at 1 to 10 °C to limit bacterial growth. Although scientific studies substantiating these requirements are lacking, these ranges are easy to achieve and will inhibit growth of most organisms. During multiple-unit transfusions, only one unit of blood at a time should be taken to the bedside, with the other units remaining in a monitored blood bank refrigerator; moreover, if it is decided not to transfuse after the blood has been issued but before the unit is entered, the blood should be returned to the blood bank refrigerator within 30 minutes, since it requires approximately 45 minutes of room temperature exposure for the temperature of blood to exceed 10 °C, the maximum allowable for shipping blood.

In addition, it is important to impose strict storage periods for blood and components that limit the potential for bacterial growth. Thus, while it appears safe to store whole blood and red blood cells prepared in a closed system for up to 42 days at 1 to 6 °C, it does not currently appear to be safe to store platelets for more than 5 days at 20 to 24 °C. In addition, any product customarily stored at 1 to 6 °C that is prepared by an open method (ie, red blood cells prepared from whole blood in a single bag) should be transfused within 24 hours or discarded; any product that is customarily stored at 20 to 24 °C after preparation or pooling (ie, platelets or thawed cryoprecipitate) should be transfused within 4 hours or discarded. These time frames have been established apparently on an arbitrary basis in the absence of data, erring on the side of safety, although they may be modified in the future based on scientific data. Thus, it appears that platelets collected by apheresis only rarely are contaminated by bacteria if stored for less than 3 days,[59] and the introduction of "sterile docking devices" may allow maintenance of a "closed" system during procedures that currently require use of open technique such as pooling platelets and cryoprecipitate or deglycerolyzing frozen red blood cells. If substantiated, the use of such devices may allow extension of the storage interval.

References

1. Borden CW, Hall WH: Fatal transfusion reactions from massive bacterial contamination of blood. *N Engl Med* 245:760–765, 1951.

2. Anderson KC, Lew MA, Gorgone BC, et al: Transfusion-related sepsis after prolonged platelet storage. *Am J Med* 81:405–410, 1986.

3. Stenhouse MAE, Milner LV: *Yersinia enterocolitica*: A hazard in blood transfusion. *Transfusion* 22:396–398, 1982.

4. Tabor E, Gerety RJ: Five cases of pseudomonas sepsis transmitted by blood transfusion (letter). *Lancet* 1:1403, 1984.

5. Wright DC, Seiss IF, Vinton, KJ, et al: Fatal *Yersinia enterocolitica* sepsis after blood transfusion. *Arch Pathol Lab Med* 109:1040–1042, 1985.

6. Rhame FS, Root RK, MacLowery JD, et al: Salmonella septicemia from platelet transfusions. *Ann Intern Med* 78:633–641, 1973.

7. Heal JM, Jones ME, Forey J, et al: Fatal salmonella septicemia after platelet transfusion. *Transfusion* 27:2–5, 1987.

8. MacFarlane RG, Mainwaring BRS, MacSween JC, Parish HJ: Technique for the filtration of human plasma and serum for transfusion. *Br Med J* 1:377–381, 1942.

9. Swedberg B, Widstrom G, Alin K: The importance of aseptic technique and the fallaciousness of chemical bacteriostatics in blood banking and plasma preserving. *Acta Med Scand* 127:480–493, 1947.

10. Whitby LEH: The hazards of transfusion. *Lancet* 1:581–584, 1942.

11. Novak M: Preservation of stored blood with sulfanilamide. *JAMA* 113:2227–2229, 1939.

12. Duma RJ, Warner JF, Dalton HP: Septicemia from intravenous infusions. *N Engl J Med* 284:257–260, 1971.

13. Maki DG, Martin WT: Nationwide epidemic of septicemia caused by contaminated infusion products: IV. Growth of microbial pathogens in fluids for intravenous infusion. *J Infect Dis* 131:267–272, 1975.

14. Steere AC, Tenney JH, Mackel DC, et al: *Pseudomonas* species bacteremia caused by contaminated normal human serum albumin. *J Infect Dis* 135:729–735, 1977.

15. Kosmin M: Bacteremia during leukapheresis. *Transfusion* 20:115, 1980.

16. Blajchman MA, Thornley JH, Richardson H, et al: Platelet transfusion-induced *Serratia marcescens* sepsis due to vacuum tube contamination. *Transfusion* 19:39–44, 1979.

17. Felsby M, Munk-Anderson G, Siboni K: Simultaneous contamination of transfusion blood with *Enterobacter agglomerans* and *Pseudomonas flurescens*, supposedly from the pilot tubes. *J Med Microbiol* 6:413–416, 1973.

18. Katz L, Johnson DL, Neufeld PD, et al: Evacuated blood-collection tubes: The backflow hazard. *Can Med Assn J* 113:208–213, 1975.

19. McLeish WA, Corrigan EN, Elder RH, Westwood JCN: Contaminated vacuum tubes (letter). *Can Med Assoc J* 112:682, 1975.

20. Rhame FS, McCullough J, Hospital Infections Branch, Bacterial Diseases Div., Bureau of Epidemiology, CDC: Nosocomial *Pseudomonas cepacia* infection. *MMWR* 28:289–290, 1979.

21. Rhame FS, McCullough J, Hospital Infections Branch, Bacterial Diseases Div, Bureau of Epidemiology, CDC: Follow-up on nosocomial *Pseudomonas cepacia* infection. *MMWR* 28:409, 1979.

22. Elliott GA, MacFarlane RG, Vaughan JM: The use of stored blood for transfusion. *Lancet* 1:384–387, 1939.

23. Braude AI, Sanford JP, Bartlett JE, Mallery OT Jr: Effects and clinical significance of bacterial contaminants in transfused blood. *J Lab Clin Med* 39:902–916, 1952.

24. Wetterlow LH, Kay FH, Edsall G: Missed contaminations in biologic products: The role of psychrophilic bacteria. *J Lab Clin Med* 43:411–421, 1954.

25. James JD, Stokes EJ: Effect of temperature on survival of bacteria in blood for transfusion, with a note on contamination by cold growing organisms. *Br Med J* 2:1389–1395, 1957.

26. Chaplin H, Chang E, Kolb RW: Report of routine tests for psychrophilic and mesophilic contaminants in banked blood. *J Appl Microbiol* 3:213–215, 1955.

27. Pittman M: A study of bacteria implicated in transfusion reactions and of bacteria isolated from blood products: *J Lab Clin Med* 42:273–288, 1953.

28. Walter CW, Kundsin RB, Button LN: New technic for detection of bacterial contamination in a blood bank using plastic equipment. *N Engl J Med* 257:364–369, 1957.

29. Geller P, Jawetz E: Experimental studies on bacterial contaminations of bank blood: I. The nature of 'toxicity' of contaminated blood. *J Lab Clin Med* 43:696–706, 1954.

30. Khabbaz RF, Arnow PM, Highsmith AK, et al: *Pseudomonas fluorescens* bacteremia from blood transfusion. *Am J Med* 76:62–67, 1984.

31. McEntegart MG: Dangerous contaminants in stored blood. *Lancet* 1:909–911, 1956.

32. Braude AI, Carey FJ, Siemienski J: Studies of bacterial transfusion reactions from refrigerated blood: The properties of cold-growing bacteria. *J Clin Invest* 34:311–325, 1954.

33. Braude AI: Transfusion reactions from contaminated blood: Their recognition and treatment. *N Engl J Med* 258:1289–1293, 1958.

34. Paxon CL: Collection and use of autologous fetal blood. *Am J Obstet Gynecol* 134:708–710, 1979.

35. Strauss RG, Crawford GF, Elbert C, et al: Sterility and quality of blood dispensed in syringes for infants. *Transfusion* 26:163–166, 1986.

36. Kahn RA, Meryman HT, Syring RL, Flinton LJ: The fate of bacteria in frozen red cells. *Transfusion* 16:215–220, 1976.

37. Myhre BA, Nakasako YY, Schott R: Studies on 4 °C stored frozen-reconstituted red blood cells: I. Bacterial growth. *Transfusion* 17:454–459, 1977.

38. Honig CL, Bove JR: Transfusion-Associated Fatalities: Review of Bureau of Biologics Report 1976–1978. *Transfusion* 20:653–661, 1980.

39. Myhre BA: Fatalities from blood transfusion. *JAMA* 244:1333–1335, 1980.

40. Heal JM, Singal S, Sardisco E, Mayer T: Bacterial proliferation in platelet concentrates. *Transfusion* 26:388–390, 1986.

41. Katz AJ, Tilton RC: Sterility of platelet concentrates stored at 25 °C. *Transfusion* 10:329–339, 1970.

42. Mallin WS, Reuss DT, Bracke JW, et al: Bacteriological studies of platelet concentrates stored at 22 °C and 4 °C. *Transfusion* 13:439–442, 1973.

43. Silver H, Sonnenwirth AC, Beisser LD: Bacteriologic study of platelet concentrates prepared and stored without refrigeration. *Transfusion* 10:315–316, 1970.

44. Buchholz DH, Young VM, Friedman NR, et al: Bacterial proliferation in platelet products stored at room temperature: Transfusion-induced enterobacteria sepsis. *N Engl J Med* 285:429–433, 1971.

45. Buchholz DH, Young VM, Freidman NR, et al: Detection and quantitation of bacteria in platelet products stored at ambient temperature. *Transfusion* 13:268–275, 1973.

46. Cunningham M, Cash JD: Bacterial contamination of platelet concentrates stored at 20 °C. *J Clin Pathol* 26:401–404, 1973.

47. Wrenn HE, Speicher CE: Platelet concentrates: Sterility of 400 single units stored at room temperature. *Transfusion* 14:171–172, 1974.

48. Goddard D, Jacobs SI, Manohitharajah SM: The bacteriological screening of platelet concentrates stored at 22 °C. *Transfusion* 13:103–106, 1973.

49. Kahn RA, Syring RL: The fate of bacteria introduced into whole blood from which platelet concentrates were prepared and stored at 22 or 4 °C. *Transfusion* 15:363–367, 1975.

50. Myhre BA, Walker LJ, White ML: Bacteriocidal properties of platelet concentrates. *Transfusion* 14:116–123, 1974.

51. Braine HG, Kickler TS, Charache P, et al: Bacterial sepsis secondary to platelet transfusion: An adverse effect of extended storage at room temperature. *Transfusion* 26:391–393, 1986.

52. Arnow PM, Weiss LM, Weil O, Rosen NR: *Escherichia coli* sepsis from contaminated platelet transfusion. *Arch Intern Med* 146:321–324, 1986.

53. Stevens AR Jr, Legg JS, Henry BS, et al: Fatal transfusion reactions from contamination of stored blood by cold growing bacteria. *Ann Intern Med* 39:1228–1239, 1953.

54. File TM Jr, Tan JS, Salstrom S-J et al: Timentin versus pipercillin or moxalactam in the therapy of acute bacterial infections. *Antimicrob Agents Chemother* 26:310, 1984.

55. Fuchs PC, Barry AL, Thornberry C, Jones RN: In vitro activity of ticarcillin plus clavulanic acid against 632 clinical isolates. *Antimicrob Agents Chemother* 16:497, 1985.

56. Freimer EH, Donabedian H, Raeder R, Ribner BS: Empirical use of imipenem as the sole antibiotic in the treatment of serious infections: *J Antimicrob Chemother* 16:497, 1985.

57. Jones RN; Review of the in vitro spectrum of activity of imipenem. *Am J Med* 78(6A):22, 1985.

58. Baltch Al, Pressman HL, Hammer MC, et al: Bacteremia following dental extractions in patients with and without penicillin prophylaxis. *Am J Med Sci* 283:129–140, 1982.

59. Szymanski IO: Sterility of single-donor apheresis platelets (letter). *Transfusion* 25:290, 1985.

13
Donor Screening Procedures and Their Role in Enhancing Transfusion Safety

Steven Kleinman, MD

Many techniques have been and continue to be utilized in an effort to protect the transfusion recipient against transfusion-transmitted disease. Although laboratory testing is the method that is probably of greatest visibility to the public, other methods have been utilized first when a new infectious disease has been found to be transmitted by transfusion.[1] In the cases of transfusion-transmitted hepatitis and AIDS, for example, the recognition of disease transmission preceded the discovery of the etiologic agent and the development of serologic tests. The etiologic agent of Creutzfeldt-Jakob disease has not yet been characterized, but policies have been implemented to decrease the risk of its transmission by transfusion.[2]

Thus, in the usual sequence of events, the possibility that there is a significant risk of transmitting an infectious disease agent necessitates that donor screening decisions be made in the absence of firm scientific data. At this point, a reasonable approach is to construct a hypothesis as to which groups of persons may be likely to transmit the disease agent and to act on that hypothesis by establishing donor selection criteria. As further knowledge of the etiologic agent is obtained, better estimates can be made about its prevalence in various groups. When appropriate serologic methods become available, donor selection criteria can be formulated based on large-scale epidemiologic studies. Such studies should produce data that will permit an evaluation of the efficacy of the donor selection criteria. Ideally, at this stage of knowledge, donor selection criteria could be appropriately modified.[1]

While this approach is theoretically sound, it must be recognized that the legal and practical limitations of liberalizing donor selection criteria in the current climate of concern about transfusion safety are formidable, especially if such procedures have been included in the Code of Federal Regulations.

Approaches to Blood Safety

The theoretical approaches to improving the safety of blood transfusion are simple and straightforward. First, if a donor is found to pose a risk of transmitting disease, the unit of blood should not be drawn. Second, after the unit of blood is collected, it can be discarded based on results of laboratory testing. At this stage, the unit may also be discarded if additional information concerning the donor has been obtained; such information may be supplied by the donor after the donation or may be obtained by checking the donor's name against a list of permanently ineligible persons (using a donor deferral registry). Third, the collected unit of blood may be modified by physical or chemical methods to remove or inactivate infectious agents that may be present in some units, despite donor screening and laboratory testing.

These methods for assuring the safety of transfused blood need to be considered as additive and not mutually exclusive. Several arguments can be made for continuing to use donor selection procedures even after the implementation of serologic testing for a particular agent. First, it is unlikely that any laboratory test (or combination of tests) will be 100% sensitive in detecting the carrier state for any infectious disease. The limitations of the test may be due to a "window period" during which the donor is infectious but the laboratory test has not yet turned positive (eg, anti-HIV) or may be due to a persistently negative carrier state (eg, HBsAg).[3,4] The possibility also exists that after some time, a donor would no longer test positive for an infectious agent or alternatively that a donor could intermittently test negative while still being infectious.[5,6] A second limitation in placing total reliance on laboratory testing is the possibility of error.[7] A technical or clerical error in a laboratory testing procedure could possibly result in the release of an infectious unit of blood if such an infectious unit has been collected by the blood bank. In an efficiently functioning blood center, such errors should be rare. However, the use of donor selection criteria to defer donors who might have a high probability of transmitting infection will provide an additional safeguard against the possibility of such an error. Furthermore, from a practical standpoint, the work load of the laboratory (in performing confirmatory testing and quarantine procedures) will be diminished if fewer units with positive laboratory test results are collected. The issues of decreased workload and the prevention of potential errors provide compelling arguments for performing laboratory testing on blood donor samples at the donation site before collection of the unit of blood. Such approaches are currently under development.

While there are distinct advantages to eliminating donors with higher probabilities of positive laboratory tests and higher risks of disease transmission, there is also a disadvantage to this approach. If donor eligibility criteria are nonspecific (as they often are), it should be expected that large numbers of persons who are perfectly safe will be eliminated as blood donors.[8] This may have a substantial impact on the amount of blood available for distribution and transfusion. While this dilemma has been universally recognized, there is no formal set of rules that can be applied to determine if

Table 13–1 Types of Donor Screening Procedures Used to Protect the Blood Supply

Procedure	Diseases That May Be Eliminated
Preselection of donor groups	Hepatitis, AIDS
Elimination of donor incentives (paid donors)	Hepatitis
Public education	AIDS
Donor "self-deferral"	AIDS
Health history interview	Hepatitis, AIDS, malaria, others
Telephone call-back	All infectious diseases
Confidential unit exclusion	AIDS
Donor deferral registries	Hepatitis, AIDS
Posttransfusion case follow-up	Hepatitis, others

the implementation of given criteria for donor eligibility is indicated. Instead, such decisions have usually been made intuitively, attempting to balance some or all of the following factors: the extent of disease transmission, the severity of the consequences of such disease to the recipients, the number of donors lost by implementation of an eligibility requirement, and the stigmatization of donors who are rejected.

In considering and evaluating interventions (both donor screening and laboratory testing) to improve the safety of blood, I believe that certain basic risk-reduction axioms will hold. (1) In a biologic system, it is unlikely that any method can be 100% effective. Therefore, if we desire to achieve zero risk, multiple methods are required. (2) The drawback to using multiple methods is that as procedures become administratively more complex the potential for error increases. (3) Successive risk reductions achieve less but cost more. (4) If the risk is already low, it will be extremely difficult to measure the effect of adding additional procedures that are designed to provide further safeguards.

Specific Methods

A number of different approaches (exclusive of laboratory testing) have been utilized in attempts to improve the safety of transfused blood (Table 13–1).

Preselection of Donor Groups

Because of the increased risk of possible disease transmission, blood banks do not collect blood at particular types of institutions, including prisons, homes for the mentally retarded, and agencies or groups that serve primarily male homosexuals.[9-11]

Removal of Self-Serving Donor Incentives

The primary example of a self-serving donor incentive that has been associated with disease transmission is the payment of cash to blood donors. To this end, the federal government instituted regulations in 1978 that required the labeling of a unit of blood with a volunteer or paid donor sticker.[12] Some states have passed laws prohibiting, except in special circumstances, the use of commercial blood donors. It is clear that the elimination of commercial blood donors has been the most important event in decreasing the risk of posttransfusion hepatitis.[13]

In the early 1970s, commercial blood donors were documented to have a greater rate of exposure to hepatitis B (anti-HBs–positive) and of the hepatitis B carrier state (HBsAg–positive).[14,15] Despite the advent of HBsAg testing, it could be predicted that this population would still be at greater risk for transmitting hepatitis B infection due to an increased prevalence of carrier donors with subdetectable HBsAg levels. Furthermore, because of the financial incentive to donate, this high-risk population of donors would be less likely to provide a truthful medical history, thereby removing the safeguard provided by the donor screening process. The combined factors of an increased prevalence of the viral carrier state and the compromised donor history contribute to the decreased safety of this group of donors.

It should be pointed out that many authors have suggested that it is not the act of payment that makes a blood donor unsafe but the fact that a particular type of person from a socioeconomic group of lower status is attracted by the financial incentive.[16,17] In contrast, it has been demonstrated that the use of paid donors from a different segment of society has not been associated with an increased risk of disease transmission.[18] Nevertheless, it must be recognized that the payment of blood donors will increase the likelihood of inaccurate donor histories and raises the risk of attracting persons from a lower-status socioeconomic background in whom the risk of hepatitis transmission (and perhaps other infectious disease agents) is greater.

A more controversial aspect of donor incentives is the providing of blood at decreased cost to recipients who supply replacement donors.[19] This nonreplacement fee is still used in some blood banks in the United States. There are no data that address the relative safety of this group of donors.

Another controversial issue that has emerged in the past several years is whether blood from autologous donors who fulfill homologous donor requirements can be "crossed over" to be used by other transfusion recipients.[20] It has been argued that because these donors have the additional incentive of donating for themselves, they may be less likely to be truthful during the medical history process. However, consistently increased infectious disease carrier rates have not been clearly documented in these donors.[21] Furthermore, it has been argued that these donors will be no less truthful than other donors if they are assured that an accurate medical history will not preclude collection of blood for their own use. Although some blood centers currently do not use blood from autologous donors for homologous use (crossover donors), there currently are no regulations that prohibit this practice.[22]

An additional mechanism of safeguarding the blood supply by removing incentives for a particular high-risk population to donate blood was the establishment of alternative testing sites for HIV antibody. This program attempted to remove the benefit of easily available, no-cost anti-HIV testing at the blood center as an incentive for donation.[23]

Selection of Donors Through Education

This approach became widely used in 1983 with the recognition that HIV could be transmitted by blood transfusion. Specific groups of individuals were identified as being at high risk of AIDS (eg, male homosexuals with multiple partners and intravenous drug users who shared needles).[24] Extensive efforts were made by blood banks through the use of the media and through discussion with gay community leaders to inform the public that individuals with such risk factors should not donate blood. Community education was augmented by distribution of written information concerning donor eligibility at the time of donor recruitment.[24] In addition to their traditional function, donor recruitment departments were given the additional task of instructing individuals with possible risk factors to refrain from blood donation.[25]

Self-Assessment Before Donation

Donor eligibility has always been routinely assessed at the time of health history interview by blood center personnel. In 1983, in response to AIDS transmission by transfusion, an additional mechanism was introduced in which predonation written material provided to blood donors at the collection site was modified to include a description of risk factors for various transfusion-transmitted diseases (AIDS, hepatitis, malaria, and syphilis). Donors were instructed that if one of the described conditions or risk factors applied to them, then they should not proceed with the donation process.[24]

Health History Interview

During the health history interview, the donor is asked questions that may lead to deferral. These questions can be broadly classified into the following categories:

1. Medical history of a specific disease (hepatitis, AIDS, malaria).
2. History of possible exposure to a disease due to specific behavior (AIDS, hepatitis).
3. History of possible exposure to a disease secondary to travel (malaria).
4. History of possible exposure to a disease secondary to country of birth (malaria, AIDS).
5. Medical symptoms compatible with a specific disease (AIDS).

Opportunity for Donor to Designate That the Blood Donation Not Be Used

Most blood centers have traditionally had procedures whereby blood donors could call the blood center after their donation and volunteer pertinent additions to their medical histories. These mechanisms were most often used when donors developed a febrile illness shortly after donation. With the advent of AIDS, this telephone call-back system became formalized as a mechanism for donors to indicate risk factors for HIV infection that they might not have freely admitted to at the time of donation.[24] In addition to the telephone call-back mechanism, the possibility of HIV transmission has led to the introduction of a system known as confidential unit exclusion. Using this procedure, the donor can designate, before phlebotomy, whether his or her blood should be used for transfusion purposes.[26]

Donor Deferral Registries

Donor deferral registries were originated in an effort to decrease the risk of transfusion-associated hepatitis. More recently their use has been extended to also include donors who could transmit HIV infection.

These registries are computer or microfiche files of donors who have been previously deferred for specified reasons. Individual blood centers have established in-house donor deferral registries to comply with a section of the Code of Federal Regulations that states that persons who have ever tested positive for HBsAg or anti-HIV should no longer be accepted as blood donors. The rationale of donor deferral registries is that individuals with a previous positive test result may revert to a negative test result at a later date despite the fact that they could still transmit disease.[1] This situation could occur because of either a biologic phenomenon or a testing error. However, in the case of anti-HIV testing by the screening ELISA method, this would most likely be due to the fact that the original reaction was false-positive.

Donor deferral registries have expanded to include the names of donors who have previously volunteered information (ie, history of intravenous drug use, hepatitis, or high-risk AIDS activity) that should have permanently excluded them as blood donors. Donors who volunteer such information at one visit may be tempted to withhold the information at a subsequent visit, especially if their self-assessment is that the history ought not to have precluded them as blood donors. While precise statistics for this phenomenon are unavailable, it has been documented to occur at the Los Angeles–Orange Counties Region of the American Red Cross despite the fact that deferred donors receive written notification of their permanent exclusion.

Since donors may not always donate to the same blood collection agency, some states have created statewide donor deferral registries that include the names of donors deferred at any blood collection agency within the state. The American Red Cross uses a system in which donors who are entered into the donor deferral registry of an individual Red Cross region also have their names included in a national registry.[1] Because of donor confidentiality concerns, donor deferral registries that extend beyond an individual blood center do not list the reason for donor entry to the registry.

The donor deferral registry is used by checking the identity of new donors against the names in the registry; if a donation has been made by a previously deferred donor, that unit is identified, quarantined, and destroyed. Large donor deferral registries encounter the problem of "false hits," ie, blood from a donor with the same name as a donor already in the registry may be misidentified as unsuitable for transfusion.

Maintenance and continued use of a statewide or national donor deferral registry is time consuming, logistically complex, and expensive. Unfortunately it has remained difficult to assess whether such massive efforts afford significant increases in safety to the blood transfusion recipient.

Donor Selection Criteria in Various Diseases

Hepatitis

General considerations.   Hepatitis was identified as a serious complication of blood transfusion in the 1800s; its serious nature was reemphasized by complications of vaccination programs during World War II.[16] Consequently, donor selection criteria for preventing hepatitis transmission were implemented before the discovery of the viral agents that cause this disease. At the time of implementation, the utility of many of these criteria could not be evaluated since no serologic testing existed. With the discovery of both the hepatitis A and hepatitis B viruses and the development of serologic tests for these two agents, data could be accumulated concerning the potential efficacy of hepatitis donor screening methods. However, it became apparent by 1975, only a few years after the development of laboratory testing to screen for hepatitis B, that a substantial amount of posttransfusion hepatitis was spread by one or more viral agents designated as the non-A, non-B virus(es).[27,28] Recently, serologic tests have been developed for a newly discovered agent of non-A, non-B hepatitis (termed *hepatitis C virus*), despite the fact that the virus has not yet been isolated or fully characterized.[29,30] Preliminary data indicate that at least 80% of post transfusion non-A non-B hepatitis is due to Hepatitis C.[34] Table 13–2 summarizes the evolution of hepatitis donor screening procedures.

Regulations.   Initial federal guidelines for preventing the transmission of hepatitis from blood donors were established in the 1950s.[17] The current guidelines (Code of Federal Regulations 640.3), which have remained unchanged in the Code of Federal Regulations since at least 1975,[31] state that individuals shall not be used as blood donors if they have:

a. a history of viral hepatitis,
b. a history of close contact within 6 months of donation with an individual having viral hepatitis,
c. a history of having received within 6 months a transfusion of 'human blood.'[32]

Section 610.41 of the Code of Federal Regulations states: "A person testing positive for HBsAg or known to have previously tested positive for HBsAg may not serve as a donor of human blood."

Table 13–2 Donor Screening Procedures to Protect Against Hepatitis Transmission

Event	Action
Recognition of transfusion transmitted hepatitis	Establishment of donor deferral criteria
Discovery of hepatitis B virus and development of HB$_s$AG testing	Validation of increased risk from commercial blood donors
	Donor deferral registries established
Discovery of Hepatitis A virus	Modification of donor deferral criteria in some countries (not USA)
Implementation of anti-HBC and ALT testing as surrogate tests for non-A, non-B hepatitis	No changes in donor deferral criteria but change in posttransfusion hepatitis follow-up at some blood centers
Development of a test for hepatitis C	Probable change of some donor deferral criteria from 6 months to 12 months

The standards of the AABB cite the following additional donor restrictions: (1) deferral of donors with a tattoo applied in the previous 6 months; (2) deferral of the donor if the donor's unit was the only unit given to a patient who developed posttransfusion hepatitis within 6 months.[33] The 1989 version of the AABB standards differs from previous versions and from the Code of Federal Regulations with regard to eligibility of donors with a history of viral hepatitis. The AABB standards permit donations by persons with a history of viral hepatitis in the event that the episode of hepatitis occurred before 10 years of age.

New data regarding hepatitis C indicate that, in some cases, seroconversion to anti-hepatitis C virus may not occur for 6 months to 1 year after exposure.[34] Since anti-hepatitis C virus positivity is correlated with HCV infectivity,[34] these data suggest that an asymptomatic seronegative HCV carrier may escape detection by anti-HCV testing for up to one year after such exposure. For this reason, the AABB standards have recently extended to 1 year the deferral period after blood transfusion or close contact with an individual having viral hepatitis.

The American Red Cross requirements for donor deferral include those required by the FDA and those recommended by the AABB.[35] In contrast to the revised AABB standards, all donors with a history of viral hepatitis are deferred from donation. In addition, Red Cross requires that (1) a question be asked concerning any history of intravenous drug use (a positive answer requires permanent deferral); (2) that persons residing in penal institutions, psychiatric hospitals, and institutions for the mentally retarded be deferred due to the high incidence of hepatitis in those institutional settings.

Deferral statistics.   In the Los Angeles–Orange Counties Red Cross region, deferral statistics for hepatitis related deferrals for a 4-month period

(January through April 1987) were compiled. During this period approximately 150,000 persons volunteered to donate blood. Deferral rates were as follows:

History of hepatitis (including case-by-case evaluation of
donors with a history of jaundice or liver disease, or a
positive blood test for hepatitis)   0.11%

History of blood transfusion (or blood injection or tattoo)
within the past 6 months   0.08%

History of close contact in the past 6 months with a patient
who has had hepatitis, jaundice, or undergoing
hemodialysis   0.06%

History of intravenous drug use: 0.06%

Total of hepatitis-related deferrals: 0.31%

The best available data indicate that 14.8 million persons volunteer to donate blood annually in the United States.[36] Using the deferral rates from the Los Angeles–Orange Counties region as representative of the entire country, it can be calculated that 45,880 persons are deferred annually for hepatitis-related reasons. Of these deferrals, 28,120 are permanent because of the possibility of a chronic carrier state (eg, history of hepatitis or intravenous drug use) and 17,760 are 6-month deferrals, because of the possibility of acute hepatitis infection. While it is unknown with what frequency persons in the latter group will make a future attempt to donate blood, data suggest that most donors who are temporarily deferred do not return at a later date.[37]

Specific deferral criteria

Commercial (paid) donors.   It had been known as early as 1959 that blood from commercial donors carried a sixfold increased risk for transmitting icteric hepatitis to transfusion recipients.[38] With the development of HBsAg testing in the early 1970s, studies confirmed that commercial donors had much higher carrier rates of the hepatitis B virus than did volunteer donors.[14,15] The most definitive study concerning disease transmission by commercial blood was performed by Alter and colleagues,[13] who demonstrated that rates of posttransfusion hepatitis were dramatically lowered because of the combined effect of eliminating commercial blood donors and the introduction of HBsAg testing. They estimated that 75% of the documented reduction was due to the elimination of the commercial donor source. In addition to posing an increased risk for hepatitis B transmission, commercial donors have also been shown to carry an increased risk for the transmission of non-A, non-B hepatitis.[39] In a review article, Aach and Kahn[40] reported the results of four studies that showed that the rate of non-A, non-B hepatitis in recipients of blood from commercial donors ranged from 17% to 53%. Since it is possible that still other hepatitis viruses are transmitted via blood transfusion, the experience with hepatitis B and non-A, non-B suggests that the use of commercial donor blood will still be likely to carry an increased risk of disease transmission.

In 1978, the FDA established requirements that the source of blood (commercial *v* volunteer) must be indicated on the label of the blood bag.[12] Virtually all blood in the United States is now collected from volunteer donors. In the past, commercial donors generally were people from lower socioeconomic classes. Although it has been suggested that volunteer donor blood collected from donors in lower socioeconomic groups (such as on selected military bases) may also carry an increased risk for hepatitis transmission,[41] these data have not been confirmed and blood collection policies based on a donor's socioeconomic status have not been seriously considered.

Donors with a history of intravenous drug use.   Both hepatitis B and non-A, non-B (including hepatitis C virus) are spread by parenteral routes and therefore can be spread between intravenous drug users who share needles.[16] Because of the potential for hepatitis transmission, persons who have ever injected intravenous drugs by needle have long been deferred as blood donors by the American Red Cross.[35] The importance of eliminating current or former intravenous drug users as blood donors has been reemphasized during the AIDS epidemic. Efforts to protect the blood supply from HIV have resulted in extending the prohibition of donation by intravenous drug users to also exclude their sexual partners.[42] This newer criterion may fortuitously also have the effect of decreasing the risk of hepatitis transmission. It has been shown that 26% of persons with clinical non-A, non-B hepatitis who had no direct hepatitis risk factors gave a history of exposure to household members who either admitted parenteral drug use, received a blood transfusion, or worked in a medical or dental field.[43] Hepatitis C virus seropositivity in intravenous drug users has recently been documented to be 70%; studies are currently in progress to determine the rate of hepatitis C virus seropositivity in their sexual partners.[44]

Donors with a history of viral hepatitis or jaundice.   In the United States, the FDA requires that all donors with a history of viral hepatitis be permanently deferred. Data to support this policy are provided by two early studies, one of which actually suggests that a 5-year deferral period would be almost as effective as permanent deferral.[45,46] These studies reflect the situation prior to HBsAg testing of donated blood and are limited by the small number of cases followed up and the use of clinical jaundice as a diagnostic sign of hepatitis.

Policies concerning history of hepatitis and deferral from blood donation vary from country to country. In a survey conducted in 1981, it was reported that while a history of hepatitis was cause for permanent deferral in 11 countries, such donors were temporarily deferred (for periods of 6 months to 5 years) in seven additional countries.[47] In 1977, a WHO expert panel recommended that deferral for a history of viral hepatitis be temporary.[48]

In at least two countries where donors with a history of viral hepatitis are not permanently deferred (the United Kingdom and the Netherlands), the rates of hepatitis B and non-A, non-B hepatitis are low.[49,50] Several studies performed in the United Kingdom have indicted that the large majority of patients with a history of hepatitis or jaundice had antibodies to the hepatitis A virus.[49,51] Since the transmission of hepatitis A by blood transfusion is extremely rare,[52] the incidence of non-A, non-B hepatitis is low, and hepatitis B transmission is prevented by HBsAg screening, the policy for deferral of such donors in the United Kingdom was modified to require only temporary deferral.[53]

Several authors have attempted to study prospective donors in the United States who admit to a history of hepatitis. In a study of 203 prospective donors with a history of hepatitis or contact with a hepatitis patient, Polesky and Hanson[54] found that 30% had antibody to hepatitis A and 14% had antibody to hepatitis B. In a second study of 138 donors with a history of hepatitis or jaundice, 41% had been exposed to hepatitis A and 23% to hepatitis B.[55] Despite serologic evidence of exposure to hepatitis A or B, it is possible that the exposure to these agents produced subclinical disease, while the clinical episode of hepatitis may have been caused by another hepatitis virus, such as hepatitis C.[28,56] In support of this hypothesis, a case-control study of patients with acute non-A, non-B hepatitis showed that these patients had an increased prevalence of antibody to hepatitis B (39% v 17% in controls), indicating that infection with multiple hepatitis agents may occur at different times in the same patient population.[57] The two previously cited studies (as well as an additional study[43]) have shown that approximately one third of donors with a history of hepatitis had negative serologic tests for antibodies to hepatitis A and B. It is possible therefore that these donors might have been previously exposed to the hepatitis C virus, and have become carriers who were capable of transmitting the infection.

Using data obtained from prospective studies of transfusion-transmitted hepatitis in the late 1970s,[39] as well as estimates of the likelihood of acute non-A, non-B infection leading to the carrier state, Alter[58] has calculated that 12.5% of individuals with a history of clinical hepatitis may be carriers of the non-A, non-B agent. Even though the introduction of surrogate testing for non-A, non-B and testing for hepatitis C virus antibody may detect most of these potential carriers, it still remains possible that, because of limitations of first-generation hepatitis C virus testing, the rate of potential transmission from this group of donors will exceed that of blood donors who do not supply such a history. Therefore, although deferral because of a history of hepatitis probably does little to protect the transfusion recipient from hepatitis B acquisition (since HBsAg and anti-HBc screening are done), it seems prudent to continue this practice for prevention of hepatitis C and any other possible agents of non-A, non-B hepatitis.

Most authorities agree that since hepatitis A is rarely transmitted by blood transfusion (except during asymptomatic acute-phase infection),[52] donors should be considered safe if their previous hepatitis can be documented to be due to hepatitis A.[28,54] Unfortunately, donors will rarely be able to provide documentation that an acute episode of hepatitis was temporally related to the development of hepatitis A antibodies.

The recent change in AABB standards that allows donation from persons with a history of viral hepatitis before age 10 is predicated on the fact that inferences about the cause of hepatitis can be made based on epidemiologic data.[57,59] Hepatitis A is extremely common in childhood, whereas hepatitis B and non-A, non-B hepatitis are rare.[16] Since both of the latter two viruses are transmitted primarily by parenteral and sexual routes, it may be more difficult to establish an origin of hepatitis acquired during adolescence, since it is conceivable that such activities might be practiced by teenagers. For this reason, 10 years of age was selected as a cutoff; individuals whose clinical hepatitis occurred before age 11 are assumed to have had hepatitis A and are acceptable as blood donors according to AABB criteria.

In the past, a history of jaundice was also cause for deferral of donors.[60] Currently, most blood collection agencies do not automatically defer a donor with a history of jaundice; rather, the history is elucidated further to establish the cause of the jaundice.[35,61] Specifically, a history of neonatal jaundice or jaundice due to biliary tract disease does not prevent persons from serving as blood donors. Furthermore, donors who have histories of hepatitis associated with anesthesia, medications, chemical exposures, or infectious mononucleosis generally are accepted as donors, since readily transmissible viral agents have been excluded as the likely cause of the clinical episode.[61]

Donors who have had close contact with a hepatitis patient. The regulation for a 6-month deferral of persons who have had close contact with a patient with hepatitis was initiated before the discovery of the hepatitis A and B viruses.

Subsequent to the availability of HBsAg testing, epidemiologic studies have strongly suggested that while hepatitis B may be transmitted by sexual contact, it is extremely rare for hepatitis B to be transmitted from an acutely infected patient to a nonintimate household contact.[62] The question of transmission of hepatitis C by sexual or household contact has not yet been fully resolved. Preliminary data suggest that sexual transmission can occur but is likely to be infrequent.[63]

While the data are sufficient to establish that persons who have had sexual contact with hepatitis patients should be temporarily deferred, there are no convincing data to support the deferral of persons who have close (nonsexual) contact with a person who has acute hepatitis B. Nevertheless, federal regulations require this deferral, which is uniformly practiced by blood collecting agencies.

The American Red Cross Blood Services Directives and a recent edition of a standard blood-banking textbook use similar definitions for close contact.[35,61] Close contact is defined as (1) the sharing of household, kitchen, and toilet facilities, or (2) living in a group setting such as a dormitory or military barracks where multiple cases of hepatitis have occurred. It should be noted that such a definition might appropriately apply to individuals at risk for acquiring hepatitis A transmission after an index case has occurred.

Attempts to define close contact raise practical problems. How should the prospective donor who occasionally visits or eats a meal with a patient who has viral hepatitis be evaluated? My opinion is that such persons should be acceptable as donors since the rationale for this entire deferral category is questionable.

The deferral of donors who may have been exposed to a person with hepatitis has been extended by the American Red Cross to include persons who reside in penal institutions, institutions for the mentally retarded, and psychiatric hospitals.[35] Since intravenous drug use and sexual encounters may occur in penal institutions, deferral of such donors seems reasonable with regard to potential hepatitis transmission, as well as with regard to HIV transmission.[9] Residents of institutions for the mentally retarded or of psychiatric institutions may engage in behaviors that permit the exchange of body fluids, and perhaps may therefore be at increased risk for transmitting hepatitis B or non-A, non-B hepatitis.[10]

American Red Cross procedures require that prospective donors be questioned as to whether or not they have been exposed (ie, nonsexually) to a hemodialysis patient. A decision as to whether or not to defer the donor is then made on a case-by-case basis. Deferral for such individuals is recommended in a standard blood-banking textbook.[61] Donors who are deferred for this reason are excluded based on the combined assumptions that a particular hemodialysis patient may be infected with hepatitis (B or C) and that transmission of such an infection may occur by nonsexual routes. In my opinion, the data do not convincingly support the deferral of such donors unless the hemodialysis patient is known to be a chronic hepatitis B carrier.

Donors who have received tattoos.   Because of the documented risk of hepatitis B transmission by the use of unsterile tattooing equipment,[64] prospective blood donors who have been tattooed are deferred for 6 months. No data exist documenting the efficacy of this procedure, although the number of donors deferred is probably minimal.

Donors who have had ear piercing or acupuncture.   Ear piercing and acupuncture are commonly performed procedures that utilize disposable sterile needles. Although, in the 1970s, there had been consideration given to deferring persons undergoing either one of these procedures,[65] such precautions seem unnecessary if such practices have been performed according to commonly established techniques.

Donors receiving hepatitis B immunoglobulin.   Hepatitis B immunoglobulin (HBIG) is administered to individuals who have suffered a possible parenteral exposure to hepatitis B. The administration of HBIG may delay the incubation period of hepatitis B for up to 12 months after exposure. For this reason, such donors are deferred for 12 rather than 6 months.[61]

Donors receiving hepatitis B vaccine.   These donors should be evaluated as to their possible exposure risk for hepatitis B. In the absence of any risks that require deferral, such donors should be accepted for blood donation.

Donors with possible occupational risk.   Using anti-HBs as a measure of past exposure, several studies conducted in the 1970s and early 1980s have demonstrated high rates of past hepatitis B infection in specific groups of health care workers, including hemodialysis staff, surgical personnel, physicians, dentists, and laboratory workers.[66-68] This led to formulation of policies that considered temporary deferral of hemodialysis workers, since they had been documented to have the highest risk of hepatitis B infection.[35,61] One rationale for such a policy was the possibility that health care personnel who had not previously developed hepatitis B infection might acquire a new case of hepatitis B that could be transmitted by blood donation during the acute phase of the infection. A second rationale for deferral of such individuals was that populations of health care workers might include an increased number of carriers with subdetectable levels of HBsAg.

Several changes have occurred since these studies were performed that make it less likely that hepatitis B will be transmitted from blood donated by health care workers. Rates of acute hepatitis B infection in health care workers are likely to have decreased in these particular occupational settings since many persons in such settings have received the hepatitis B vaccine. In addition, anti-HBc testing of donated blood should decrease the already low rate of hepatitis B transmission from persons who might be hepatitis B carriers but who have subdetectable HBsAg levels.[4]

There currently are no data to establish the relative risk of health care workers acquiring or transmitting hepatitis C; therefore, deferral of such personnel for this reason can only be speculative.

Blood-banking practices still include deferral of some health care workers in the previously discussed high-risk settings. The donor eligibility requirements of the American Red Cross suggest that individuals who deliver health care to hemodialysis patients, hemophiliacs, oncology patients, and trauma and emergency room patients be evaluated for possible temporary deferral.[35] All prospective donors are questioned as to whether they have been exposed to patients undergoing hemodialysis. A hemodialysis worker who responds affirmatively to this health history question might be temporarily deferred. However, since other specific questions about health care activities are not asked, it is unlikely that a history of other potential occupational exposures will routinely be elicited during the health history interview.

Health care workers who give a history of parenteral exposure (eg, needle-stick injury) within the past 6 months to body fluids from a patient with hepatitis B infection should be temporarily deferred.[61] In practice, since it may be difficult to obtain documentation of the hepatitis B infectivity of hospitalized patients, a parenteral exposure to body fluids of any patient may lead to a 6-month temporary deferral.

Donors with a history of transfusion.   Both the Code of Federal Regulations and AABB standards require that prospective donors who within the past 6 months received transfusion of blood or human blood components or derivatives known to be possible sources of hepatitis be deferred from blood donation.[32,33] Although there is a study demonstrating an association between a history of transfusion and hepatitis transmission, it was performed before HBsAg testing and furthermore, correlated hepatitis transmission with a lifetime history of transfusion rather than transfusion during the previous 6 months.[45] Given the rarity of hepatitis B transmission by blood transfusion since the implementation of HBsAg testing and the expected further decrease with the implementation of anti-HBc testing, such a requirement does not seem to be supportable for decreasing the risk of hepatitis B transmission.

However, in the case of hepatitis C, data indicate that the issue is somewhat different. Seroconversion may not occur for up to 1 year after exposure.[34] Therefore, newer policy recommendations require deferral for a period of 1 year after a transfusion episode.[34]

The issue of whether individuals who had ever previously received a blood transfusion should be allowed to donate blood can be considered with regard to potential for non-A, non-B transmission.[60] It had previously been estimated from hepatitis cases occurring after single-unit transfusions that as many as 2% of blood donors may be carriers of the non-A, non-B hepatitis virus.[58] Tabor et al[69] have provided the only data on the question of whether a lifetime history of transfusion may increase the risk of hepatitis transmission to recipients. In a study conducted after the routine use of HBsAg testing, they found that of 128 donors implicated in 1- or 2-unit cases of posttransfusion hepatitis (presumed to be non-A, non-B), only eight (6.2%) had a history of transfusion. Therefore, the large majority of non-A, non-B hepatitis was transmitted by donors without such a history. Unfortunately, the transfusion history of control donors (those donors not implicated in posttransfusion hepatitis) was not presented in this study.

Data for a history of previous transfusion can be obtained for comparison purposes from other sources. In the Los Angeles–Orange Counties Red Cross region in June 1986, we established that 4.5% of 32,000 interviewed donors had a history of transfusion; this percentage is similar to that found among the donors implicated in posttransfusion hepatitis in Tabor and colleagues'[69] study.

Since a significant portion of the donor population has previously received a blood transfusion, deferral of such donors would have a major impact on the blood supply. The available data fail to implicate donors with a lifetime history of transfusion as being less safe than other donors. Therefore, the current practice of accepting persons with a lifetime history of transfusion should be continued.

Posttransfusion hepatitis case investigations.   The rationale for posttransfusion hepatitis case investigation is to use evidence of clinical hepatitis in recipients to identify donors who might transmit hepatitis to additional recipients. In the 1950s and 1960s, such transmission occurred more frequently than at present and little else could be done to prevent future cases of hepatitis transmission. Currently, according to AABB criteria, if a patient receives a 1-unit transfusion and develops posttransfusion hepatitis, the donor of that unit must be deferred from future donations.[33] Such cases are rare, since almost all transfusion recipients receive multiple units of blood components. When the recipient has received multiple blood units, it is, of course, not possible to identify which donor transmitted the disease. Therefore, in cases of posttransfusion hepatitis B infection, some blood banks have attempted to investigate further a group of possibly implicated donors by recontacting them and retesting them for serologic evidence of hepatitis B infection.[70] This course of action has usually been unproductive. Given the current practice of screening blood for anti-HBc, this procedure would be expected to be even less productive than in the past.

In cases of posttransfusion non-A, non-B hepatitis, the lack of adequate tests has not allowed for postdonation donor follow-up. It is possible, however, that newer approaches may be adopted with the advent of hepatitis C testing. As part of their current investigations of transfusion-related hepatitis cases, most blood centers have adopted the approach of creating lists of suspect donors.[71] Donors can continue to donate while on this list. In some blood centers, if the donor subsequently becomes a suspect in a second case of posttransfusion hepatitis, he or she is assumed to be a hepatitis carrier and is deferred from further donation. The problem with this approach is that if there were numerous donations (eg, 100 units) in both transfusion-induced hepatitis cases, then a donor who made frequent donations might by chance be implicated in two cases and be deferred from further donations.[28,71] To alleviate the problem of falsely implicating a donor as a hepatitis carrier, two approaches have been developed. The American Red Cross has adopted a policy of placing donors' names on suspect lists only if the recipient received blood from ten or fewer donors.[72] If the recipient received more than ten donations, no suspect list is created. In another approach, practiced in some other blood centers, each donor in a case of posttransfusion hepatitis is assigned a risk factor that may be calculated as one divided by the number of donors in the case.[70] If the donor is implicated in a second case, he or she is assigned a second risk factor. The donor is deferred only if the cumulative sum of the risk factors exceeds a previously designated number. A third, more conservative algorithm based on a different statistical approach and leading to the deferral of an increased number of potentially implicated donors has also been advocated.[73]

Posttransfusion hepatitis case investigations are time consuming and often are logistically complex. First, such investigations are dependent on adequate reporting from community physicians or hospital blood banks to the blood center. Second, an assessment must be made to determine whether the patient's hepatitis should be attributed to transfusion. In some cases the blood center physician may find it difficult to obtain all the necessary data to make such an assessment.[70] Only limited data are available concerning the outcome of posttransfusion case investigations. The data do not permit a cost-benefit analysis of the utility of this approach in enhancing blood transfusion safety.

HIV and AIDS Transmission

General considerations.   In late 1982 and early 1983, at a time when evidence for the infectious origin of AIDS was not yet conclusive, it was recognized that AIDS might be transmitted by transfusion.[74,75] Because of the high mortality rate associated with AIDS, donor-screening policies deigned to safeguard the blood supply were rapidly implemented, despite the fact that the risk of AIDS transmission via transfusion at that time was estimated to be very low.[75] These policies were based on epidemiologic data that had established high-risk groups for AIDS. The newly implemented donor screening procedures were intended to protect the blood supply while simultaneously addressing two sensitive social issues: (1) avoiding falsely labeling persons as possible AIDS carriers, and (2) developing an acceptable strategy for questioning prospective donors about sexual orientation or sexual behavior. It should be realized that such intimate questioning had not been previously conducted at blood collection sites and quite probably had never been attempted in as broad a public health context (8 million persons annually) as would be done in blood donor screening programs.

As knowledge about the risks of transfusion-transmitted AIDS increased, it became evident that the extent of the problem was greater than was previously recognized. As further epidemiologic data accumulated concerning risk factors for AIDS, modifications of donor screening criteria were rapidly adopted.[76] The speed of implementation of these policy modifications can be appreciated when contrasted against the slow evolution of donor-screening criteria for hepatitis and malaria. Indeed, the discovery of transfusion-transmitted AIDS can be seen to be a focal point for transfusion medicine, leading to increased scrutiny of donor screening criteria used for all transfusion-transmitted diseases.[6]

In 1985, the development of the HIV antibody test led to screening of all donated blood in the United States.[77,78] Within a short time, it became possible to identify failures of donor-screening procedures (ie, those blood donors who tested anti-HIV–positive) and to use this information to further modify these procedures.[78] Because of the window period of HIV infectivity before the appearance of detectable antibody, it was realized that even with laboratory testing, vigilance in regard to proper donor screening procedures was still an important element in protecting the safety of the blood supply.[3,8]

Another potential use of data gained from the experience with anti-HIV blood donor testing might have been to substantiate that persons who had been at epidemiologic risk in the remote past (ie, well beyond the 6-month window period) could be considered safe as blood donors. In 1986, the application of a 6-month deferral period (to cover the HIV "window") was used in formulating deferral criteria for one group of persons at risk (those with prostitute contact).[79] However, the high mortality of AIDS and the fear of its transmission has thus far precluded the liberalization of permanent donor deferral criteria for other HIV risk factors (ie, male homosexual partners in the distant past).

Formal recommendations for donor screening (and related procedures) in the United States.   In January 1983, the three major United States blood banking organizations (the American Red Cross, the AABB, and the Council of Community Blood Centers)[11] issued a joint statement on AIDS related to transfusion. The document stated that efforts to prevent transfusion-transmitted AIDS needed to focus in two major directions: (1) the cautious use of homologous blood and blood products, and (2) reasonable attempts to limit blood donation from individuals in groups that may have an unacceptably high risk of AIDS. Specific recommendations as to how to limit such blood donations included the following: (1) not targeting donor recruitment efforts towards groups that might have a high incidence of AIDS, (2) asking donors specific questions related to the symptoms of AIDS and carefully evaluating those donors who gave positive answers, (3) meeting with the leadership of groups that included individuals at high risk of AIDS.

In March 1983, the FDA issued a document to all blood collection establishments entitled *Recommendations to Decrease the Risk of Transmitting Acquired Immunodeficiency Syndrome (AIDS) from Blood Donors.*[42] This document stated that educational programs, including donor-screening procedures, should be implemented to inform persons at increased risk of AIDS that they should refrain from blood donation. The FDA also recommended that donors be directly questioned concerning symptoms that might be associated with AIDS.

In December 1984, the FDA issued an updated set of recommendations that revised the definitions of persons at risk for AIDS, enlarged on the symptoms associated with AIDS, and stated that blood collection establishments should consider a confidential means whereby after the donor's blood was collected, he or she could confidentially indicate that it should not be transfused.[80]

In the spring of 1985, with the wide-scale implementation of anti-HIV testing at blood banks throughout the United States, the US Public Health Service, in conjunction with state and local health departments, established a program of alternative test sites for anti-HIV testing.[23] At the same time, some states (New York, Illinois, and California) passed legislation that prohibited notifying anti-HIV positive blood donors of their test results until alternative test sites were functioning.

In September 1985, an additional FDA memorandum further modified the description of groups at risk for HIV infection.[81] In October 1986, the FDA suggested further modifications of these definitions and advocated a specific method to be used at the blood collection site by which a donor could confidentially exclude his or her unit from transfusion use.[79] In February 1988, the FDA recommended changes in donor screening procedures designed to protect the blood supply against HIV-2 transmission.[82]

Public education.   In 1983, in many communities, blood center staff members worked closely with gay community leaders to deliver the message that sexually active male homosexuals should no longer donate blood. This was publicized through articles appearing in gay community publications and general interest print and electronic media. Educational efforts were also implemented at blood collection sites through distribution of pamphlets to prospective donors. In most blood centers, this pamphlet discussed the signs and symptoms of AIDS and indicated which groups of people were at high risk for acquiring AIDS; the recommendation was made that such individuals not donate blood. In addition, the written material also provided information concerning the risks of donors transmitting hepatitis, syphilis, malaria, or other infectious disease.

Establishment of alternative test sites. Establishment of alternative test sites for free and anonymous anti-HIV testing was instituted in many parts of the United States at the time of implementation of routine blood bank anti-HIV screening. The primary purpose of such sites was to decrease the likelihood that individuals with a high risk for HIV infection would donate blood to learn their anti-HIV status. An influx of such persons into blood centers would have increased the likelihood of transfusing blood from individuals who were in the HIV antibody–negative window period and thus capable of transmitting HIV infection. This risk was considered to be great enough to motivate federal and state governments to fund these public health programs.

HIV data obtained from alternative test sites indicate that the rate of seropositivity among the large number of persons tested is significantly higher than at blood collection agencies.[83] While it is not certain how many of these individuals would have donated blood had alternative test sites not been available, studies have indicated that some percentage would have done so.[83,84] Therefore, it seems reasonable to conclude that the alternative test site program has been an important adjunct to blood transfusion safety.

Health history interview

Signs and symptoms of AIDS. In 1983, the health history interview was modified to include questions relating to symptoms that could possibly be compatible with AIDS. Initially such symptoms included unexplained fevers, night sweats, unexpected weight loss, evidence of lymphadenopathy (lumps in the axilla or groin), Kaposi's sarcoma, or a diagnosis of AIDS. As the range of symptoms associated with HIV infection became better understood, additional symptoms were added to the list of questions, including a history of persistent cough, shortness of breath, and persistent unexplained diarrhea.

These symptoms, although possibly associated with AIDS, could also be associated with many other kinds of illness. However, because of the severity of AIDS, the donor loss associated with using these nonspecific deferral criteria was never seriously considered as an impediment to their use. In practice, these policies necessitated informing prospective donors that their symptoms precluded them from donating blood because of the fact that these symptoms could possibly be compatible with infection with an agent that caused AIDS. Because of the potential anxiety caused by this type of message, medical staff members at the Los Angeles–Orange Counties Red Cross adopted a policy of carefully reviewing all health history deferrals for AIDS-related symptoms. This review process was used to educate blood collection staff in accurately assessing the significance of such nonspecific symptoms.[85]

Possible exposure to HIV (AIDS) carriers. In March 1983, the FDA identified the following groups as being at increased risk of AIDS: persons with symptoms and signs suggestive of AIDS, sexually active homosexual or bisexual men with multiple partners, Haitian entrants to the United States, present or past users of intravenous drugs, and sexual partners of persons at increased risk of AIDS.[42] In December 1984, the FDA revised these definitions to state that "males who have had sex with more than one male since 1979 and males whose male partner has had sex with more than one male since 1979 were at risk."[80] Other changes recommended at that time were that Haitian entrants be deferred if they entered the country since 1977 and that patients with hemophilia and their sexual partners be deferred.

With the implementation of anti-HIV testing in the spring of 1985, anti-HIV–positive blood donors were identified, notified of their test results, and interviewed. As a result of these interviews, evidence was accumulated that allowed for an objective assessment of the effectiveness of donor education efforts. Interviews with anti-HIV–positive donors revealed that although many were men who had sex with other men, they had not considered themselves to be at risk for HIV infection.[78] It became apparent that a person might respond very differently if asked whether he were a member of a specific group (ie, a homosexual man) as opposed to being asked if he had ever engaged in a specific activity (ie, having sex with another man). The FDA therefore recommended in September 1985 that "any male who has had sex with another male since 1977" should not donate blood.[81] The recommendation emphasized that individuals who had had only a single homosexual experience should refrain from donating.

Deferral by country of origin.   Because of the high rates of HIV infection in some geographic locations and the common mode of transmission of HIV through heterosexual routes in these locales, donor deferral policies have been adopted based on country of origin. Although such policies are clearly nonspecific and will defer many uninfected persons, the severity of posttransfusion HIV infection has led to this approach. In 1983, early in the recognition of the AIDS epidemic, FDA recommendations included deferral of those persons from Haiti who had entered the United States after 1979.[42] Subsequently, in 1986, the FDA recommended deferral of persons from many central African nations where HIV infection was found to be endemic.[79] In 1988, the deferral recommendations were modified, this time in response to the discovery of HIV-2 in western Africa.[82] Although not yet demonstrated as a problem in the United States, the potential for HIV-2 infection via transfusion is of some concern because of the fact that HIV-2 may have existed in human populations for a longer time than has HIV-1, and because some HIV-2–infected persons will escape detection using anti–HIV-1 assays.[86] For these reasons, FDA recommendations have been extended to include deferral of all natives of sub-Saharan Africa.

Visitors to Africa or Haiti are acceptable as blood donors (with regard to HIV risk) provided that they have not engaged in sexual activities with members of the native population and that they have not received a blood transfusion in that country. The health history interview conducted by the American Red Cross inquires as to whether individuals have visited Africa or Haiti;

an affirmative answer is explored further by asking more specific questions concerning sexual activities and medical treatment.

Another group of people that must be evaluated are persons who have resided in Africa for long periods. One approach is to evaluate such individuals in the same fashion as visitors to African countries. Another approach is to assume that residence in such countries might increase a person's potential for sexual exposure or exposure to nonsterile needles during medical procedures, and furthermore to assume that these events might not be accurately recalled at the time of the health history interview. These assumptions would lead to deferral of such individuals.

Heterosexual risk of HIV exposure.   The initial FDA recommendations had established several potential heterosexual exposures to HIV as causes for donor deferral, including sexual activity with intravenous drug users, hemophiliacs, or bisexual men.[42] In October 1986, with the increased recognition of potential transmission of HIV by heterosexuals who were not intravenous drug users, the FDA recommended that additional deferral criteria be implemented so that a person would be deferred from donating if (1) he or she had immigrated to the United States from a country in which heterosexual activity played a major role in transmission of HIV infection (this included Haiti and many Central African countries), (2) he or she had engaged in prostitution, (3) and he or she had been a heterosexual partner of a prostitute within the preceding 6 months.[79] Thus far, surveillance of anti-HIV–positive donor populations has failed to reveal an increased number of persons with heterosexual risk (or no identified risk) for HIV infection.[87] Continued monitoring of anti-HIV–positive donors will be necessary to assess whether the risk of HIV transmission from seronegative heterosexuals might require the consideration of additional nonspecific donor-deferral criteria.

Casual exposure to HIV-infected (AIDS) patients.   It is well established that HIV is not transmitted by casual contact; therefore, persons who have had close contact with individuals who are anti-HIV positive or who have AIDS should not be deferred as blood donors.[88] If a person admits to living in the same household as an HIV-infected person, the potential for sexual contact with that individual should be determined; if no sexual contact has occurred the donor should not be deferred.

Occupational exposure to HIV-infected (AIDS) patients.   Occupational exposure to a patient with AIDS or HIV infection is not cause for deferral from blood donation since HIV is spread only by parenteral, sexual, or transplacental routes. On the other hand, there is a small but real risk of HIV infection if the health care worker has been parenterally exposed by a needle stick or contact with blood or body fluids from a person with a high likelihood of HIV infection. Such individuals should be temporarily deferred from blood donation. Recent data from the CDC suggest that seroconversion in this group will occur within 6 months, although such persons continue to be monitored for 12 months after exposure.[89] Therefore, it is my opinion that a 12-month deferral period should assure that a potentially exposed individual would be a safe blood donor. However, in the absence of firm data a more conservative deferral approach may be adopted by blood-collection agencies.

Mechanisms for excluding the transfusion of a donated unit.   Soon after the initiation of donor-deferral procedures for HIV infection, it was recognized that some persons at high risk for HIV infection might continue to donate blood because deferral in the presence of coworkers or other peers might be interpreted as an admission of homosexual behavior. For this reason, blood centers provided donors with a mechanism to exclude their donated blood from transfusion. In most blood centers, donors were provided with a telephone number that they could call after they had left the blood center to indicate that their blood should not be utilized. An alternative approach, now known as confidential unit exclusion, was introduced by the New York Blood Center.[26] In this procedure, each blood donor was required to complete an additional form before donating blood in which he or she indicated if the donated blood should be transfused to others. This form was confidential in that it was not seen by blood center personnel nor did it contain the donor's name.

In late 1986, the FDA issued a recommendation that stated that, at the time of donation, donors be offered a procedure by which they could designate confidentially whether their blood should not be transfused to others.[79] Most blood centers implemented this recommendation by establishing confidential unit exclusion procedures that either used a manual form or required the application of a bar-coded sticker to the health history record. Before the FDA recommendation, some blood centers using the confidential unit exclusion procedure had designated the two available options as "transfuse my blood," or "use my blood for research."[26] Subsequent to the FDA recommendation, most blood centers established the categories of "transfuse (use) my blood" or "do not transfuse (use) my blood." Despite this attempt to clarify the wording of the options, evidence has accumulated that many donors find the confidential unit exclusion process to be confusing. Follow-up interviews conducted with donors who selected the "do not transfuse" option have revealed that a significant percentage of donors (67% in one study, 65% in a second study that may have had a selection bias) who chose this option did so by mistake.[90,91]

It is difficult to establish whether the use of the confidential unit exclusion option appreciably increases transfusion safety. Data from three separate studies indicate that persons who choose confidentially to exclude their units are statistically different from the remainder of the donor population in that they have an increased rate of anti-HIV positivity as well as an increased rate of positivity to other infectious disease markers.[26,92,93] It should be noted, however, that this increased rate might be partially explained by the increased numbers of first-time donors in the confidentially excluded group. More pertinent to establishing the efficacy of the confidential unit exclusion procedure is knowing whether or not donors who donate in the window period for HIV infection choose to exclude their blood from transfusion. At the Los Angeles–

Orange Counties Regional Red Cross, none of eight seronegative donors who tested seropositive on subsequent donations chose this option.[94]

Evaluating the effectiveness of donor screening policies.   Before the implementation of anti-HIV testing, several attempts were made to evaluate the effectiveness of donor screening policies. Since there were no accurate estimates as to the number of high-risk individuals (primarily homosexual men) who had donated blood either before or after the initiation of AIDS-related donor screening procedures, such studies used indirect evidence to measure efficacy. In one study, a 12% decrease in donations among men from 21 to 31 years of age was noted in Manhattan after the implementation of donor screening procedures in 1983.[26] In Los Angeles, it was demonstrated that there was an additional 6% decrease in the rate of donation from young men in zip codes with large numbers of reported AIDS cases (as compared with low AIDS–risk zip codes) in the year after implementation of FDA recommendations.[8]

Although these studies suggested that many high-risk individuals did refrain from blood donation, the introduction of anti-HIV testing established that some high-risk individuals continued to donate blood despite the existence of donor screening procedures. Interviews with 41 anti-HIV–positive donors indicated that most had risk factors for HIV infection that should have precluded them from donating blood.[78] These data resulted in the implementation of changed wording in the information pamphlets used by blood banks. A study performed in late 1985, shortly after the implementation of the new wording suggested by the FDA, indicated that fewer anti-HIV–positive donors were identified in a comparable period of time, suggesting that this modification was helpful.[95] However, other factors might also have contributed to this decreased anti-HIV positivity rate; such rates would have been anticipated to decrease because of notification of previously identified anti-HIV–positive donors and their removal from the blood donor pool.

Several additional studies have continued to obtain interview information from newly identified anti-HIV–positive donors.[87,94,96] These studies uniformly have found that the majority of anti-HIV–positive donors do have HIV risk factors that should have precluded them from blood donation. When questioned concerning their motivations for donating, several reasons were cited. The most common was that the donor had not believed himself to be at risk for HIV infection at the time of donation despite receiving information from the blood center concerning HIV risk. Other reasons less frequently cited for blood donation were the desire to obtain anti-HIV test results and the necessity to donate because of peer pressure. These data indicate that it is still important for blood centers to explore approaches to more effectively deliver the deferral message to high-risk donors. However, it should be recognized that the denial exhibited by this group of donors may meet deep psychological needs and may be difficult to influence by any modifications in blood center procedures.

In 1983 most, if not all blood centers, felt that it was inappropriate to question blood donors directly concerning their sexual activity.[24] Instead, reliance was placed on the donor to accurately evaluate himself after reading the information pamphlet or when filling out the donor history card. Verbal questioning did not define risk groups but generally followed a format similar to the following question: "Have you ever had AIDS or had intimate contact with someone who has had AIDS or is at risk of acquiring AIDS?"

In the early years of the AIDS epidemic, there were no available data to indicate that more explicit questioning might result in deferral of an increased number of high-risk persons; indeed, one hypothesis was that direct questioning about a person's sexual orientation might lead to untruthful answers because of concerns about maintaining the confidentiality of information. A more direct approach also posed the possibility of embarrassing or offending potential blood donors as well as presenting implementation problems for the nursing staff.

As the AIDS epidemic has evolved, society has been forced to discuss issues of sexual orientation and sexual behavior more openly. Parallelling this general change of attitude in society, and with the more precise FDA recommendations concerning HIV risk behavior, there has been a trend during the past several years for workers at blood centers to ask donors verbally explicit questions about sexual orientation and sexual behavior. Data to support the efficacy and acceptance of this approach have been recently reported. One study has indicated that an increased number of donors admitted to having HIV risk factors when a policy was implemented to ask all prospective donors explicit verbal questions concerning HIV risk factors during the health history interview.[97] A second study, conducted in 1988, surveyed blood donors and determined that most donors felt that explicit questioning concerning sexual behavior should be undertaken to protect the blood supply further.[98]

Malaria

Policy recommendations.   Policies for the prevention of transfusion-transmitted malaria are based on determining whether a prospective donor may have been exposed to malaria because of travel to or immigration from an area in which malaria is endemic.[99] In the United States, where transfusion-transmitted malaria is rare (estimated at 0.25 cases per 1 million donated units for 1972 through 1981),[100] decisions on donor deferral are based solely on information obtained when eliciting a medical history.[101] In Europe, where travel to and immigration from malaria-endemic areas is more common, the medical history is supplemented by serologic testing for antibodies to plasmodial (primarily *P falciparum*) antigens.[99] Results of serologic testing are used for two distinct purposes: (1) to provide an additional measure of safety before accepting donors with a history of exposure or (2) to permit acceptance of donors after a shorter deferral period than would otherwise be permitted.[102-104] It has been shown that with the use of such serologic testing, only about 5% of persons with a history of possible exposure need to be deferred.[99]

In most countries, two critical waiting periods for deferral have been defined: 6 months and 3 years (5 years in some countries). In the United

States, most blood collecting agencies follow the policies recommended in 1974 in the seventh edition of the AABB standards:[105]

1. Travelers who have been in areas considered endemic for malaria by the CDC may be accepted as blood donors 6 months after return to the nonendemic area, providing they have been free of symptoms and have not taken antimalarial drugs.
2. Persons who have had malaria shall be deferred for 3 years after becoming asymptomatic or after cessation of therapy.
3. Persons who have taken antimalarial prophylaxis shall be deferred for 3 years after cessation of therapy or after departure from the area if they have been asymptomatic in the interim.
4. Immigrants or visitors from endemic areas may be accepted three years after departure from the area if they have been asymptomatic in the interim.

The AABB standards differ in some respects from the recommendations of the Council of Europe's Sixth Meeting of the Select Committee of Experts on Blood Transfusion and Immunohematology (1983).[102] The European recommendations are more stringent in that they recommend permanent deferral for persons with a history of malaria. There is a 3-year deferral for persons who were born in malaria-endemic areas and subsequently visited endemic areas; however, it is recommended that these donors be accepted for donation only if results of serologic tests for plasmodial antibodies are negative. One of the recommendations of the Council of Europe Committee is less stringent than the United States criteria: travelers from nonendemic areas are acceptable as blood donors 6 months after their visit to malaria-endemic areas whether or not they have taken chemoprophylaxis.

Policies instituted in European countries may vary from the Council of Europe recommendations. In one country, for example, donors with a previous history of *P falciparum* or *P ovale* malaria are deferred for 5 years and those with a history of *P vivax* or *P malariae* are permanently deferred. In some countries, travelers to endemic areas are accepted as donors 4 months after their return provided that results of serologic tests for antibody are negative.[104]

It is of historical interest that before 1974, policies in the United States were more restrictive than at present. All immigrants or visitors from malaria-endemic areas, as well as persons with a history of malaria, were permanently deferred.[106]

The above recommendations apply to transfusion of cell-containing blood components. There are no deferral requirements if a donation is to be used solely for the preparation of frozen plasma or fractionated plasma derivatives.

Rationale.   Travelers to endemic areas are deferred for 6 months because nonimmune persons who have not received antimalarial prophylaxis will develop clinical symptoms within 6 months of initial infection.[101] The extended deferral period (3 years) in the United States for persons receiving chemoprophylaxis has been selected because of the possibility that clinical symptoms after infection may be markedly delayed; it seems, however, that the lack of an extended deferral secondary to chemoprophylaxis in European countries reflects a difference in opinion as to the likelihood of this occurrence.[101,102] The use of serologic testing to shorten the deferral period for travelers is based on the premise that antibody development will occur within a few months of infection.[107] The 3-year deferral period for persons with previous infection is based on the general consensus of opinion that *P falciparum* organisms will be cleared within 2 years and that *P vivax* or *P ovale* will generally not persist for more than 3 years after the cessation of symptoms.[107] The 3-year deferral period for immigrants or for persons born in an endemic area who once again visit such an area is based on the premise that these individuals may have acquired some immunity to malaria because of previous exposure; hence, upon reinfection they do not develop symptoms of malaria for a prolonged period.[101]

These policies represent a compromise between prevention of transfusion-transmitted malaria and acceptable levels of donor deferral. It is well known that *P malariae* infection may result in a chronic carrier state that can persist for decades; therefore, if the aim were to prevent all possible cases of malaria, permanent deferral based on possible exposure would be required.[108] The extent of donor loss due to current deferral policies can be illustrated by our experience at the Los Angeles–Orange Counties Red Cross, where 0.75% of potential donors are deferred because of possible malaria exposure.

Practical aspects of applying deferral criteria. Successful application of donor-screening procedures for malaria requires obtaining an accurate travel history. Since, in the United States, deferral for visiting a malaria-endemic area may be for a period of 3 years, donors should be questioned about trips outside the country during the previous 3 years. It is necessary for the blood collection staff to be knowledgeable about areas of the world in which malaria is endemic. In the United States, this information is distributed by the CDC in a publication entitled *Health Information for International Travel.*[109] In other countries, similar information can be obtained from a WHO publication. Two authors have recommended that maps should be available to eliminate any confusion concerning which countries have been visited.[101,102]

The CDC publication *Health Information for International Travel* indicates which areas within a given country are believed to be free of malaria.[109] If travelers have confined their visit to these nonendemic areas, they can be accepted as blood donors. At least one author has stressed that the length of time spent in a malaria endemic area is not pertinent, since infection can occur even during a very brief visit.[101]

In a review of posttransfusion malaria cases in the United States from 1972 to 1981, Guerrero et al[100] found that 12 of 17 implicated donors were foreign-born. Three of these donors had lived in the United States for many years but had donated their implicated units from 6 months to 1 year after visiting a malaria-endemic area. The authors recommend that blood collection staff members make a distinction between travelers who are native to the

United States (6-month deferral) and travelers who have previously resided in malaria-endemic areas (3-year deferral).[100]

Creutzfeldt-Jakob Disease

Creutzfeldt-Jakob disease is an untreatable, fatal, degenerative neurologic disease with a long, asymptomatic incubation phase. The causative agent is thought to be a viruslike particle termed a *prion* (for "small proteinaceous particle").[2,110] The disease has been experimentally transmitted to rodents in three cases through the transfusion of blood obtained post mortem from patients with Creutzfeldt-Jakob disease.[111-113] Furthermore, transmission between humans has apparently occurred after transplantation of cornea and dura mater from infected donors.[114] Although no cases of Creutzfeldt-Jakob disease have been transmitted by transfusion, the data indicate that such transmission could theoretically occur if a person infected with the Creutzfeldt-Jakob agent were to donate blood.

Creutzfeldt-Jakob disease is rare and has occurred primarily in elderly persons on a sporadic basis. However, it has recently become recognized that seven cases of this disease have occurred among approximately 16,000 recipients of pituitary-derived human growth hormone administered in the 1970s and early 1980s.[115,116] These preparations were utilized to treat growth hormone deficiency but were also sometimes used by athletes as muscle-building agents. Attempts have been made to publicize the need for such persons to refrain from blood donation.[116] However, since it is doubtful that all such growth hormone recipients can be notified of this information and since recipients of human growth hormone appear to be at increased risk of harboring the Creutzfeldt-Jakob agent, the FDA recommended in early 1988 that prospective blood donors be asked whether they have ever received pituitary-derived human growth hormone.[117] This policy has been incorporated into the donor screening procedures of the American Red Cross and has been adopted as an AABB standard.[2] An affirmative answer should permanently disqualify an individual as a blood donor.

Bacterial Disease

Bacterial agents can be transmitted to patients from transfused blood. If a unit of blood contains bacteria at the time of collection, prolonged storage of platelet concentrates at room temperature[118,119] or of red blood cells in the refrigerator (for cold-growing bacterial species)[120,121] can provide a good growth environment. Transfusion of such bacterially contaminated units to debilitated patients can cause sepsis and death.[118-121]

Bacteria can be introduced into the bag of collected blood under several circumstances: if the donor is bacteremic at the time of blood donation, if there is an abscess adjacent to venous structures in the antecubital fossa, or through contamination from the skin at the collection site.[119,120,122]

Information obtained along with the health history is used to reduce the risk of transfusion-transmitted bacterial infection. Blood is not collected from persons who are febrile at the time of donation or who state that they do not feel well.[61] In addition, many blood centers will temporarily defer donors who have had a dental extraction within the previous 72 hours because of the high frequency of bacteremia following this procedure. At one time, it was recommended that donors be temporarily deferred for even more minor dental procedures. Subsequently, it has been documented that bacteremia in these situations is transient and is no more common than after other traumas to mucous membranes that are not evaluated when the health history is obtained.[123]

Examination of the skin at the venipuncture site is conducted before phlebotomy and strict requirements for assuring the sterility of the site are adhered to by the phlebotomist.

HTLV-I and HTLV-II Infection

HTLV-I is a retrovirus known to cause adult T-cell leukemia and the neurologic disease termed tropical spastic paraparesis or HTLV-I–associated myelopathy.[124] HTLV-I infection occurs with high frequency in some parts of Japan, the Caribbean, and Africa. HTLV-I infection, or infection with a closely related retrovirus (HTLV-II) of unknown disease potential, has been documented to occur frequently in populations of intravenous drug users in the United States.[125] In a study of approximately 40,000 US blood donors, intravenous drug use or sexual contact with an intravenous drug user was the risk factor for HTLV-I and HTLV-II infection in four of seven seropositive donors.[126] Country of origin was not implicated as a risk factor for any of these donors.

According to these data, deferral policies to protect against HTLV-I and HTLV-II transmission should logically be directed against intravenous drug users and their sexual contacts. Intravenous drug users are already deferred from donating because of AIDS and hepatitis risks while their sexual partners should be deferred under the criterion of intimate contact with a person at risk for HIV infection. Data obtained at the Los Angeles–Orange Counties Red Cross indicate that an increased number of prospective donors will be deferred as sexual contacts of intravenous drug users if this question is explicitly asked during the health history interview.

The current data on US blood donor populations do not suggest that deferral for country of origin would provide protection against transfusion-transmitted HTLV-I and HTLV-II infection.

Practical Problems in Donor Screening at the Donation Site

The successful application of donor screening procedures requires good communication between the blood donor and the blood center. This is accomplished by providing the donor with written material and by conducting a health history interview. Both of these methods have some practical difficulties.

Limitations to the use of written material involve the clarity of presentation, the reading comprehension skills of the donor, and the willingness of the donor to take the time to read the material. Furthermore, even if the donor reads and understands the material, there is no guarantee that he or she will carefully consider the information presented.[25]

Several difficulties may also arise at the time of the health history interview. It may be difficult to assure the quality of the interview since the interview skills of blood center staff members will almost certainly vary. The donor is asked questions of a sensitive social nature and not every donor may be comfortable in revealing such information to an interviewer. If the interview is being conducted at a busy bloodmobile with limited privacy, concerns about confidentially may preclude donors from sharing this sensitive information. Furthermore, donors may not consciously withhold such information but may for psychological reasons deny their risks to themselves.

Another practical problem in blood donor screening is that policies written in the procedure manual may be difficult to apply to an individual case at the blood collection site. For example, blood donor interviewers may need to evaluate whether a donor has had close contact with a hepatitis patient, whether the cities visited in a malaria-endemic country require deferral, and whether a person's sexual partners might have put him or her at risk for transmission of HIV. While it is difficult to anticipate all possible situations in a written procedure manual, attempts should be made to provide clear definitions to staff members. In addition, feedback should be obtained from blood collection staff members as to how well policies function at the blood collection site.

References

1. Dodd RY: Donor screening and epidemiology, in Barker LF, Dodd RY (eds): *Infection, Immunity, and Blood Transfusion.* New York, Alan R Liss, 1985, pp 389–405.

2. Holland PV: Why a new standard to prevent Creutzfeldt-Jakob disease? *Transfusion* 28:293–294, 1988.

3. Ward JW, Holmberg SD, Allen JR, et al: Transmission of human immunodeficiency virus (HIV) by blood transfusions screened negative for HIV antibody. *N Engl J Med* 318:473–478, 1988.

4. Hoofnagle JH, Seeff LB, Bales B, et al: Type B hepatitis after transfusion with blood containing antibody to hepatitis B core antigen. *N Engl J Med* 298:1379–1383, 1978.

5. Farzadegan H, Polis MA, Wolinsky SM, et al: Loss of human immunodeficiency virus type 1 (HIV-1) antibodies with evidence of viral infection in homosexual men. *Ann Intern Med* 108:785–790, 1988.

6. Alter HJ: You'll wonder where the yellow went: A 15 year retrospective of post transfusion hepatitis, In Moore SB (ed): *Transfusion Transmitted Viral Diseases.* Arlington, VA, American Association of Blood Banks, 1987, pp 53–86.

7. Zuck TF: Greetings: A final look back with comments about a policy of zero-risk blood supply. *Transfusion* 27:447–448, 1987.

8. Kaplan HS, Kleinman SH: AIDS: Blood donor studies and screening methods, in Barker LF, Dodd RY (eds): *Infection, Immunity and Blood Transfusion*. New York, Alan R Liss, 1985, pp 297–308.

9. Schafer IA, Mosley JW: A study of viral hepatitis in a penal institution. *Ann Intern Med* 149:1162–1177, 1958.

10. Krugman S, Friedman H, Latimer C: Hepatitis A and B: Serologic survey of various population groups. *Am J Med Sci* 275:249–255, 1978.

11. American Association of Blood Banks, American Red Cross, Council of Community Blood Centers: *Joint Statement on Acquired Immune Deficiency Syndrome Related to Transfusion*. January 13, 1983.

12. *Fed Reg* 43:2142, 1978.

13. Alter HJ, Holland PV, Purcell RH, et al: Post transfusion hepatitis after exclusion of commercial and hepatitis B antigen positive donors. *Ann Intern Med* 77:691–699, 1972.

14. Cherubin CE, Prince AM: Serum hepatitis specific antigen (SH) in commercial and volunteer sources of blood. *Transfusion* 11:25–27, 1971.

15. Szmuness W, Prince AM, Brotman B, Hirsch RL: Hepatitis B antigen and antibody in blood donors: An epidemiologic study. *J Infect Dis* 127:17–25, 1973.

16. Mosley JW, Galambos JT: Viral hepatitis, in Schiff L (ed): *Diseases of the Liver*. Philadelphia, JB Lippincott, 1975, pp 500–594.

17. Kahn RA: Donor screening to prevent posttransfusion hepatitis, in Keating LJ, Silvergleid AJ (eds): *Hepatitis*. Washington, DC, American Association of Blood Banks, 1981, pp 99–125.

18. Taswell HA: Directed, paid and self donors, in Clark GM (ed): *Competition in Blood Services*. Arlington, VA, American Association of Blood Banks, 1987, pp 137–148.

19. Morris JP: International Forum: Which criteria must be fulfilled for a donation or a donor to be considered voluntary? *Vox Sang* 34:362–371, 1978.

20. Polesky HF: Is blood from autologous donors safe for others? *Transfusion* 28:204, 1988.

21. Kruskall MS, Popovsky MA, Pacini DG: Autologous versus homologous donors: Evaluation of markers for infectious disease. *Transfusion* 28:286–288, 1988.

22. AuBuchon JP, Dodd RY: Analysis of the relative safety of autologous blood units available for transfusion to homologous recipients. *Transfusion* 28:403–405, 1988.

23. Mason JO: Alternative sits for screening blood for antibodies to AIDS virus. *N Engl J Med* 313:1157–1158, 1985.

24. Dodd RY: Donor screening for HIV in the United States, in Madhok R, Forbes CD, Evatt BL (eds): *Blood, Blood Products and AIDS*. London, Chapman & Hall, 1987, pp 143–160.

25. Kleinman SH, Shapiro A; The agreement to donate blood: Presenting information to blood donors and obtaining consent, in Smith DM, Carlson KB (eds): *Current Scientific-Ethical Dilemmas in Blood Banking*. Arlington, VA, American Association of Blood Banks, 1987, pp 29–54.

26. Pindyk J, Waldman A, Zang E, et al: Measures to decrease the risk of acquired immunodeficiency syndrome transmission by blood transfusion. *Transfusion* 25:3–9, 1985.

27. Feinstone SM, Kapskian AZ, Purcell RH et al: Transfusion associated hepatitis not due to viral hepatitis type A or B. *N Engl J Med* 292:767–770, 1975.

28. Alter HJ: Discussion: Transfusion associated hepatitis, in Polesky HF, Walker RH (eds): *Safety in Transfusion Practices*. Skokie, IL, College of American Pathologists, 1980, pp 32–40.

29. Choo Q-L, Kuo G, Weiner AJ, et al: Isolation of a cDNA clone derived from a blood borne non-A, non-B viral hepatitis genome. *Science* 244:359–362, 1989.

30. Kuo G, Choo Q-L, Alter HJ, et al: An assay for circulating antibodies to a major etiologic virus of human non-A, non-B hepatitis. *Science* 244:362–364, 1989.

31. Tabor E: Hepatitis B as a complication of a blood transfusion, in Tabor E (ed): *Infectious Complications of Blood Transfusion*. New York, Academic Press, 1982, pp 1–27.

32. US Food and Drug Administration: *Code of Federal Regulations*. 1988, vol. 21.

33. Holland PV, (ed): *Standards for Blood Banks and Transfusion Services*, ed. 13. Arlington, VA, American Association of Blood Banks, 1987.

34. Alter HJ, Purcell RH, Shih JW, et al: Detection of antibody to hepatitis C virus in prospectively followed transfusion recipients with acute and chronic non-A, non-B hepatitis. *N Engl J Med* 321:1494–1500, 1989.

35. American Red Cross: *Blood Services Directive 5.29*, revised 1988.

36. Cumming PD, Schorr JB, Wallace EL: Annual blood facts. *American Red Cross Blood Services Letter* 87–82, 1987.

37. Piliavin JA: Temporary deferral and donor return. *Transfusion* 27:199–200, 1987.

38. Allen JG, Dawson D, Saymor WA, et al: Blood transfusion and serum hepatitis: Use of monochloroacetate as an antibacterial agent in plasma. *Ann Surg* 150:455–468, 1959.

39. Aach RD, Szmuness W, Mosley JW, et al: Serum alanine aminotransferase of donors in relation to the risk of non-A, non-B hepatitis in recipients. *N Engl J Med* 304:989–994, 1981.

40. Aach RD, Kahn RA: Post-transfusion hepatitis: Current perspectives. *Ann Intern Med* 92:539–546, 1980.

41. Goldfield M, Bill J, Colosimo F: The control of transfusion associated hepatitis, in Vyas GN, Cohen SN, Schmid R (eds): *Viral Hepatitis*. Philadelphia, Franklin Institute Press, 1978, pp 405–414.

42. Director, Office of Biologics Research and Review, Food and Drug Administration: Recommendations to decrease the risk of transmitting acquired immune deficiency syndrome (AIDS) from blood donors. Memorandum to all establishments collecting human blood for transfusion. March 24, 1983.

43. Alter MJ, Hadler SC, Francis DP, Maynard JE: The epidemiology of non-A, non-B hepatitis in the United States, in Barker LF, Dodd RY (eds): *Infection, Immunity, and Blood Transfusion*. New York, Alan R Liss, 1985, pp 71–79.

44. Esteban JI, Esteban R, Viladomiu L, et al: Hepatitis C virus antibodies among risk groups in Spain. *Lancet* 2:294–297, 1989.

45. Egoz N, Brachott D, Mosley JW, Yekutrel P: Viral hepatitis in Israel. *Transfusion* 12:12–22, 1972.

46. Mathes M, Riderer V: Blood donation after hepatitis. *Germ Med Monthly* 2:107–110, 1957.

47. Tabor E, Hoofinagle JH, Barker LF, et al: Antibody to hepatitis B core antigen in blood donors with a history of hepatitis. *Transfusion* 21:366–371, 1981.

48. World Health Organization Expert Committee on Viral Hepatitis: *Advances in Viral Hepatitis.* Geneva, World Health Organization, 1977.

49. Follett H, Barr A, Crawford RJ, Mitchell R: Viral hepatitis markers in blood donors and patients with a history of jaundice. *Lancet* 1:246–249, 1980.

50. Reesnick HW: International Forum: Should donors with a history of jaundice still be rejected? *Vox Sang* 41:110–127, 1981.

51. Hopkins R, Robertson AE, Ravie A, McClelland DBL: Blood donors with a history of jaundice. *Lancet* 1:596, 1980.

52. Sherertz RJ, Russell BA, Reuman PD: Transmission of hepatitis A by transfusion of blood products. *Arch Intern Med* 144:1579–1580, 1984.

53. Bird GWG: International Forum: Should donors with a history of jaundice still be rejected? *Vox Sang* 41:110–127, 1981.

54. Polesky HF, Hanson M: Tests for viral hepatitis markers in blood donors, in Polesky HF, Walker RH (eds): *Safety in Transfusion Practices.* Skokie, IL, College of American Pathologists, 1980, pp 17–26.

55. Tegtmeier G: Transfusion associated hepatitis, in Polesky HF, Walker RH (eds): *Safety in Transfusion Practices.* Skokie, IL, College of American Pathologists, 1980, pp 32–40.

56. Seeff LB: International Forum: Should donors with a history of jaundice still be rejected? *Vox Sang* 41:110–127, 1981.

57. Alter MJ, Gerety RJ, Smallwood LA, et al: Sporadic non-A, non-B hepatitis: Frequency and epidemiology in an urban U.S. population. *J Infect Dis* 145:886–893, 1982.

58. Alter HJ: International Forum: Should donors with a history of jaundice still be rejected? *Vox Sang* 41:110–127, 1981.

59. Trepo C: International Forum: Should donors with a history of jaundice still be rejected? *Vox Sang* 41:110–127, 1981.

60. Aach RD: International Forum: Should donors with a history of jaundice still be rejected? *Vox Sang* 41:110–127, 1981.

61. Huestis DW, Bove JR, Case J: *Practical Blood Transfusion,* ed 4. Boston, Little Brown and Co, 1988.

62. Perillo RP, Gelb L, Campbell C, et al: Hepatitis B antigen, DNA polymerase activity, and infection of household contacts with hepatitis B virus. *Gastroenterology* 76:1319–1325, 1979.

63. Everhart JE, Di Bisceglie AM, Murray LM, et al: Risk for non-A, non-B (type C) hepatitis through sexual or household contact with chronic carriers. *Ann Intern Med* 112:544–545, 1990.

64. Mowat NAG, Brunt DW, Albert-Recht F, Walker W: Outbreak of serum hepatitis associated with tattooing. *Lancet* 1:33–34, 1973.

65. Huestis DW, Bove JR, Busch S: *Practical Blood Transfusion,* ed 2. Boston, Little Brown & Co, 1976.

66. Maynard JE. Viral hepatitis as an occupational hazard in the health care profession, in Vyas GN, Cohen SN, Schmid R (eds): *Viral Hepatitis*. Philadelphia, Franklin Institute Press, 1978, pp 321–331.

67. Froesner GG, Peterson DA, Holmes AW, Deinhardt FW: Prevalence of antibody to hepatitis B surface antigen in various populations. *Infect Immunol* 11:732–736, 1975.

68. Grady GF: Hepatitis B immunity in hospital staff targeted for vaccination. *JAMA* 248:2266–2269, 1982.

69. Tabor E, Hoofnagle JH, Smallwood LA, et al: Studies of donors who transmit post-transfusion hepatitis. *Transfusion* 19:725–731, 1979.

70. Polesky HF, Hanson M: Transfusion associated hepatitis. *Lab Med* 14:717–720, 1988.

71. Walker RH: Discussion: Transfusion associated hepatitis, in Polesky HF, Walker RH (eds): *Safety in Transfusion Practices*. Skokie, IL, College of American Pathologists, 1980, pp 32–40.

72. American Red Cross Blood Services Directive 4.9, revised 1985.

73. Ladd DJ, Hillis A: A new method for evaluating the hepatitis risk of the multiply implicated donor. *Transfusion* 24:80–82, 1984.

74. Ammann AJ, Cowan MJ, Wara DW, et al: Acquired immunodeficiency in an infant: possible transmission by means of blood products. *Lancet* 1:956–958, 1983.

75. Curran JW, Lawrence DL, Jaffe H, et al: Acquired immunodeficiency syndrome (AIDS) associated with transfusions. *N Engl J Med* 310:69–75, 1984.

76. Zuck TF: Transfusion transmitted AIDS reassessed. *N Engl J Med* 318:511–512, 1988.

77. Provisional Public Health Service interagency recommendations for screening donated blood and plasma for antibody to the virus causing acquired immunodeficiency syndrome. *MMWR* 34:1–5, 1985.

78. Schorr JB, Berkowitz A, Cumming PD, et al: Prevalence of HTLV-III antibody in American blood donors. *N Engl J Med* 313:384–385, 1985.

79. Director, Office of Biologics Research and Review, Food and Drug Administration: Additional recommendations for reducing further the number of units of blood and plasma donated for transfusion or for further manufacture by persons at increased risk of HTLV-III/LAV infection. Memorandum to all registered blood establishments. Oct 30, 1986.

80. Acting Director, Office of Biologics Research and Review, Food and Drug Administration: Revised recommendations to decrease the risk of transmitting acquired immunodeficiency syndrome (AIDS) from blood and plasma donors. Memorandum to establishments collecting blood, blood components or source plasma and all licensed manufacturers of plasma derivatives. Dec 14, 1984.

81. Director, Office of Biologics Research and Review, Food and Drug Administration: Revised definition of high risk groups with respect to acquired immunodeficiency syndrome (AIDS) transmission from blood and plasma donors. Memorandum to all registered blood establishments. Sept 3, 1985.

82. Director, Office of Biologics Research and Review, Food and Drug Administration: Recommendations concerning persons at increased risk of HIV-1 and HIV-2 infection. Memorandum to all registered blood establishments. April 6, 1988.

83. Forstein M, Page PL, Coburn TJ: Alternative sites for screening blood for antibodies to AIDS virus. *N Engl J Med* 313:1158, 1985.

84. Snyder AJ, Vergeront JM: Safeguarding the blood supply by providing opportunities for anonymous HIV testing. *N Engl J Med* 319:374–375, 1988.

85. Kleinman S, Thompson PR, Kaplan H: Evaluation of donor screening procedures for AIDS prevention in a high risk area. *Transfusion* 24:434, 1984.

86. Clavel F, Mansinho K, Chamaret S: Human immunodeficiency virus type 2 infection associated with AIDS in West Africa. *N Engl J Med* 316:1180–1185, 1987.

87. Ward JW, Kleinman SH, Douglas DA, et al: Epidemiologic characteristics of blood donors with antibody to human immunodeficiency virus. *Transfusion* 28:298–301, 1988.

88. Friedland GH, Saltzman BR, Rogers MF, et al: Lack of transmission of HTLV-III/LAV infection to household contacts of patients with AIDS or AIDS related complex with oral candidiasis. *N Engl J Med* 314:344–349, 1986.

89. Marcus R, CDC Cooperative Needlestick Surveillance Group: Surveillance of health care workers exposed to blood from patients infected with the human immunodeficiency virus. *N Engl J Med* 319:1118–1123, 1988.

90. Swenke P, Aufenthie J, Nelson C, et al: Unnecessary loss of blood donors due to confidential unit exclusion program. *Transfusion* 28(suppl):15, 1988.

91. Kleinman S, Crawley P: An assessment of HIV related donor screening procedures. *Transfusion* 28(suppl):42, 1988.

92. Nusbacher J, Chiavetta J, Naiman R, et al: Evaluation of a confidential method of excluding blood donors exposed to human immunodeficiency virus. *Transfusion* 26:539–541, 1988.

93. Rutter P, Herman A, Kilroy Forman P: Confidential unit exclusion and other infectious disease markers in the donor population. *Transfusion* 28(suppl):29, 1988.

94. Kleinman S, Secord K, Doyle M: Demographic profile and motivations for donation in donors who have seroconverted for HIV. *Transfusion* 28(suppl):29, 1988.

95. Kalish RI, Cable RG, Roberts SC: Voluntary deferral of blood donations and HTLV-III antibody positivity. *N Engl J Med* 314:1115–1116, 1986.

96. Kleinman S, Sohner S, Wilke D: Analysis of HTLV-III antibody positive donors: Donor deferral policies and infection prevalence. *Transfusion* 26:576, 1986.

97. Silvergleid AJ, Watrin G: Impact of explicit questions about high risk activities on donor deferral patterns. *Transfusion* 28(suppl):54, 1988.

98. Leparc GF, Schmidt PJ: Direct questioning of donors about high risk behavior for AIDS: A survey of donor attitudes. *Transfusion* 28(supp): 29, 1988.

99. Hassig A: International Forum: Which are the appropriate modifications of existing regulations designed to prevent transmission of malaria by blood transfusion, in view of the increasing frequency of travel to endemic areas? *Vox Sang* 52:138–148, 1987.

100. Guerrero IC, Weniger BC, Schultz MG: Transfusion malaria in the United States, 1972–1981. *Ann Intern Med* 99:221–226, 1983.

101. Kark JA: Malaria transmitted by blood transfusion, in Tabor E (ed): *Infectious Complications of Blood Transfusion*. New York, Academic Press, 1982, pp 93–126.

102. Emmanuel JC: International Forum: Which are the appropriate modifications of existing regulations designed to prevent transmission of malaria by blood transfusion, in view of the increasing frequency of travel to endemic areas? *Vox Sang* 52:138–148, 1987.

103. Perrin LH: International Forum: Which are the appropriate modifications of existing regulations designed to prevent transmission of malaria by blood transfusion, in view of the increasing frequency of travel to endemic areas? *Vox Sang* 52:138–148, 1987.

104. Soulier JP: International Forum: Which are the appropriate modifications of existing regulations designed to prevent transmission of malaria by blood transfusion, in view of the increasing frequency of travel to endemic areas? *Vox Sang* 52:138–148, 1987.

105. Oberman HA (ed): *Standards for Blood Banks and Transfusion Services of the American Association of Blood Banks*, ed 7. Chicago, Gunthorp-Warren, 1974.

106. Perkins HA (ed): *Standards for Blood Banks and Transfusion Services of the American Association of Blood Banks*, ed 5. Chicago, Twentieth Century Press, 1970.

107. Deroff P, Reguer M, Simitzis AM, et al: Screening blood donors for plasmodium falciparum malaria: Application of ready to use homologous antigens. *Vox Sang* 45:392–396, 1983.

108. Bruce-Chwatt LJ: International Forum: Which are the appropriate modifications of existing regulations designed to prevent transmission of malaria by blood transfusion, in view of the increasing frequency of travel to endemic areas? *Vox Sang* 52:138–148, 1987.

109. *Health Information for International Travel*. HHS Publication No. (CDC) 85–8280. US Department of Health and Human Services, Washington, DC, 1990.

110. Prusiner SB: Prions and neurodegenerative diseases. *N Engl J Med* 317:1571–1581, 1987.

111. Manuelidis EE, Manuelidis L, Pincus JH, Collins WF: Transmission from man to hamster of Creutzfeldt-Jakob disease with clinical recovery. *Lancet* 2:40, 1978.

112. Manuelidis EE, Kim JH, Mericangas JR, Manuelidis L: Transmission to animals of Creutzfeldt-Jakob disease from human blood. *Lancet* 2:897–898, 1985.

113. Tateishi J: Transmission of Creutzfeldt-Jakob disease from human blood and urine into mice. *Lancet* 2:1074, 1985.

114. Rapaport EB: Iatrogenic Creutzfeldt-Jakob disease. *Neurology* 37:1520–1522, 1987.

115. Gibbs CJ Jr, Joy A, Heffner R, et al: Clinical and pathologic features and laboratory confirmation of Creutzfeldt-Jakob disease in a recipient of pituitary derived human growth hormone. *N Engl J Med* 313:734–738, 1985.

116. NIDDK Fact Sheet: Human growth hormone and Creutzfeldt-Jakob disease. Washington DC, National Institutes of Health, NIH Publication No. 86–2793, December 1987.

117. Director, Office of Biologics Research and Review, Food and Drug Administration: Deferral of donors who have received human pituitary derived growth hormone. Memorandum to all registered blood establishments. Nov 25, 1987.

118. Heal JM, Jones ME, Forey J, et al: Fatal salmonella septicemia after platelet transfusion. *Transfusion* 27:2–5, 1987.

119. Braine HG, Kickler TS, Charache P, et al: Bacterial sepsis secondary to platelet transfusion: An adverse effect of extended storage at room temperature. *Transfusion* 26:391–393, 1986.

120. Wright C, Seiss IF, Vinton KJ, Pierce RN: Fatal *Yersinia enterocolitica* sepsis after blood transfusion. *Arch Pathol Lab Med* 109:1040–1042, 1985.

121. Scott J, Boulton FE, Govan JRW, et al: A fatal transfusion reaction associated with blood contaminated with *Pseudomonas fluorescens*. *Vox Sang* 54:201–204, 1988.

122. Anderson KC, Gorgone BC, Leu M: Transfusion related sepsis after prolonged platelet storage. *Blood* 66(suppl 1):273a, 1985.

123. Ness PM, Perkins HA: Transient bacteremia after dental procedures and other minor manipulations. *Transfusion* 20:82–85, 1980.

124. Rosenblatt JD, Chen ISY, Wachsman W: Infection with HTLV-I and HTLV-II: Evolving concepts. *Semin Hematol* 25:230–246, 1988.

125. Robert-Guroff M, Weiss SH, Giron JA, et al: Prevalence of antibodies to HTLV-I, II, and III in intravenous drug abusers from an AIDS endemic region. *JAMA* 255:3133–3137, 1986.

126. Williams AE, Fang CT, Slamon E, et al: Seroprevalence and epidemiological correlates of HTLV-I infection in U.S. blood donors. *Science* 240:643–646, 1988.

14
Donor Testing and its Impact on Transfusion-Transmitted Infection

Roger Y. Dodd, PhD

Testing is the second of the three lines of defense against transfusion-transmitted infection. Although donor selection is clearly the most effective measure in terms of the overall impact on blood safety, there is no question that laboratory testing is a critical link in the chain. The final step to assuring product safety is the inactivation of residual viruses, which is an effective procedure for pooled plasma products but, as yet, only a dream for single-donor components.

Laboratory testing has proved to be extremely effective in virtually eliminating transfusion-associated infection with the hepatitis B virus and the AIDS virus, HIV. The use of surrogate testing to identify donor populations believed to be at increased risk of transmitting the virus(es) responsible for non-A, non-B hepatitis has been accompanied by a significant decline in the reported frequency of acute posttransfusion hepatitis and it is anticipated that the recently described test for antibodies to hepatitis C virus will shortly lead to further improvement in this area. The finding that there was a significant prevalence of infection with HTLV-I and HTLV-II among blood donors in the United States[1] contributed to the decision to initiate testing for antibodies to this class of retrovirus. The efficacy of this screening measure has been shown to be high, at least in Japan. Finally, although logistically difficult, screening for antibodies to CMV has proved to be an effective intervention in the prevention of CMV disease in some immunocompromised groups. In contrast, testing for syphilis has continued for many years without any current evaluation of efficacy or indeed, even need. At the same time, recognition of additional blood-transmissible viruses generates new pressures for further testing.

Each new test adds to the process of blood collection and distribution. Obviously, as additional infections and interventions are recognized, more

Manufacturer	Viral Isolate	Sensitivity, %	Specificity, %*
Abbott	HTLV-III	100	99.85
Cellular Products	PI†	100	99.85
Ortho Diagnostics (formerly DuPont)	HTLV-III	99.3	99.7
Electronucleonics	HTLV-III	100	99.7
Genetic Systems	LAV	100	99.8
Organon Teknika	HTLV-III	100	99.97
Ortho Diagnostics	HTLV-III	99.3	99.7
United Biomedical (Olympus)	Synthetic peptide	100	99.71

*Performance claims from product insert.

†Proprietary isolate of HIV.

tests must be performed, but this is accompanied by increases both in record keeping and in the proportion of blood components that must be held in quarantine. It is not clear whether these measure have themselves affected the adequacy of the blood supply, but there is evidence that the complexities of managing the process may have affected the ability of blood centers to minimize or avoid all errors.

Testing for HIV

Tests

HIV antibody testing.   Recognition of the causative agent of AIDS by Barre-Sinoussi et al,[2] Gallo et al,[3] and others[4] was accompanied by the development of simple ELISA tests for antibodies to HIV.[5] Since HIV is a retrovirus, infection is persistent and essentially lifelong. Thus, the presence of antibodies implies the presence of virus and antibody tests may be used to identify potentially infectious blood donations. In May 1984, virus and cell lines were made available to a group of American companies with the ability to manufacture screening tests and in March 1985, after less than 1 year, anti-HIV tests were first licensed for use. At the time of this writing, nine manufacturers are licensed in the United States, and eight ELISA tests are currently available (Table 14–1).

ELISA tests for antibodies to HIV almost all have the same basic design, with a solid-phase capture reagent bearing HIV antigens and a probe consisting of an enzyme-linked antiglobulin reagent. The test sample is serum or plasma and it is generally diluted before initiation of the test. Antibodies to HIV, if present, adhere to the solid phase. After washing, the adherent antibodies can be detected with the probe, which is itself detected by a suitable chromogenic substrate. The variations between those tests that are currently licensed and available in the United States are relatively trivial. All of the eight initially licensed tests use a capture reagent based on lysed HIV grown in tissue culture. The majority of the manufacturers use the prototype virus, HTLV-III, grown in H9 cells. At least one manufacturer uses a test based on the LAV isolate,[2] grown in CEM cells, and one manufacturer uses a third isolate and cell substrate. As will be discussed, there is very little difference in the performance characteristics of these tests, so the source of the virus appears to have little practical relevance. In fact, it seems that the nature of the parent cell is of more importance, since this may contribute to the specificity of the test, particularly when cell-derived HLA antigens are incorporated into the virus.[6,7] The source of the antiglobulin reagent and the enzyme used (horseradish peroxidase or alkaline phosphatase) also differ between tests, but again have little or no impact on performance. The other major difference between tests available in the United States is the format, either bead or microplate, of the capture reagent. Absorbance is read by a suitable instrument. A cutoff value is defined, usually as some simple function of the value obtained by testing positive or negative controls. All samples giving values equal to or above the cutoff are regarded as reactive.[8]

Although variation between tests is limited in the United States, there are other important differences in test formulations that are available in other parts of the world. For example, at least one manufacturer has developed an inhibition test in which the capture reagent is solid-phase viral antigen and the probe is enzyme-conjugated human anti-HIV.[9] This procedure offers advantages of specificity. Another important variation is the use of viral antigens prepared by recombinant DNA technology[10] or by direct synthesis of immunodominant peptides.[11] One ELISA test, licensed in the United States, uses synthetic HIV peptides as the capture reagent. These variant procedures enjoy extensive use in Europe and are apparently at least equivalent to those in use in the United States, where they have not yet been licensed by the FDA.

Rapid tests for anti-HIV have also been developed, using latex agglutination[12] or membrane-based visualization[13] procedures. These techniques offer considerable promise in circumstances where rapid testing is required or, if affordable, in third world countries. Although it would be anticipated that both sensitivity and specificity would suffer, these rapid tests are reported to be similar to conventional methods on both counts.[12] It is unlikely that they will be used to any extent in the screening of donors or donor blood. One latex agglutination test is licensed for use in the United States; it uses recombinant HIV antigens.

Screening tests for donated blood are usually conducted according to a simple algorithm. Each sample is tested singly and all those found to be nonreactive are considered to be negative for HIV antibodies. The components may be released for transfusion. Samples that generate a reactive value are retested in duplicate, preferably using the original sample, plus another sample. If either or both of these replicate tests are reactive, the blood unit and all components are recorded as repeatably reactive and must be discarded. The final stage in the algorithm is confirmatory testing to determine the extent and nature of donor notification that is required. This protocol was developed on the basis of demonstrated experience that forward sandwich–type immunoassays are susceptible to nonrepeatable false-positive results. Careful evaluation clearly suggests that these nonrepeatable reactive findings are not associated with increased risk of infectivity.[14] Neither does it appear that a repeatable ELISA-reactive result with a negative Western blot offers any excess risk of infectivity.[15]

The key performance characteristics of tests for anti-HIV are sensitivity and specificity. Since the tests were designed for qualitative screening, and because the actual quantitation of naturally occurring antibodies is neither simple nor really meaningful, the epidemiologic definitions of sensitivity and specificity are used and are defined for repeatably reactive values. Thus, the sensitivity of a test is the frequency of positive results in a population known to have the true presence of the disease or factor under test. In the case of tests for anti-HIV, product performance claims were developed and approved on the basis of testing known AIDS patients. Because some AIDS patients lose detectable antibodies at the end of their illness, not all tests have a claimed sensitivity of 100%, although all are better than 99.3%.[16] However, as will be discussed below, this is not necessarily the most effective way of considering the sensitivity of a test for blood screening. Perhaps the most pertinent characteristic is the ability to detect asymptomatic carriers, particularly at a very early stage in the infection.

The specificity of an anti-HIV test is the proportion of negative results found when testing a population in which the disease or factor is known to be absent. In developing product claims, manufacturers defined specificity by testing populations of blood or plasma donors. In most cases, specificities are better than 99.8%. The specificity of tests can be readily confirmed on the basis of donor screening and can be corrected to account for the presence of true-positive results in the donor population. Experience shows that the product claims in the package insert are reliable predictors of test specificity in routine use. However, even though a specificity of 99.8% is very high and is exceeded by few, if any, tests, it must be recognized that the prevalence of true HIV-positive results is extremely low in the donor population. After 5 years of continuous testing, for example, the frequency of true-positives is 0.01% in the Red Cross donor population.[17] A specificity of 99.8% necessarily implies that 0.2% of samples will yield false-positive results. Consequently, at current detection rates, only one repeatedly reactive value in every 20 actually represents a true-positive; the positive predictive value of the test is only 5%. This predictive value is dependent on the prevalence of the marker in the test population, and should not be confused with specificity, which is an inherent property of the test. Manufacturers have recognized the problems associated with lower levels of specificity and have improved the performance of tests to better than 99.95% in some cases.

Thus, while repeatedly reactive ELISA test results are considered to be adequate for a decision to discard a blood unit, they must not be used to notify a donor or other individual that he or she has been infected with HIV. Confirmatory testing must be performed to differentiate the true-positive from the false-positive results. Before discussing these supplementary procedures, it is appropriate to comment on the possible reasons for the occurrence of false-positive results in anti-HIV tests. First, as noted above, the virus that is used to prepare the capture reagent is grown in tissue culture and the mature virus incorporates cell membrane material. This material cannot be fully purified away from the other viral components, and in some cases it expresses HLA antigens. Consequently, complementary antibodies, if present in the donor serum, will adhere to the solid phase and generate a repeatable reactive test result. Although this mechanism has been discussed in the literature,[6,7] manufacturers of test kits appear to have resolved this problem and there is little evidence that it continues to cause difficulties. However, the final steps of the tests are nonspecific inasmuch as they are designed to detect immunoglobulins. Thus, nonspecifically "sticky" immunoglobulins, or those with an affinity for polystyrene surfaces, will also generate false-positive results. Finally, it is clear that there is a more troublesome form of false-positive reaction in which there are antibodies that react with polypeptide sequences that are coded by the viral genome, but that do not reflect actual infection with HIV[18]; these will be discussed in more detail below.

Western blot testing.   Implementation of blood donor screening for anti-HIV generated a number of ethical and operational problems that had to be resolved. It became standard practice to notify donors of the result of a truly positive test. Since the message is extremely serious to the recipient, it is clearly necessary to confirm the ELISA result. There are a number of methods available for this purpose, including the use of indirect immunofluorescence[19] and radioimmunoprecipitation,[20,21] but the procedure that is most commonly employed in association with blood collection is the western blot. This procedure permits the identification of antibodies to individual viral polypeptides and careful interpretation of the patterns can result in extremely specific and suitably sensitive identification of truly infected individuals. In addition, the absence of any reactivity in the Western blot is clear evidence that the sample does not come from a person infected with HIV.

The Western blot procedure[5] involves the lysis of purified HIV and the electrophoresis of the resulting polypeptides on polyacrylamide gel in the presence of SDS. Viral polypeptides migrate at a rate that is inversely proportional to their molecular weight. Once the electrophoresis is complete, the polypeptide pattern is transferred (blotted) to a sheet of nitrocellulose paper. The transfer is accomplished by placing the paper on the face of the acrylamide gel and applying an electric field across the gel. As a result, the band pattern migrates electrophoretically into the nitrocellulose. The nitrocellulose may be dried and cut into narrow strips. To perform an assay, the strip is incubated in a dilution of the sample to be tested. Antibodies to viral polypeptides, if present, adhere at characteristic positions on the strip. After incubation, the strip is washed and adherent antibodies are detected by means of an appropriately labeled antiglobulin. Usually, the antiglobulin is conjugated to an enzyme and its presence is detected by a suitable color reaction.

The Western blot provides additional information as it permits the separate identification of antibodies to individual viral polypeptides. However, interpretation of a blot is not particularly easy and well-defined criteria must be used to read a blot. Currently accepted criteria also require that the blot system must, as a minimum, be able to detect antibodies to the major structural polypeptides of the virus. More specifically, these are the *gag* products p17, p24, and the parent p55, the *pol* products, p31, p51, and p66, and the *env* products gp41, gp120 and gp160. The absence of any visible bands in a properly performed blot signifies that the donor or patient is not infected with HIV. Conversely, the presence of certain combinations of bands is regarded as a positive reading and defines infection with HIV for diagnostic purposes and for notification of donors.[22] The criterion used by the American Red Cross is the presence of antibodies to at least one product of each of the three structural genes. Use of this approach does not appear to have resulted in any false-positive notifications, although it is also sensitive. A subset of this criterion is used in the licensed blot kit jointly manufactured by Biotech and Dupont. In this case, the presence of p24, p31, and gp41 or gp120/160 are required to define a sample as positive. This is highly specific, but lacks sensitivity relative to other criteria, as antibodies to p31 are not always present. The criterion for positivity proposed by the Association of State and Territorial Public Health Laboratory Directors[23] and endorsed by the CDC[24] requires the presence of antibodies to at least two of p24, gp41, or gp120/160, and a criterion proposed by a consensus group[22] relies on the presence of antibodies to p24 or p31, plus gp41 or gp120/160. In general, when applied to donor samples, the three criteria described above give similar results.[25]

Unfortunately, patterns other than those that are clearly positive or negative are also seen when samples are subjected to Western blot testing. When a large population of blood donor samples that are repeatedly reactive in anti-HIV ELISA test are subjected to the Western blot test, about 10% to 20% are positive, about 60% to 80% are negative, and 10% to 20% have indeterminate patterns. Indeterminate patterns cannot be interpreted without further clinical or virologic information. This is because at least some patterns, notably the presence of isolated reactions to *gag* peptides, may be due to cross-reacting antibodies apparently unassociated with HIV infection,[18] or may represent the early stages of seroconversion in an infected individual.[20] Among blood donors, it appears that fewer than 5% of indeterminate patterns reflect true infection. Indeterminate plot patterns that do not progress towards a full pattern over 6 months signify the absence of HIV infection.[26,27] Thus, the status of the majority of indeterminate patterns can be resolved by testing the donor again after 3 to 6 months.

Although it may be operationally desirable to notify donors with repeatedly reactive ELISA test results that they cannot give blood again, it is critical to note that an ELISA test result is not diagnostic of HIV infection. Neither is an indeterminate blot pattern. Therefore, every effort must be made to establish the absence (or presence) of HIV infection before completing the notification process.

HIV antigen testing.   As has been indicated above, infection with HIV is not immediately accompanied with the development of detectable levels of antibodies. Nevertheless, there is evidence that HIV infection may be transmitted by blood drawn in the period between infection and antibody detection.[28] It has also been shown that sensitive techniques, such as the PCR for HIV genome, can, in rare cases, show the presence of HIV some time before antibody development or after the apparent disappearance of HIV antibodies.[29,30] These findings have generated concern about the sensitivity of ELISA tests for anti-HIV as a donor screening measure. Recently, it has been shown that a soluble antigen with the specificity of the p24 *gag* polypeptide may be found in the circulation during certain phases of HIV infection. In particular, the antigen is transiently present during the early infection stage, and before the development of overt disease.[31,32] It has therefore been suggested that blood donors should be tested for the HIV p24 antigen to detect early infection. However, limited trials suggest that the antigen test results are positive only for a relatively brief period within a week or two of the appearance of antibodies detectable by conventional tests. It is apparent that relatively few additional samples would be detected: data from Bavaria, for example, showed that there were no samples that were positive only for the HIV antigen when 600,000 successive donations were tested.[33] A similar study, with identical findings, has been completed in the United States.[34] It is also possible that antibody tests of greater sensitivity, particularly for envelope antigens, would be equally effective in detecting this early phase.[20,35]

A number of different HIV antigen tests are available. All are antigen-capture procedures, in which the solid phase is antibody to the HIV antigen and the captured analyte is detected by a labeled antibody system. In at least some configurations, the probe is a sequence of antibodies, which presumably increases the sensitivity of the method. Based on studies described above, a specific decision has been made to avoid the routine use of HIV antigen tests for blood and plasma donors.

A second AIDS virus, termed HIV-2, has been identified and is known to be the predominant cause of AIDS in parts of West Africa. This agent is responsible for a significant number of cases of AIDS in a small number of Western European countries. As of early 1990, however, only about 17 infections with HIV-2 had been recognized in the United States. ELISA tests for antibodies to HIV-1 detect some, but not all, infections with HIV-2, suggesting that additional measures may be needed to prevent HIV-2 transmission by transfusion. Such measures are not currently indicated in the United States. Should such need become apparent, the most appropriate method will be to use a single test with the ability to detect infection with both HIV-1 and HIV-2. Such tests have been developed and are used in parts of Europe.

Impact of Testing on the Blood System

Impact on safety.   In the first year of HIV antibody testing, the American Red Cross identified about 1,600 donations that were confirmed to be positive

Table 14–2   Testing for Anti-HIV Among 41 Selected Red Cross Blood
Services Regions*

| | Confirmed Positives/100,000 Donors | | |
Year[†]	First-Time	Repeat	All
1985	51.7	23.1	27.3
1986	41.8	12.0	16.6
1987	35.6	8.8	12.8
1988	24.6	7.0	9.2

*Regions selected as having complete data from the initiation of testing. (Data compiled by Paul Cumming, PhD.)

†Starting in April.

by Western blot analysis.[36,37] A similar number of positive results was identified among all other collections. Since it is clear that almost all such donations are infectious for HIV,[38,39] screening clearly prevented a substantial number of cases of posttransfusion AIDS. In subsequent years, the total number of detected positive results has decreased substantially, largely as a result of the continued elimination of seropositive individuals from the pool of repeat donors. Table 14–2 outlines these findings. In addition, the prevalence of HIV infection among new donors is decreasing, and there has been no significant increase in incidence rates among repeat donors.[17] It is also important to note that the frequency of positive test results among donors is much lower than that seen among other tested groups, such as military recruits,[40] inner city emergency room patients,[41] or randomly selected newborns.[42] In addition, the current rate of approximately ten per hundred thousand is 40-fold lower than would be expected in a random sample of the US population based on the assumption that there are approximately 1 million infected persons in the United States.[43,44] Donor selection procedures have been successful in maintaining a safe and healthy donor population and it is reasonable to expect continued improvement.

Although it is obvious that laboratory testing has identified a large number of infectious donations, it is not quite so easy to define the efficacy of the testing. In other words, what proportion of all potentially infectious blood units have been identified? The proportion of AIDS cases attributable to blood transfusion is approximately 2% and this proportion did not change significantly over the 3 years following the introduction of donor testing. This appears to be a result of the lengthy incubation period for AIDS and the extent of infection that occurred before initiation of testing.[45] In fact, reports from the CDC suggest that, by the beginning of 1990, only seven cases of transfusion-associated AIDS were linked to transfusion that took place after anti-HIV testing started. There were no cases among pediatric transfusion recipients.[46] James Allen, MD (personal communication, 1988) has compared risk factors in two comparable birth cohorts of infants with AIDS, representing

2-year periods before and after testing. In the first group, a total of 78 patients were shown to have maternal infection as a risk factor and nine had transfusion as the sole risk factor. In contrast, in an exactly comparable cohort studied after the initiation of donor screening, 258 infants with AIDS had maternal infection as a risk factor, whereas only one (which has not been fully investigated) may have been infected via transfusion.[47] Taken together, these reports suggest that, as a result of testing, there has been a highly meaningful decrease in the frequency of transfusion-transmitted AIDS.

At the same time, there is certainly evidence that infectious but seronegative blood units are present in the blood supply. Ward and colleagues[28] discussed 13 blood recipients who had been infected with HIV as a result of receipt of products from seven donors, most of whom were shown to have engaged in AIDS-risk behavior 3 to 4 months before the donation. This article was accompanied by a worst-case estimate suggesting that the frequency of this type of event might be of the order of one infectious product for every 40,000. It is possible that this estimate is unduly high, as it is based on an overestimate of the incidence of new infections among donors, and a refinement of this model suggests that the nationwide frequency is roughly one in 150,000.[17] Another estimate of the frequency of seronegative but infectious donors has been made by Kleinman and Secord,[48] who evaluated the frequency of HIV infection among recipients of the last seronegative donation from donors who were subsequently found to be seropositive. They showed that 50% of recipients of donations made less than 6 months before the positive donation were infected, but none was infected if blood was given more than 6 months before a positive finding was made. The data were interpreted to suggest that, in Los Angeles, about one donation in 67,000 might be infectious but seronegative. Since prevalence rates in Los Angeles are considerably higher than rates nationwide, this estimate is probably too high for the United States overall. Finally, prospective studies on blood recipients in Baltimore and Houston found one HIV infection among the recipients of about 38,000 units transfused since the initiation of testing.[49]

In summary, it appears reasonable to suggest that the minimum infectivity of the blood supply immediately before the start of donor screening for HIV was about 35 per 100,000, which was the seropositivity rate at that time.[37] This contrasts with the current rate, which is believed to be approximately 0.7 to two per 100,000 or better.

Impact on supply.   As discussed above, tests for anti-HIV are highly specific, generating 0.2% or fewer false-positive results. Thus, discarding blood units that are repeatedly reactive in anti-HIV test has had a relatively trivial effect on the adequacy of the blood supply. However, since the advent of AIDS, there has been an unusually high frequency of shortages of supply. At least anecdotally, these shortages have been linked to the popular perception of a relationship between AIDS and blood. There have also been surveys that have clearly shown that many individuals believe that AIDS can be contracted as a result of giving blood. It is not, however, certain if this perception affects established blood donors or potential donors.

Blood shortages, whether or not associated with public fears of AIDS, can be offset by trends in blood usage that have developed as a result of concern about transfusion-transmitted AIDS. Increased use of autologous transfusion, intraoperative salvage and hemodilution, plus a decrease in willingness to transfuse are all leading to a reduction in the need for transfusion with homologous blood.

Testing for HTLV-I and HTLV-II

HTLV-I was the first human retrovirus to be described.[50] It is known to be the cause of adult T-cell leukemia and almost certainly is the causative agent of tropical spastic paraparesis, otherwise known as HTLV-associated myelopathy. Studies in Japan have shown that this virus is transmissible by transfusion, and some cases of HTLV-associated myelopathy are attributed to infection by this route. Studies in the United States also show that HTLV-I can be transmitted by this route.[50,51] Williams and colleagues showed that the overall prevalence rate for HTLV-1 antibodies in the United States was about 0.025%.[1] The virus appears to be exclusively cell-associated and it does not appear to be necessary to test plasma used for further manufacture.

Because of the association of HTLV-I with disease, the seroprevalence rate, and the potential to interrupt transmission, routine testing for antibodies to HTLV-I was introduced in the United States at the end of 1988. Test methods are essentially identical to those used for HIV, that is, ELISA tests designed to detect antibodies to the virus. The capture reagent is derived from a lysate of cultured virus, and the detection reagent is an enzyme-labeled antiglobulin. Licensed procedures are available from three sources; Abbott Laboratories, Cellular Products, and Ortho Diagnostics. In the latter case, the reagents are those previously distributed through Dupont.

Confirmation testing for HTLV-I is more complex than for HIV. The criterion for a positive confirmatory test is the presence of antibodies to the *gag* gene product p24 and to an *env* product, such as gp46.[51] Unfortunately, although antibodies to the envelope glycoproteins may be present, they cannot always be detected on a Western blot. Consequently, samples with Western blot patterns that include a p24 band but lack envelope bands must be tested further by radioimmunoprecipitation, a fairly complex research technique.

An additional complication is that serologic tests for antibodies to HTLV-I also detect the closely related HTLV-II. This virus is not known to be the causative agent of any known disease at present, although it was first isolated from patients with hairy cell leukemia. In practice, it is probably not desirable to transfuse blood that may be infectious with such a retrovirus, so the broad specificity of test methods is a benefit. However, differentiation between infection with the two viruses is difficult and requires the use of gene amplification techniques. Thus, it is not possible to provide accurate information to donors about the nature or clinical importance of their test result. More subtly, it is not really possible to define the actual sensitivity of current HTLV-

I screening tests for HTLV-II, since there is no readily accessible independent test.

The majority of donors found positive for HTLV-I and HTLV-II have been found to be nonwhite, with a female predominance. Risk factors for infection appear to be geographic (generally Caribbean) origin or contact or a history of use of illicit drugs or sexual contact with a drug user. Current detection rates across the American Red Cross system are approximately 0.017%.

Testing for Hepatitis

Specific Test

HBsAg.   Recognition of the relationship between a circulating antigen, now known as HBsAg, and one form of viral hepatitis[52,53] was the direct predecessor of all current laboratory screening of donor blood. It is now well known that HBsAg is excess coat material from the hepatitis B virus, released into the blood from infected liver cells. HBsAg particles are approximately 22 nm in diameter and are essentially lipoproteins. They do not themselves contain any nucleic acid and are thus noninfectious. In general, HBsAg particles are present in far greater numbers than the infectious virions of hepatitis B; the ratio may be as great as 1 in 10^6. This vast excess permits the detection of HBsAg by relatively simple assays that are, nevertheless, sensitive indicators of HBV infectivity.

HBsAg was first identified using simple agar gel diffusion techniques, with antibodies derived from human recipients of numerous transfusions. Simple agar gel diffusion, however, was insensitive and very slow and second-generation tests were developed in which an electric field or directed diffusion were used to drive the antigen and antibody reagents together. In particular, the counterelectrophoresis procedure was routinely used in blood screening for a number of years before the development of a radioimmunoassay for HBsAg.[54] Since then, enzyme immunoassays have become the predominant screening procedure used in the United States. The solid-phase capture reagent consists of antibodies to HBsAg bound to a plastic bead, tube, or microwell. Sample is applied to the solid phase and HBsAg, if present, is bound to the antibodies. The detection reagent is an enzyme-conjugated antibody to HBsAg. The conjugate is detected by means of an appropriate color reaction. A variety of antibodies are used both as probe and capture reagent. The selection of appropriate pairs of monoclonal antibodies directed against different HBsAg epitopes permits the use of single-addition formats, in which both sample and conjugate can be applied simultaneously. However, use of capture and probe antibodies from the same animal species can compromise the specificity of the test, since naturally occurring antiglobulins readily generate false-positive results.[55,56]

Tests for HBsAg should be able to detect the antigen at an approximate concentration of 1 ng/mL in serum or plasma, and most current tests do have this level of analytic sensitivity.[16] The tests are able to detect the predominant subtypes of HBsAg, adw, ayw, adr, and ayr, with the same sensitivity. In fact, unlike tests for anti-HIV, the performance characteristics of HBsAg tests are generally expressed in terms of this type of analytic sensitivity. The specificity of HBsAg tests is 99.9% or better, with approximately 0.05% of donors found to be truly positive for HBsAg and approximately 0.1% repeatedly reactive. The algorithm for screening is essentially the same as that described for anti-HIV, with all samples tested singly; nonreactive values are interpreted as negative and the unit is issued. Reactive values are repeated in duplicate and if one or both of the duplicates are reactive, the unit is discarded. Repeatedly reactive samples must be confirmed before the donor is notified; a simple inhibition test is used for this purpose. A characterized anti-HBs is incubated with the sample and if reactivity is inhibited by 50% or more relative to an appropriate control, then the sample is regarded as a true positive.

Antibody to HBcAg.   The hepatitis virus is relatively complex, consisting of the outer lipoprotein coat with the characteristic HBsAg reactivity and an inner capsid incorporating the circular, partially double stranded DNA and the DNA polymerase. The capsid component includes a structural polypeptide with its own characteristic "core" antigen, HBcAg. This antigen was originally identified by immuno–electron microscopy of detergent-treated HBV from plasma.[57] The antigen is not found free in the plasma or serum, but is expressed in the nucleus of a proportion of infected hepatocytes. During infection with HBV, the antibody to the core antigen (anti-HBc) is the first to appear and may be the only antibody detectable in chronic carriers of HBsAg or during the period during which an acute infection is resolving, when HBsAg disappears and is eventually replaced by anti-HBs. In some cases anti-HBc may be the only marker remaining many years after the resolution of an HBV infection. Thus, the presence of anti-HBc is a reliable marker of current or past HBV infection, although it may be absent in about 4% of HBsAg-positive donors who are presumed to be in the very early stage of infection.[58] Anti-HBc is not found in recipients of the hepatitis B vaccine, which is prepared from natural or recombinant HBsAg.

Diagnostic tests for anti-HBc were developed many years ago. The first format was radioimmunoassay, which has now largely been replaced by enzyme immunoassays. The majority of available tests are competitive inhibition tests in which the capture reagent is a solid-phase preparation of the HBcAg and the probe is a labeled preparation of human, chimpanzee, or animal anti-HBc. Thus, the presence of anti-HBc in a test sample is denoted by a low signal level in the test, and its absence results in a high signal level. Early tests were developed using antigen derived directly from infected chimpanzee liver or plasma. Because of the difficulty of preparing this material, it was presumably more economical to configure the test as a competitive inhibition procedure. Now, however, anti-HBc tests are invariably prepared using HBcAg prepared by recombinant technology and other formats may soon be available.[16]

The performance characteristics of tests for anti-HBc are not easy to define, since there is no meaningful standard or confirmatory test. Approximately 2.9% of donor samples were found to be reactive on initial screening of a very large donor population. On repeated testing, the frequency of reactive values dropped to 2.6%.[59] Anecdotal reports suggest that a substantial proportion of donors found to be reactive at one donation may be nonreactive at a subsequent donation. A number of factors account for this. First, inhibition tests are sensitive to the volumes of critical reagents, so that there may be variations between tests performed at different times. Second, there is clearly lot-to-lot variation in the reagents, and finally, there is variation from manufacturer to manufacturer. Careful review of the distribution of test signals also suggests that there is no clear differentiation between populations of reactive and nonreactive samples. In some cases, presumptive confirmation of a reactive result may be obtained by testing for other markers of HBV infection, particularly anti-HBs, since its presence provides additional evidence of previous HBV infection. However, the absence of anti-HBs is not necessarily informative. Some authors have suggested that the radioimmunoassay procedure for anti-HBc may be used for confirmation of the ELISA test, and one experimental, immunoadsorption-based confirmatory procedure has been published.

In addition to its use as a surrogate test for the identification of populations presumptively at increased risk of non-A, non-B infectivity, the anti-HBc test is also used in the evaluation of unexpected results in tests for HBsAg. The FDA has issued a protocol for the reentry of donors with nonconfirmable ELISA test results for HBsAg, in which a reactive result in a test for anti-HBc is interpreted as supportive evidence for HBV infection and results in permanent deferral of the donor. Conversely, if the ELISA test for HBsAg is nonreactive on a subsequent donation and the donor is nonreactive for anti-HBc, then the unit is acceptable.

Antibody to hepatitis C virus.   During 1989, it became apparent that the long search for a serologic test for a causative agent of non-A, non-B hepatitis had been rewarded. In a collaboration between Daniel Bradley, PhD, at the CDC and Michael Houghton, PhD, and his team at Chiron Corporation in Emeryville, CA, nucleic acids from the serum of a chimpanzee infected with non-A, non-B hepatitis were cloned and expressed in bacteria and an antigenic protein was isolated. This protein reacted with antibodies from persons known to have been infected with non-A, non-B hepatitis.[60,61] It is clear that antibodies to this protein are strongly associated with the predominant form of non-A, non-B hepatitis among blood recipients. In a prospective study of transfusion recipients and their donors, Alter and colleagues[62] evaluated 20 recipients who developed posttransfusion hepatitis. Of the 15 patients with biopsy-proven chronic non-A, non-B hepatitis, all seroconverted for anti-HCV, whereas three of five recipients with acute, resolving hepatitis demonstrated anti-HCV seroconversion. Anti-HCV was found in samples of donor serum given to 14 of the 16 anti-HCV–positive recipients for whom all donor samples were available.[62] Commercial test procedures for antibodies to HCV were licensed and implemented early in 1990; Ortho Diagnostics has entered into a joint agreement with Chiron to develop the test and the antigen has been licensed to Abbott Laboratories for independent development. These tests will be valuable in further reducing the incidence of posttransfusion non-A, non-B hepatitis. Data from clinical trials suggest that approximately 0.6% of donors will be found to be repeatedly reactive. There is no validated confirmatory test that will be available at the time of implementation.

Surrogate Tests

A number of studies performed during the late 1970s established that liver dysfunction, as defined by abnormal levels of alanine aminotransferase (ALT), were a frequent sequel to transfusion,[63,64] affecting 7% to 12% of recipients. These events were defined as hepatitis and, in 95% of cases, were not associated with evidence of infection by known hepatitis-causing agents. Although the vast majority of these cases of hepatitis were subclinical, at least in the acute phase, it became apparent that 20% or more of the cases resulted in chronic liver disease, as defined by prolonged ALT level elevation and pathologic changes evident in biopsy specimens. Careful evaluation of the characteristics of blood donors in these studies revealed that posttransfusion hepatitis was more frequently associated with donors who themselves had elevated ALT levels or anti-HBc. As a consequence, it was suggested that screening donors for these two markers would be likely to reduce the incidence of posttransfusion non-A, non-B hepatitis and such testing was implemented in 1986.

ALT testing.   The enzyme ALT (formerly known as serum glutamate pyruvate transaminase) catalyses the transfer of an amino group from alanine to pyruvic acid to generate glutamic acid. It is present in relatively high concentrations in liver cells and is released into the circulation when hepatocytes are damaged. It is also present in other cells, including red blood cells and some muscle cells. Consequently, elevated serum levels of ALT are not necessarily a specific sign of liver damage.

The enzyme is usually assayed by a kinetic spectrophotometric method[65] using linked reactions. The primary reaction is, in fact, the reverse of the physiologic reaction; the substrates are glutamate and 2-oxo-glutarate. The conditions are such that the reaction is pseudo first order and the enzyme concentration is rate-limiting. The products of the reaction are alanine and pyruvate. To determine the rate of this reaction, the generation of pyruvate is assessed by a secondary reaction. In most cases, the secondary reaction is the reduction of pyruvate by lactate dehydrogenase, which is linked to the oxidation of NADH. NADH can be detected by its absorbance at 340 nm.

Thus, the amount of ALT in the initial sample is proportional to the rate of decrease of absorbance at 340 nm. The rate of decrease is usually measured over a period of a few minutes. A number of aspects of the test must be carefully controlled, including sample and reagent volumes, time, and temperature. In addition, endogenous sample pyruvate must be consumed before the reading is started and the reaction rate must be tested for linearity. Consequently, testing is generally performed using an automated, or semiautomated analyzer designed for clinical chemistry. Results are expressed as international units per liter (IU/L), where one IU is the quantity of enzyme required to catalyze the reaction of 1 μmol of substrate per minute.

In any population, there is continuous distribution of ALT levels and there is no intuitive way to define a cutoff for establishing which samples have elevated levels. For diagnostic purposes, such a cutoff is conventionally defined as the 97.5th percentile value of a carefully screened normal population from which outlying values have been excluded. Posttransfusion follow-up studies suggested that such cutoff values were probably appropriate for donor screening, although one of the studies[63] recommended that a value equivalent to the 98.4th percentile had the best overall efficacy. The American Red Cross has elected to use the 97.5 percentile value of the overall donor population as a single, system-wide cutoff. This cutoff is derived after correcting locally obtained values for variations attributable to instrument, reagents or methodology. Cutoff values are best derived by simple, nonparametric methods, since it is not clear whether the distribution of ALT values in a donor population can be transformed to a strictly gaussian form.[66]

It is widely recognized that there are many factors influencing ALT levels in populations and individuals[67] and that mild elevations are often temporary. Consequently, it is conventional to establish two cutoff values for donor screening, the first, or lower of which is a signal to discard the blood unit, while the second, or higher level is a trigger to notify the donor that there may be some medical problem requiring attention. The lower cutoff is the value discussed above, while the upper cutoff is approximately twice this value. Typically, for tests performed at 37 °C, lower cutoff values range from 50 to 60 IU/L and the upper cutoff is 100 to 120 IU/L. If a donor's ALT value is between the lower and upper cutoff, the blood is discarded but the donor may return at a later time. If two such moderate elevations occur within a single year, the donor is permanently deferred and notified. In contrast, if a donor has an ALT level above the upper cutoff, the donation is discarded and the donor is permanently deferred and notified. Higher ALT levels offer a greater risk of infectivity for non-A, non-B hepatitis and a higher presumption of liver disease. In general, ALT testing results in the discarding of 1% to 3% of collected blood, depending on the selected cutoff, location, and demographic structure of the donor population and a variety of other factors.

Antibody to HBcAg. Additional analysis of two key posttransfusion hepatitis studies performed in the late 1970s revealed that there was an association between the presence of anti-HBc in a donor and risk of transmitting non-A, non-B hepatitis to recipients.[68,69] This relationship seemed to relate to a different donor population from that identified by ALT testing. The findings were tentatively interpreted as reflecting similar risk and transmission routes for the hepatitis B and non-A, non-B viruses. Ultimately, these observations led to the implementation of anti-HBc testing as an additional surrogate measure to reduce the incidence of posttransfusion non-A, non-B hepatitis.

Table 14–3   Posttransfusion Hepatitis Cases Reported to the American Red Cross*

	No. of Cases			
Fiscal Year[†]	Hepatitis B	Non-A, Non-B Hepatitis	Others	Total
1981-1982	222	434	318	974
1985-1986	166	401	276	843
1986-1987	141	353	190	684
1987-1988	108	194	113	415

*Data compiled by Sharon Benavides.
[†]Starting in July.

Impact of Testing on the Blood System

Impact on safety.   There is no question that laboratory testing for HBsAg has been singularly effective in increasing the safety of the blood supply. A few thousand positive donors are identified each year, and it is clear that the majority of these would offer risk of infection to recipients of their blood. Again, however, the key question is the failure rate of the test. Even in 1984, it was apparent that reporting rates for clinically obvious posttransfusion hepatitis B were similar to those for the general population.[70] From 1986 through 1988 this rate dropped even further. It is thus possible that a high proportion of so-called posttransfusion hepatitis B might have occurred in the absence of the transfusion. It should also be noted that the percentage of hepatitis B cases epidemiologically linked to transfusion has dropped dramatically, to 1% of the total (Miriam Alter, PhD, personal communication, 1989).[71] Although it is tempting to attribute these improvements in safety to the implementation of testing for anti-HBc, it must be recognized that there have been many other changes in the donor population as a result of AIDS-related screening. In addition, reporting rates for hepatitis are notoriously unreliable.[72] On the other hand, data from prospective, posttransfusion studies have suggested that 0.5% or fewer of blood recipients may seroconvert and develop HBV markers, although there are no recent data.

Surrogate testing for non-A, non-B hepatitis was introduced with the expectation that it would be of value and in the absence of any experimental demonstration of efficacy. By extension from the posttransfusion studies, it was anticipated that the two tests might reduce the posttransfusion incidence of non-A, non-B hepatitis by up to 60%. Table 14–3 shows the reporting rates for posttransfusion hepatitis for the American Red Cross for the three most recent years, plus a comparable statistic for 1982. It is clear that the reporting rates for non-B forms of hepatitis have declined by about 50% over the past 2 years, with the major change in 1987 and 1988. However, there has also been an overall decline in the frequency of all forms of non-A, non-B hepatitis in the United States (Miriam Alter, personal communication 1989), so it is again possible that the observed decreases merely reflect a coincidence. Data that are now available as a result of the development of the assay for anti-HCV confirm that these surrogate tests may well have been efficacious. For example, in Alter's study, 33% of HCV-positive donors had elevated ALT levels and 54% were positive for anti-HBc. It was estimated that the use of the surrogate tests could have prevented about 50% of the cases in this NIH study.[62]

Impact on supply.   HBsAg testing has little effect on the blood supply, with reactive rates of 0.1% or less; furthermore, it has been a routine aspect of blood collection for many years. In contrast, tests for ALT and anti-HBc have had a significant impact on the supply, classifying some 4% to 6% of units as unsuitable for transfusion. It is not clear whether this rejection rate has contributed to some of the blood shortages that have been discussed above. What is apparent, however, is that the implementation of these additional tests, along with the high rejection rates, have placed a real burden on the operations of blood centers. Although there is an economic cost, perhaps the greatest problems are associated with the increase in the number of blood components that must be quarantined. This increases the risk of erroneous release. One way to manage this problem may be to implement mechanisms to test donors for ALT and anti-HBc before a decision is made to accept or reject the individual as a donor.

Testing for Syphilis

Tests

Historically, testing for syphilis was the first form of laboratory screening applied to blood destined for transfusion and was implemented in the 1920s after recognition of transfusion-transmitted syphilis, first described in 1915. Subsequently, the value of this procedure has been essentially eliminated because *T pallidum* is effectively killed by the processes currently used to prepare and store blood. In addition, infectivity is most likely to be associated with the early phases of infection, when spirochetes are present in the blood, but before the development of detectable antibodies. Nevertheless, testing continues to be done since it is required by Federal regulation.

In the United States, essentially all donor testing is performed using tests based on the nontreponemal cardiolipin antigen; that is, the rapid plasma reagin or VDRL tests. These tests are agglutination or flocculation tests and must, in general, be performed manually. Less than 0.1% of donations are found to be reactive and the blood is discarded, although the plasma may be fractionated. Syphilis tests of this type are not specific for infection with the organism and reactive tests must be confirmed. Such confirmation is traditionally performed by public health laboratories, using *T pallidum*–specific procedures such as the FTA or FTA-ABS tests.[65] In some countries, treponema-specific tests, such as a passive hemagglutination test, are being used for laboratory testing of donated blood. This offers opportunities for automation, although the reagents are much more expensive than the cardiolipin tests. Recently, a particle agglutination test for syphilis was approved for use with the Olympus PK7100 automated blood typing instrument.

There seems to be very little direct benefit from syphilis testing in terms of protecting recipients from infection with *T pallidum*. In fact, the requirement for such testing has been deleted from current editions of the standards issued by the AABB. However, this is overridden by the federal requirement to test. It has been postulated that testing for reagins may have some value in identifying a group at increased risk of sexually transmitted disease and thus at increased risk of HIV infection. The efficacy of this proposal has not been proven but may, nevertheless be a barrier to abandonment of testing.

Testing for CMV

Numerous studies have shown that CMV may be transmitted from seropositive blood donors to seronegative recipients and, in the case of immunocompromised recipients, the outcome may be serious morbidity or even death. Consequently, it is considered appropriate to provide screened, CMV antibody–negative blood to selected recipients at risk. However, because the prevalence rates for anti-CMV frequently exceed 50%, such prescreening must necessarily be limited. There appear to be two strategies for the provision of CMV-seronegative products. The first is to collect routinely and then test the products for antibodies; in cases where special product formulations, such as quadruple packs, are required, this implies a need to overcollect for this category of product. The alternate strategy is to develop a prescreened panel of seronegative donors; this strategy may, surprisingly, generate a need to screen almost all presenting donors for a lengthy period to develop a panel large enough to support ongoing needs. In general, blood centers distribute about 1% of their products as CMV-seronegative units for the support of neonates, but other applications may well increase this proportion substantially.

Tests for Donor Screening

Total antibody to CMV.   Currently, all laboratory testing of donor blood uses procedures designed to detect all classes of antibody directed against CMV. While there are numerous available methods, including classical reference procedures such as complement fixation and indirect immunofluorescence, the majority of blood center testing is done by particle agglutination or ELISA procedures.[65] ELISA procedures are essentially the same as those described for anti-HIV, with a solid-phase capture reagent prepared from viral proteins and a labeled antiglobulin probe. Performance and interpretation of these tests is conventional and they are available in bead and microplate formats. These procedures are of value in blood centers, particularly when objective interpretations and consistency of test instrumentation is desirable. Particle agglutination tests for anti-CMV are however, increasingly popular. Passive hemagglutination tests were developed some years ago, but were found to take too long and were somewhat inconsistent. A rapid latex agglutination procedure is now available; it may be completed in less than 10 minutes. The procedure is simple, rapid and has comparable sensitivity and specificity to other methods.[65] It can be used for rapid screening of collected products and, in some situations, can be used before collection. A particle agglutination test for anti-CMV has also been developed and approved for use on the Olympus PK 7100.

Tests for other CMV-related antibodies. Although the prevalence rate for CMV antibodies in donor populations is approximately 50%, review of the outcome of transfusion of seropositive units suggests that only a small proportion of them are actually infectious. It would be desirable to use a test that had the capability of detecting only those units which are infectious. Two candidate systems have been described: tests for IgM antibodies to CMV[74] and tests for antibodies to the so-called early antigens of CMV.[75] ELISA procedures to detect IgM anti-CMV do not appear to be readily available in the United States, although some procedures have been developed in Europe. Lamberson and colleagues[74] used an indirect immunofluorescence assay to show that, in a population of 1535 blood donors, 38% were reactive for CMV total antibodies in ELISA and 6% were reactive for IgM antibodies. In studies to determine the potential value of donor screening for IgM anti-CMV, this group showed that the incidence of CMV among neonatal recipients of unscreened blood was 3.2%, whereas the incidence was 0.7% among infants receiving only IgM anti-CMV nonreactive blood, representing a single case in which the implicated unit did have a positive ELISA test and detectable levels of IgM anti-CMV by another test. Results of these studies had not been confirmed at this writing and it may be too early to make a specific recommendation about this approach.

Another study by Lentz and associates[75] (including Lamberson) compared the results of various serologic tests with viral isolation from urine among 500 donors. Three of the donors (0.6%) were viruric; all three were positive in an immunofluorescent assay test for antibodies to CMV early antigen and in conventional ELISA and latex agglutination tests. One of the viruric donors was identified by immunofluorescent assay, and two by an ELISA, for IgM anti-CMV. Among all donors, 35% were positive by conventional ELISA, 16% were positive in the test for antibodies to early antigens, and 3% were positive by the ELISA for IgM anti-CMV. It was suggested that tests for antibodies to the early antigens might have some value in identifying infectious donors. Again, it is too early to make any specific recommendations.

Is Testing Necessary?

The major blood-banking organizations in the United States have recognized the risk of morbidity or mortality among CMV-seronegative, immunocompromised recipients of CMV-seropositive blood. The benefit of using screened, CMV-seronegative blood for transfusion of seronegative, low birth weight infants (weighing less than 1250 g) has been clearly established and this procedure is recommended. Clearly, it would also be desirable to transfuse seronegative blood to a seronegative pregnant woman. There has been some concern about the indiscriminate use of seronegative products in seropositive infants however, since dilutional effects may result in increased morbidity.[76] The benefits of using seronegative blood products for other patient groups are not so clear and must be weighed against the availability of an adequate supply. Organ transplant recipients are at risk of reactivation of intrinsic infection and may also be infected via the transplanted organ. It is possible that CMV infection among seronegative recipients of seronegative organs may be controlled by the use of CMV immune globulin, provided granulocytes are not transfused.[77] However, recipients of liver transplants may warrant special attention. In addition, bone marrow recipients are at extraordinarily high risk of death from CMV infection and it is considered appropriate to use granulocytes from CMV-seronegative donors for these patients.[65] It has also been suggested that AIDS patients should be considered at risk of transfusion-associated CMV disease.[78] It is important to note, however, that there is no evidence that immunocompetent recipients are at any major risk of disease from CMV-positive transfusions and that the process of testing blood for anti-CMV should be considered more in the light of a compatibility assessment to match an appropriate product to the special needs of a selected patient. Recently, it has become apparent that leukocyte filters may be an effective means of interrupting transfusion-transmitted CMV infection.[79,80] It is possible that this approach could obviate the need for donor test.

Financial Implications of Laboratory Testing

In general, the direct costs of laboratory testing are relatively modest, as indicated in Table 14–4, which shows the general range of the costs of test reagents and the direct labor costs for each of the tests discussed. The reagent costs are for 1988, are approximate, and are based on the assumption that reagents are available under negotiated supply contracts with substantial volume discounts. List prices for spot purchase of test kits are substantially higher, by a factor of between 2 and 5. These direct costs constitute 10% to 15% of the total value of a unit of blood or a red blood cell product. Indirect costs have not been estimated, since they are dependent on numerous factors that vary locally.

The rate at which reactive values are determined will affect the frequency with which it is necessary to repeat tests and perform confirmatory assays. The frequency of true-positive findings will directly influence the time and

Test	Costs: Supplies Plus Labor, $
ALT	0.25–0.50
anti-HBc	1.40–1.75
anti-HIV	1.25–1.55
anti HTLV-I	1.25–2.25
HBsAg	1.05–1.45
Syphilis	0.50–1.00
Anti-HCV	. . .*
Total	5.70–8.50

*No data available before licensure.

resources required for notification and counseling of positive donors. In addition, most test results are available after the blood product is fully processed and ready for issue. Consequently, resources have been committed and the cost of producing the discarded unit must be absorbed. Simplistically, every 1% of products discarded loads the cost of acceptable units by 1%.

Quality control and proficiency testing are key components of an effective program for laboratory screening of blood donations.[81] In addition, recent Federal legislation makes it essentially mandatory to participate in an approved proficiency program. Thus, it is necessary to budget for the program itself, and for the reagents and staff time to perform the relatively small amount of additional testing. It is also appropriate to consider the addition of a run control with each day's testing. The control should be a sample that has a defined, but low, level of positive reactivity in the test system with which it is used. It is desirable to establish a range of expected values for the sample and to assure that each run generates results that are in control. This type of reagent may also be used to review the performance of new master lots of each reagent.

Future Testing

Other Retroviruses

A number of other human retroviruses transmissible by blood transfusion have already been recognized and there is no reason to suppose that others will not be identified in the future. Tests for HIV-2 have already been developed, since it is clear that current HIV tests are incapable of detecting all HIV-2 seropositive persons. Presumably, it will make most sense to attempt to supplement HIV tests with HIV-2–related antigens to assure detection of infection with either virus in a single test.

Other Infectious Agents

New laboratory tests have always been implemented in response to an existing need and it is apparent that current needs relating to blood safety are being met by tests that are either in hand, or which will shortly be available. The example of AIDS has shown that it is practically impossible to predict the appearance of a major threat to the blood supply, so it is difficult to predict the need for, or nature of, future tests. In addition, there is real hope that the development of viral inactivation or depletion procedures for blood components may reduce the future need for testing. Two possible areas of concern may be identified at this time. The first is the possibility that *Trypanosoma cruzi*, the causative agent of Chagas' disease, may be present among populations that have emigrated from Central or South America. Tests are available and may, perhaps, be selectively applied to donor populations at risk as has been proposed in Europe for donors from malaria-endemic populations. Second, it has been known for some time that the B19 human parvovirus may cause aplastic crisis in certain anemia patients and that it is transmissible by transfusion. Viremia is extremely infrequent in donor populations and it seems unlikely that there will be any real pressure to implement testing until more information about pathogenicity is available.[82]

References

1. Williams AE, Fang CT, Slamon DJ, et al: Seroprevalence and epidemiological correlates of HTLV-1 infection in US blood donors. *Science* 240:643–646, 1988.

2. Barre-Sinoussi F, Chermann J-C, Rey F, et al: Isolation of a T-lymphotropic retrovirus from a patient at risk for acquired immune deficiency syndrome (AIDS). *Science* 220:868–871, 1983.

3. Gallo RC, Salahuddin SZ, Popovic M, et al: Frequent detection and isolation of cytopathic retroviruses (HTLV-III) from patients with AIDS and at risk for AIDS. *Science* 224:500–503, 1984.

4. Levy JA, Hoffman AD, Kramer SM, et al: Isolation of lymphocytopathic retroviruses from San Francisco patients with AIDS. *Science* 225:840–842, 1984.

5. Sarngadharan MG, Popovic M, Bruch L, et al: Antibodies reactive with human T-lymphotropic retroviruses (HTLV-III) in the serum of patients with AIDS. *Science* 224:506–508, 1984.

6. Kuhnl P, Seidl S, Holzberger G: HLA Dr4 antibodies cause positive HTLV III antibody ELISA results. *Lancet* 1:1222–1223, 1985.

7. Sayers MH, Beatty PG, Hansen JH: HLA antibodies as a cause of false-positive reactions in screening enzyme immunoassays for antibodies to human T-lymphotropic virus type III. *Transfusion* 26:113–115, 1986.

8. Dodd RY: Testing for HTLV-III/LAV, in Menitove JE, Kolins J (eds): *AIDS*. Arlington, VA, American Association of Blood Banks, 1986, pp 55–78.

9. Mortimer PP, Parry JV, Mortimer JV: Which anti-HTLV-III/LAV assays for screening and confirmatory testing? *Lancet* 2:877–878, 1985.

10. Burke DS, Brandt BL, Redfield RR, et al: Diagnosis of human immunodeficiency virus infection by immunoassay using a molecularly cloned and expressed virus envelope polypeptide: Comparison to western blot on 2707 consecutive serum samples. *Ann Intern Med* 106:671–676, 1987.

11. Wang JJG, Steel S, Wisniewolski R, Wang CY: Detection of antibodies to human T-lymphotropic virus type III by using a synthetic peptide of 21 amino acid residues corresponding to a highly antigenic segment of gp41 envelope protein. *Proc Natl Acad Sci USA* 83:6159–6163, 1986.

12. Quinn TC, Riggin CH, Kline RL, et al: Rapid latex agglutination assay using recombinant envelope polypeptide for the detection of antibody to the HIV. *JAMA* 260:510–513, 1988.

13. Carlson JR, Mertens SC, Yee JL, et al: Rapid, easy and economical screening test for antibodies to HIV. *Lancet* 1:361–362, 1987.

14. Ward JW, Grindon AJ, Feorino PM, et al: Laboratory and epidemiologic evaluation of an enzyme immunoassay for antibodies to HTLV-III. *JAMA* 256:357–361, 1986.

15. Grindon AJ, Critchley SE, Ward JW: Risk of HIV infection in recipients of untested blood from donors now anti-HIV-positive. *Transfusion* 28:419–421, 1988.

16. Dodd RY: Selection of methods for HBsAg, anti-HIV and anti-HBc testing, in Dixon MR, Ellisor SS (eds): *Selection of Methods and Instruments for Blood Banks.* Arlington, VA, American Association of Blood Banks, 1987, pp 91–108.

17. Cumming PD, Wallace EL, Schorr JB, Dodd RY: Exposure of patients to human immunodeficiency virus through the transfusion of blood components that test antibody-negative. *N Engl J Med* 321:941–946, 1989.

18. Dock NL, Lamberson HV, O'Brien TA, et al: Evaluation of atypical human immunodeficiency virus immunoblot reactivity in blood donors. *Transfusion* 28:412–418, 1988.

19. Carlson JR, Yee J, Hinrichs SH, et al: Comparison of indirect immunofluorescence and Western blot for detection of anti-human immunodeficiency virus antibodies. *J Clin Microbiol* 25:494–497, 1987.

20. Saah AJ, Farzadegan H, Fox R, et al: Detection of early antibodies in HIV infection by enzyme-linked immunosorbent assay, western blot, and radioimmunoprecipitation. *J Clin Microbiol* 25:1605–1610, 1987.

21. Handsfield HH, Wandell M, Goldstein L, et al: Screening and diagnostic performance of enzyme immunoassay for antibody to lymphadenopathy-associated virus. *J Clin Microbiol* 25:879–884, 1987.

22. Carlson JR: Serological diagnosis of human immunodeficiency virus infection by western blot testing. *JAMA* 260:674–679, 1988.

23. Hausler WJ: Report of the Third Consensus Conference on HIV Testing sponsored by the Association of State and Territorial Public Health Laboratory Directors. *Infect Control Hosp Epidemiol* 9:345–349, 1988.

24. Interpretation and use of the western blot assay for serodiagnosis of human immunodeficiency virus type 1 infections. *MMWR* 38(suppl 5–7):1–7, 1989.

25. Dodd RY, Fang CT: The western immunoblot procedure for HIV antibodies and its interpretation. *Arch Pathol Lab Med* 114:240–245, 1990.

26. Jackson JB, MacDonald KL, Cadwell J, et al: Absence of HIV infection in blood donors with indeterminate western blot tests for antibody to HIV-1. *N Engl J Med* 322:217–222, 1990.

27. Genesca J, Shih JW-K, Jett BW, et al: What do western blot indeterminate patterns for human immunodeficiency virus mean in EIA-negative blood donors. *Lancet* 2:1023–1025, 1989.

28. Ward JW, Holmberg SD, Allen JR, et al: Transmission of human immunodeficiency virus (HIV) by blood transfusions screened as negative for HIV antibody. *N Engl J Med* 318:473–478, 1988.

29. Farzadegan H, Polis MA, Wolinsky SM, et al: Loss of human immunodeficiency virus type 1 (HIV-1) antibodies with evidence of viral infection in asymptomatic homosexual men. *Ann Intern Med* 108:785–790, 1988.

30. Wolinsky S, Rinaldo C, Farzadegan H, et al: Polymerase chain reaction (PCR) detection of HIV provirus before HIV seroconversion, in *Abstracts of IVth International Conference on AIDS*, Stockholm, Sweden, 1988, vol 1, p 137.

31. Allain J-P, Laurian Y, Paul DA, et al: Serological markers in early stages of human immunodeficiency virus infection in haemophiliacs. *Lancet* 2:1233–1236, 1986.

32. Goudsmit J, DeWolf F, Paul DA, et al: Expression of human immunodeficiency virus antigen (HIV-Ag) in serum and cerebrospinal fluid during acute and chronic infection. *Lancet* 2:177–180, 1986.

33. Backer U, Weinauer F, Gathof G, Eberle J: HIV antigen screening in blood donors (letter). *Lancet* 2:1213–1214, 1987.

34. Alter HJ, Epstein JS, Swenson SG, et al: Collaborative study to evaluate HIV antigen (HIV-Ag) screening of blood donors (abstract). *Transfusion* 29(suppl 7):56S, 1989.

35. Stramer SL, Heller JS, Coombs RW et al: Markers of HIV infection prior to IgG antibody seropositivity. *JAMA* 262:64–69, 1989.

36. Kuritsky JN, Rastogi SC, Faich GA, et al: Results of nationwide screening of blood and plasma for antibodies to human T-cell lymphotropic III virus, type III. *Transfusion* 26:205–207, 1986.

37. Schorr JB, Berkowitz A, Cumming PD, Katz AJ, Sandler SG: Prevalence of HTLV-III antibody in American blood donors. *N Engl J Med* 313:384–385, 1985.

38. Ward JW, Deppe DA, Samson S, et al: Risk of human immunodeficiency virus infection from blood donors who later developed the acquired immunodeficiency syndrome. *Ann Intern Med* 106:61–62, 1987.

39. Peterman TA, Lui K-J, Lawrence DN, Allen JR: Estimating the risks of transfusion-associated acquired immune deficiency syndrome and human immunodeficiency virus infection. *Transfusion* 27:371–374, 1987.

40. Burke DS, Brundage JF, Herbold JR, et al: Human immunodeficiency virus infections among civilian applicants for United States military service, October 1985 to March 1986: Demographic factors associated with seropositivity. *N Engl J Med* 317:131–136, 1987.

41. Baker JL, Kelen GD, Siverston KT, Quinn TC: Unsuspected human immunodeficiency virus in critically ill emergency patients. *JAMA* 257:2609–2611, 1987.

42. Hoff R, Berardi VP, Weiblen BJ, et al: Seroprevalence of human immunodeficiency virus among childbearing women: Estimation by testing samples of blood from newborns. *N Engl J Med* 318:525–530, 1988.

43. Curran JW, Jaffe HW, Hardy AM, et al: Epidemiology of HIV infection and AIDS in the United States. *Science* 239:610–616, 1988.

44. Human immunodeficiency virus infection in the United States: A review of current knowledge. *MMWR* (Suppl S6):1–48, 1987.

45. Peterman TA, Stoneburner RL, Allen JR, et al: Risk of human immunodeficiency virus transmission from heterosexual adults with transfusion-associated infections. *JAMA* 259:55–58, 1988.

46. *HIV/AIDS Surveillance Report.* Atlanta, Centers for Disease Control, April 1990, pp 1–18.

47. Dodd RY: Research in progress workshop. *Trans Med Rev* 2:299–300, 1988.

48. Kleinman S, Secord K: Risk of human immunodeficiency virus (HIV) transmission by anti-HIV negative blood: Estimates using the lookback methodology. *Transfusion* 28:499–401, 1988.

49. Cohen ND, Munoz A, Reitz BA, et al: Transmission of retroviruses of screened blood in patients undergoing cardiac surgery. *N Engl J Med* 320:1172–1176, 1989.

50. Minamoto GY, Gold JWM, Scheinberg DA, et al: Infection with human T-cell leukemia virus type 1 in patients with leukemia. *N Engl J Med* 318:219–222, 1988.

51. Licensure of screening tests for antibody to human T-lymphotropic virus type I. *MMWR* 37:736–745, 1988.

52. London WT, Sutnick AI, Blumberg BS: Australia antigen and acute viral hepatitis. *Ann Intern Med* 70:55–59, 1963.

53. Prince AM: An antigen detected in the blood during the incubation period of serum hepatitis. *Proc Natl Acad Sci USA* 60:814–821, 1968.

54. Ling CM, Overby LR: Prevalence of hepatitis B virus antigen as revealed by direct radioimmune assay with 125-I-antibody. *J Immunol* 109:834–841, 1972.

55. Thompson RJ, Jackson AP, Langlois N: Circulating antibodies to mouse monoclonal immunoglobulins in normal subjects: Incidence, species specificity, and effects on a two-site assay for creatine kinasc-MB isoenzyme. *Clin Chem* 32:476–481, 1986.

56. Zweig MH, Csako G, Benson CC, et al: Interference by anti-immunoglobulin G antibodies in immunoradiometric assays of thyrotropin involving mouse monoclonal antibodies. *Clin Chem* 33:840–844, 1987.

57. Almeida JD, Rubenstein D, Stott EJ: New antigen-antibody system in Australia-antigen positive hepatitis. *Lancet* 2:1225–1227, 1971.

58. Bastiaans MJS, Nath N, Dodd RY, Barker LF: Hepatitis-associated markers in the American Red Cross volunteer blood donor population: IV. A comparison of HBV-associated serologic markers in HBsAg-positive first-time and repeat blood donors. *Vox Sang* 42:203–210, 1982.

59. Kline WE, Bowman RJ, McCurdy KKE, et al: Hepatitis B core antibody (anti-HBc) in blood donors in the United States: Implications for surrogate testing programs. *Transfusion* 27:99–102. 1987.

60. Choo Q-L, Kuo G, Weiner AJ, et al: Isolation of a cDNA clone derived from a blood borne non-A, non-B viral hepatitis genome. *Science* 244:359–362, 1989.

61. Kuo G, Choo Q-L, Alter HJ, et al: An assay for circulating antibodies to a major etiologic virus of human non-A, non-B hepatitis. *Science* 244:362–364, 1989.

62. Alter HJ, Purcell RH, Shih JW, et al: Detection of antibody to hepatitis C virus in prospectively followed transfusion recipients with acute and chronic non-A, non-B hepatitis. *N Engl J Med* 321:1494–1500, 1989.

63. Alter HJ, Purcell RH, Holland PV, et al: Donor transaminase and recipient hepatitis: Impact on blood transfusion services. *JAMA* 246:630–634, 1981.

64. Aach RD, Szmuness W, Mosley JW, et al: Serum alanine aminotransferase of donors in relation to the risk of non-A, non-B hepatitis in recipients: The Transfusion-Transmitted Viruses Study. *N Engl J Med* 304:989–994, 1981.

65. Swenson S: Syphilis serology, cytomegalovirus testing and alanine aminotransferase testing, in Dixon MR, Ellisor SS (eds): *Selection of Methods and Instruments for Blood Banks*. Arlington, VA, American Association of Blood Banks, 1987, pp 51–90.

66. Zuck TF, Sherwood WC, Bove JR: A review of recent events related to surrogate testing of blood to prevent non-A, non-B posttransfusion hepatitis. *Transfusion* 27:203–206, 1987.

67. Sherman KE, Dodd RY, American Red Cross Alanine Aminotransferase Study Group: Alanine aminotransferase levels among volunteer blood donors: Geographic variation and risk factors. *J Infect Dis* 45:383–386, 1982.

68. Stevens CE, Aach RD, Hollinger FB, et al: Hepatitis B virus antibody in blood donors and the occurrence of non-A, non-B hepatitis in transfusion recipients: An analysis of the Transmission-Transmitted Viruses Study. *Ann Intern Med* 101:733–738, 1984.

69. Koziol DE, Holland PV, Alling DW, et al: Antibody to hepatitis B core antigen as a paradoxical marker for non-A, non-B hepatitis agents in donated blood. *Ann Intern Med* 104:488–495, 1986.

70. Dodd RY: Donor screening and epidemiology, in Dodd RY, Barker LF (eds): *Infection, Immunity, and Blood Transfusion*. New York, Alan R Liss, 1985, pp 389–405.

71. Changing patterns of groups at high risk for hepatitis B in the United States. *MMWR* 37:429–437, 1988.

72. Alter MJ, Mares A, Hadler SC, Maynard JE: The effect of underreporting on the apparent incidence and epidemiology of acute viral hepatitis. *Am J Epidemiol* 125:133–139, 1987.

73. Dodd RY, Diala C, Kline L, et al: Evaluation of a predonation test for hemoglobin, anti-HBc and ALT (abstract). *Transfusion* 29(suppl 7):43S, 1989.

74. Lamberson HV, McMillan JA, Weiner LB, et al: Prevention of transfusion-associated cytomegalovirus (CMV) infection in neonates by screening blood donors for IgM to CMV. *J Infect Dis* 157:820–823, 1988.

75. Lentz EB, Dock NL, McMahon CA, et al: Detection of antibody to CMV-induced early antigens and comparison with four serologic assays and presence of viruria in blood donors. *J Clin Microbiol* 26:133–135, 1988.

76. Yeager AS, Palumbo PE, Malachowski N, et al: Sequelae of maternally derived cytomegalovirus infections in premature infants. *J Pediatr* 102:918–922, 1983.

77. Winston DJ, Ho WG, Cheng-Hsien L, et al: Intravenous immune globulin for prevention of cytomegalovirus infection and interstitial pneumonia after bone marrow transplantation. *Ann Intern Med* 106:12–18, 1987.

78. Tegtmeier GE: Blood transfusion and the transmission of cytomegalovirus, in Moore SB (ed): *Transfusion-Transmitted Viral Diseases*. Arlington, VA, American Association of Blood Banks, 1987, pp 87–118.

79. Gilbert GL, Hudson IL, Hayes K, et al: Prevention of transfusion-associated cytomegalovirus infection in infants by blood filtration to remove leucocytes. *Lancet* 1:1228–1231, 1989.

80. De Graan-Hentzen YCE, Gratama JW, Mudde GC, et al: Prevention of primary cytomegalovirus infection in patients with hematologic malignancies by intensive white cell depletion of blood products. *Transfusion* 29:757–760, 1989.

81. Fang CT, Dodd RY: Immunoassays, in Vengelen-Tyler V, Baldwin ML (eds): *Understanding Technology New to the Blood Bank*, Arlington, VA, American Association of Blood Banks, 1988, pp 17–30.

82. Anderson MJ: Human parvovirus infections. *J Virol Meth* 17:175–181, 1987.

15
Preventing Transfusion-Transmitted Infections in Persons With Hemophilia

Jeanette K. Stehr-Green, MD
Bruce L. Evatt, MD
Dale N. Lawrence, MD

Hemophilia and other coagulation disorders result from reduced levels or defective structures of specific clotting factors in the blood that are necessary to maintain the normal hemostatic mechanism. These clotting factors are plasma proteins; therefore, patients with hemophilia do not normally receive cellular blood components during replacement therapy, but instead receive cell-free blood components that contain clotting factors, including plasma, cryoprecipitate, and commercially prepared concentrated clotting factors. Depending on the severity of the patient's bleeding disorder, intermittent transfusions of these blood products are required throughout the patient's life in response to acute bleeding episodes, for treatment before, during, and after surgery, or prophylactically to prevent bleeding episodes and related complications during periods of heavy physical demands.

Persons with hemophilia constitute a unique population for studying transfusion-transmitted infections. They differ from other patients who receive transfusions for acute blood loss or anemia with respect to specific infectious agents and risk of blood-transmitted infections. Because the hemophilic patient is treated with cell-free blood components, infectious agents of concern are those transmitted in the plasma. Those transmitted in red blood cells (such as malaria and babesiosis) or white blood cells (such as EBV, CMV, or toxoplasmosis) are not a major problem, because they are not usually associated with transfusion of plasma or plasma-derived components.[1-3] In addition, because of the large number of donors to which the hemophilic patient is exposed (through multiple transfusions and concentrated clotting factor that is prepared from plasma pools collected from hundreds to thousands of donors), the risk of infection with a particular agent in the hemophilic population is very high, even if the prevalence of infection in the donor population is low.

In this chapter we will review the infectious agents and risk of infection associated with cryoprecipitate and concentrated clotting factors in the hemophilic population. Because the use of fresh-frozen plasma is not unique to the hemophilic patient and plasma is the starting material for cryoprecipitate and commercially produced concentrated clotting factors, we will not discuss fresh frozen plasma separately. Infectious agents associated with plasma are identical to those associated with cryoprecipitate and concentrated clotting factors; however, plasma used over a brief period poses a much lower risk of infection than concentrated clotting factors. We will also review the available data on virally inactivated concentrated clotting factor. Virally inactivated factor products have received renewed attention since the identification of HIV as the causative agent of AIDS. The inactivation procedures are varied and include heat treatment (dry heat, wet heat or pasteurization, and steam), β-propriolactone and ultraviolet irradiation, mechanisms to disrupt the hydrophobic interactions of the viral coat (detergent treatment), and immunosorbent procedures for purification.[4] However, there has been only limited experience with these products. Results of *in vitro* inactivation of virus purposely inoculated into factor concentrates and chimpanzee studies may not be indicative of infectivity in humans. Published reports of human studies consist of small numbers of patients followed up for relatively short periods. Therefore, much more must be learned about these products before conclusions regarding the risk of various infections from virally inactivated products can be reached.

Hepatitis B

Prevalence of Infection

Hepatitis B was one of the first infectious agents associated with the transfusion of blood and blood components.[5] Although other infections have superseded hepatitis B in relative morbidity and mortality, it remains a serious threat to patients requiring frequent therapy with blood products. Studies of the prevalence of hepatitis B in persons with hemophilia have relied upon serologic detection of HBsAg, HBsAb, and HBcAB.

Early studies suggest that 0% to 37% of patients treated exclusively with cryoprecipitate have serologic evidence (HBsAg or HBsAb) of infection with hepatitis B.[6-8] Seroprevalence increased with increasing severity of the coagulation disorder and the number of transfusions received. These early studies, however, used less sensitive methods of antibody detection, including complement fixation and counterimmunoelectrophoresis,[9] and may have underestimated seroprevalence. With radioimmunoassay, much higher rates of seroprevalence have been reported.[9-10]

Seroprevalence in patients treated with concentrated clotting factor is generally much higher than that reported in cryoprecipitate users, ranging from 20% to 100%.[10-16] If studies using less sensitive techniques of antibody detection are excluded, reported seroprevalence ranges from 73% to 100%. Again, seroprevalence increased with increasing severity of hemophilia and the number of transfusions received. From 1% to 12% of hemophilic patients have been found to be chronic hepatitis B carriers.[11,13-16]

Results of trials with virally inactivated factor concentrates have been promising but are preliminary because the number of susceptible patients treated has been small. In three separate trials, none of 12 patients exposed to dry-heated factor VIII,[17] none of 15 patients exposed to factor VIII lyophilized in the presence of *N*-heptane,[18] and none of ten patients exposed to pasteurized factor VIII[19] developed serologic evidence of infection with hepatitis B. In contrast, four of 14 patients treated with factor VIII exposed to hot vapor developed HBsAb.[20] These results suggest that, although the risk of hepatitis B decreases with virally inactivated factor concentrate, a risk of infection still exists.

Prevalence of Disease

Because clinical status and transaminase levels are not good indicators of severity of liver damage[21,22] and liver biopsy is contraindicated in the hemophilic patient, the prevalence of liver disease in this population has not been well established. However, it is believed to be a common cause of morbidity and mortality. Twelve percent to 26% of hemophilic patients treated with concentrated clotting factor have a history of overt hepatitis and jaundice.[12,15] Biopsy studies suggest that even more patients are affected. Hay et al,[21] studying patients with persistently elevated transaminase levels, found that 38% had progressive liver disease (26% had chronic active hepatitis and 12% had cirrhosis). Schimpf,[22] studying patients needing surgery (in most cases orthopedic), found that 29% had progressive liver disease (16% chronic active hepatitis and 13% cirrhosis). The difference in disease prevalence between these two studies probably results from different selection criteria for liver biopsy. The etiology of liver disease was not determined in either study; however, other studies suggest that non-A, non-B hepatitis (see below) rather than hepatitis B accounts for the major proportion of liver disease in hemophiliacs.[23,24]

Prevention

Prevention of hepatitis B includes screening of donor blood, using hepatitis B vaccine, and using virally inactivated clotting factor products. Because none of these measures is 100% effective, all three should jointly be employed in prevention strategies.

All donated blood is screened for HBsAg; however, hemophilic patients receiving concentrated clotting factors still develop evidence for hepatitis B infection.[11,12] This may be due, in part, to the so-called window period (time after the clearance of HBsAg from the blood and before the appearance of HBsAb in which the donor is infectious but has no detectable HBsAg). Using HBcAg or antibody or ALT (as a general indicator of liver disease) may improve the sensitivity of hepatitis screening.

Hemophilic patients without serologic markers for hepatitis B should be vaccinated against hepatitis B before receiving any blood products. To avoid hemorrhagic complications, vaccination should be given subcutaneously, rather than intramuscularly as in the nonhemophilic patient. Unfortunately, HIV infection may reduce the effectiveness of hepatitis B vaccine. Drake et al,[25] studying 12 HIV-seropositive hemophilic patients and 29 HIV-seronegative hemophilic patients, noted that 50% of HIV-seropositive patients did not respond to hepatitis vaccination compared with 7% of HIV-seronegative patients. Such findings could foreshadow future problems in this population, which has a high prevalence of HIV infection (see below), and underscore the importance of virally inactivated factor products. Household contacts of patients with hemophilia, particularly sexual contacts or those administering clotting factor transfusions, should also be vaccinated against hepatitis B.[26-28]

Non-A, Non-B Hepatitis

Prevalence of Infection

Non-A, non-B hepatitis was recognized as early as 1974 as a clinical entity distinct from hepatitis A and hepatitis B. Recently, a virus believed to cause non-A, non-B hepatitis was identified and cloned from a chimpanzee with chronic non-A, non-B hepatitis.[29] This single stranded viral RNA molecule, designated hepatitis C (HCV) is not related to other hepatitis viruses and is found only in non-A, non-B hepatitis infections. A commercial EIA serological assay has been developed using viral antigen expressed by the clone. Investigators have shown that as much as 80% of post-transfusion non-A, non-B hepatitis patients have antibodies detected by this EIA.[30] However, more than one agent may be responsible for non-A, non-B hepatitis, so the impact of this discovery on preventive measures may be limited to a percentage of the cases.

Studies of the prevalence and incidence of non-A, non-B hepatitis in the hemophilic population and the safety of virally inactivated products have been inhibited by the inability to identify and isolate an etiologic agent and by the lack of an adequate animal model. Non-A, non-B hepatitis is a diagnosis of exclusion that can only be made prospectively, since no persistent serologic markers are presently available. For these reasons, studies of non-A, non-B hepatitis and the safety of blood products require specific guidelines, such as those proposed by the International Committee on Thrombosis and Hemostasis (Table 15–1). These studies define non-A, non-B hepatitis as a rise in AST or ALT levels exceeding 2.5 times the upper limit of normal in a patient who has not previously received blood products and has no serologic evidence of hepatitis A, hepatitis B, CMV, EBV virus infection, or any other known cause of hepatitis. The requirement that studies must be conducted among previously untreated patients (since previous infections may protect against future infections) seriously limits the number of patients available for these studies.

Table 15–1   International Committee on Thrombosis and Hemostasis
Criteria for the Prospective Study of the Safety of Factor
Concentrates for Hepatitis Virus

Enrollment

Patients should have no previous treatment with any blood products, including
single-donor derived units.

Patients should have no serologic markers for hepatitis B virus infection (except
for HBsAb in patients vaccinated against hepatitis B).

Pretreatment levels of aminotransferases (ALT and AST) must be normal.

Follow-up

Follow-up testing and clinical evaluation must be frequent and regular: ALT
testing every 2 weeks for the initial 4 months, then every month until one
year; hepatitis B markers at 4, 6, and 12 months.

Interpretation

Hepatitis B virus infection is diagnosed by the finding of any newly detected
hepatitis B marker (HBsAg, HBsAb, HBcAb).

Non-A, non-B hepatitis is diagnosed by finding an elevation of ALT more than
2.5 times the upper limit of normal on two successive occasions after
excluding other causes of hepatitis including Epstein-Barr virus and
cytomegalovirus.

No information is available on the incidence of non-A, non-B hepatitis
in patients using cryoprecipitate exclusively. In patients receiving factor concentrate (not virally inactivated) for the first time, the incidence of non-A,
non-B hepatitis approaches 100%.[31,32] Hepatitis risk appears to vary between
the different virally inactivated factor products. In a study by Colombo et al,
11 (85%) of 13 previously untreated patients treated with dry-heated factor
VIII developed non-A, non-B hepatitis.[17] Nine (24%) of 37 patients treated
with lyophilized factor VIII suspended in N-heptane in two separate studies
developed non-A, non-B hepatitis.[18,33] In contrast, in previously untreated
patients, none of 26 receiving pasteurized factor VIII,[19] none of 15 patients
receiving solvent-detergent–treated factor VIII,[34] and none of 28 patients
receiving factor VIII exposed to hot vapor[20] developed non-A, non-B hepatitis.
However, the number of patients treated with each product has been small,
and further studies should be undertaken.

Prevalence of Disease

Liver disease is a common cause of morbidity and mortality in the hemophilic
population; however, there are a number of causes. A study of liver biopsy
specimens from 157 hemophilic patients from hemophilia treatment centers
in the United States and Western Europe suggests that non-A, non-B hepatitis
may be the predominant cause of liver disease in hemophilic patients.[23] Based
on histologic features, 80% of biopsy specimens were considered to show

evidence of possible non-A, non-B hepatitis infection and 18 were considered to show evidence of possible hepatitis B infection. Biopsies were not done randomly and criteria for biopsy differed by treatment center; therefore, these results should not be considered indicative of the prevalence of disease in the general hemophilic population but rather of the relative occurrence of disease due to non-A, non-B hepatitis and hepatitis B.

Prevention

Because no etiologic agent has been identified for non-A, non-B hepatitis, no screening measures or vaccines have been developed specifically for this infection. Recent discovery of one of the responsible viruses should allow the development of serologic screening methods. However, because the proportion of non-A, non-B hepatitis attributable to this new virus is unknown, the impact of the discovery on prevention and control remains to be determined. At this point, prevention rests on the development and use of virally inactivated factor products. Screening donor blood for elevations in the ALT level (a general indicator of liver disease) may also be of benefit.

Delta Hepatitis Infection

Prevalence of Infection

The delta agent, first described by Rizzetto et al[35] in 1977, is a defective virus that needs hepatitis B virus as a helper for replication. Infection by the delta agent can occur as a coinfection with hepatitis B or as superinfection of a hepatitis B carrier. Because hemophilic patients are at risk of infection with hepatitis B and hepatitis B carrier state, they are at high risk of infection with the delta agent.

No information is available on the prevalence of delta virus infection in patients using cryoprecipitate exclusively. Forty to 48% of concentrated clotting factor users who are HBsAg-positive have antibody to the delta agent.[13,36,37] The prevalence is higher in adults than in children. No information is available on the risk of infection with delta agent in patients receiving virally inactivated concentrated factor.

Prevalence of Disease

As with hepatitis B and non-A, non-B hepatitis, the proportion of liver disease attributable to delta hepatitis in the hemophilic population is unknown. However, coinfection with hepatitis B and delta hepatitis is associated with a higher frequency of fulminant hepatitis than hepatitis B infection alone and therefore could have more serious implications.

Prevention

No specific means of prevention are being used for delta hepatitis. However, because the delta agent needs hepatitis B virus to replicate, prevention of hepatitis B (through screening, vaccination, or use of virally inactivated products) should also prevent infection with the delta agent.

HIV

Prevalence of Infection

The first AIDS patient with an underlying coagulation disorder was diagnosed with *Pneumocystis carinii* pneumonia in 1981.[38] As of Jan 1, 1990, 1312 cases of hemophilia-associated AIDS had been reported to the CDC. However, serologic studies suggest that many more hemophilic patients have been infected with HIV and are, therefore, at risk of AIDS.

Among patients treated exclusively with cryoprecipitate, 0% to 40% have been shown to have antibody to HIV.[39-44] Seroprevalence among patients treated with concentrated factor product has been much higher: in hemophilia treatment center–based studies, 56% to 100% of persons with hemophilia A and 30% to 52% of persons with hemophilia B have been shown to have antibody to HIV.[40-47] Patients with severe hemophilia, who received larger and more frequent doses of concentrated clotting factor, were more likely to be seropositive than less severely affected patients.

Clinically significant control of HIV infection in patients with hemophilia did not begin until after 1984, when HIV was demonstrated to be very heat-labile in vitro. Studies showed that HIV, which had been added to factor VIII concentrate test samples, was effectively inactivated at 60 °C without significantly altering the plasma recovery or half-life of clotting factors.[48] In October 1984, the National Hemophilia Foundation recommended using heat-treated factor concentrates to prevent further infection with HIV.[49] By the end of 1985, these recommendations had been almost universally adopted.

Studies of small numbers of seronegative patients have documented a lack of HIV seroconversion with American-made, heat-treated factor VIII concentrates;[46,50-52] however, reports of six seroconversions have been published.[53-55] To examine the risk of infection, the CDC surveyed 13 hemophilia treatment centers located in Western Europe, Canada, and Australia[56] to better determine the risk of seroconversion in patients receiving heat-treated products. Centers outside of the United States were chosen because of their longer history of use of heat-treated products. Products initially in use had been manufactured from donated blood that had not been screened for antibody to HIV (unscreened). As of June 1987, the 13 hemophilia treatment centers reported on 1512 patients who were seronegative when unscreened heat-treated concentrates were introduced. Twenty-three patients were known to have seroconverted after changing to unscreened heat-treated products. Only three had documented seroconversions that seemed attributable to the heat-treated factor product. These three patients represented 0.2% of the seronegative patients at these centers. Follow-up of the remaining 1489 seronegative patients from these centers since switching their therapy to *donor-screened*, heat-treated products has disclosed no further seroconversions.[57]

Table 15–2   CDC Criteria for the Relationship Between HIV
Seroconversion and Heat-Treated Factor Concentrates

Confirmation of HIV seropositivity.

Confirmation that the patient was previously negative.

No use of unheated concentrates before the last seronegative test for at least 6 months.

No other untreated, unscreened blood product exposure during the relevant periods.

No recognized or suspected gaps in therapy records.

No other risk factors.

In addition to coordinating the study of non-US centers, the CDC has maintained a surveillance system for seroconversions in hemophilic patients. Through January 11, 1988, the CDC had evaluated more than 75 reports, worldwide, of possible HIV seroconversion associated with heat-treated factor product. Of these, 18 met CDC operational criteria for a probable association with heat-treated factor concentrate (Table 15–2); nine additional reports are still under investigation. The factor concentrate associated with ten of the 18 patients had been produced from plasma collected before the initiation of donor screening. Nearly all of these seroconversions occurred in patients receiving concentrate produced by a single US manufacturer. Eight of the seroconversions are associated with use of donor-screened, heat-treated products.[57] One seroconversion occurred in the United States in a patient with an inhibitor to factor VIII who had received extremely large doses of concentrate.[58] The implicated product had been heated in the dry state at 60 °C for 24 hours. The other seven seroconversions were reported from Canada.[59] The seroconversions occurred at one hemophilia treatment center in mid-1987. A strong statistical association was demonstrated between seroconversion and reccipt of one or more of three lots of heat-treated factor VIII concentrate made from a single plasma pool produced by a single manufacturer. This product had been heated in the dry state at 60 °C for 30 hours. The company has now withdrawn these products from the market.

These data indicate that concentrated factor VIII products currently available in North America, Europe, and Australia have a high degree of safety for HIV. Based on data available from the National Hemophilia Foundation, FDA collaborative project, the Transfusion Safety Study, and CDC surveillance, the annual rate of HIV seroconversion on the donor-screened, virally inactivated factor products currently available seems to be well below one per 1000.

Prevalence of Disease

HIV infection has a spectrum of clinical manifestations ranging from asymptomatic infection (with only laboratory evidence of infection) to severe immunodeficiency with life-threatening secondary infections and cancers. National surveillance of AIDS encompasses only the severe manifestations believed to be very specific for HIV, which are included in the CDC AIDS case definition.[60] However, many persons infected with HIV have manifestations not included in the case definition.

National AIDS surveillance suggests that approximately 7% of all men with hemophilia in the United States have developed AIDS. However, hemophilia treatment center–based studies suggest that the cumulative incidence of AIDS in seropositive patients is as high as 25% in some populations.[61] The total number of patients with HIV-related illnesses, including illnesses not meeting the case definition for AIDS, exceeds these statistics substantially.

Prevention

Prevention of further HIV infection in the hemophilic population relies on screening of donor blood for antibody to HIV, self-exclusion of donors at risk of HIV infection, and viral inactivation procedures. Tests available for detecting antibody to HIV include the ELISA, western blot technique, immunofluorescence, and radioimmunoprecipitation. Most experience has been gained with the ELISA and the western blot. Clinical data submitted to the FDA by manufacturers indicate that the sensitivity and specificity of the seven licensed anti-HIV ELISA kits exceed 99%.[62] The specificity is increased to 99.8% if an initially reactive test is repeated. Use of the western blot as a confirmatory test increases the specificity even further. False-positive and false-negative reactions do occur. The former usually occur in uninfected persons who have immunologic disturbances or who have received multiple transfusions. False-negative reactions are observed in persons who have recently become infected with HIV and have not developed detectable antibody. Improvement of ELISA kits and the use of tests that measure viral antigen may help detect infectious blood donors during this period.

Sex partners and offspring of HIV-seropositive men are also at risk of infection with HIV. Counseling and public health interventions, such as the use of "safe" sexual practices and the deferral of pregnancy, should prevent further spread of the infection.

Other Infections

Several other infectious agents, though not studied as extensively as those listed above, deserve brief comment.

Parvovirus causes a febrile illness in hematologically normal people and aplastic crisis in patients with hemolytic anemia. Because the viremic phase of parvovirus infection is very short, transmission of parvovirus by blood transfusion is probably extremely rare;[3] however, use of pooled plasma products probably increases the risk. Mortimer et al[63] demonstrated an increased prevalence of antibody to parvovirus among children and young adults receiving factor concentrates, although no patient had a history of clinical manifestations. Because another report suggests that concurrent infection with HIV and parvovirus may lead to aplastic anemia,[64] this infection may be of clinical importance in the hemophilic population.

HTLV-I has been associated with adult T-cell leukemia and two similar, if not identical diseases: tropical spastic paraparesis and endemic myelopathy.[65] Retrospective studies suggest that HTLV-I can be transmitted by blood transfusion; however, only blood components containing cells have been implicated.[66] These findings have been supported in two serologic studies of patients with hemophilia. In these studies, only one of 135 hemophilic patients has been found to have antibody to HTLV-I.[67,68]

HIV-2 is a retrovirus closely related to HIV. It has been associated with an AIDS-like illness in west Africa, with modes of transmission similar to that of HIV. The CDC, FDA, and collaborating investigators have screened 22,699 serum samples collected in the United States with anti–HIV-2 enzyme immunoassay and HIV-2–specific Western blot.[69] Of these specimens, 10,766 were from persons whose activities placed them at increased risk of HIV infection. Although some samples were ELISA-positive, none were confirmed by Western blot, suggesting that the prevalence of HIV-2 infection in the United States is very low. No specific studies of HIV-2 in the hemophilic population have been published. Pasteurization has been shown to be effective in inactivating HIV-2 added experimentally to concentrated clotting factor,[70] however, continued research is needed to confirm these findings.

In summary, improvements in viral inactivation procedures have greatly reduced the risk of bloodborne infection in the hemophilic population, and the risk of withholding therapy far outweighs the risk of infection. The National Hemophilia Foundation has issued guidelines[57] for treating hemophilic patients to reduce the risk of infection in this population to an absolute minimum. These guidelines include the following recommendations:[56]

A. General recommendations: Health care providers should educate patients to use appropriate doses of clotting factor to minimize overuse and contain costs.
B. Factor VIII deficiency: Desmopressin should be used whenever possible by patients with mild or moderate hemophilia A.

   1. HIV. Products that are heated in aqueous solution (pasteurized), detergent-solvent treated, monoclonal antibody–purified, heated in suspension in organic media, or dry heated at high temperatures for long periods are preferred for treating hemophilia A.

   2. Hepatitis. Hepatitis B vaccine is essential for patients with hemophilia and its administration is recommended at birth or at diagnosis of hemophilia. Preliminary data suggest that products that are heated in aqueous solution (pasteurized), detergent-solvent treated, or monoclonal antibody–purified may be at a reduced risk of transmitting hepatitis viruses. When feasible, an alternative to concentrates may be the use of cryoprecipitate prepared from a single, well-screened and repeatedly tested donor, or from a small number of such donors.

C. Factor IX deficiency: For patients with severe factor IX deficiency, the National Hemophilia Foundation continues to recommend virally attenuated factor IX concentrate. For patients with mild or moderate factor IX deficiency, when feasible, an alternative would be fresh-frozen plasma prepared from a single or small number of well-screened and repeatedly tested donors.

References

1. Chorba TL, Evatt BL: Transfusion-associated AIDS, in Madchok R, Forbes CD, Evatt BL (eds): *Blood, Blood Products and AIDS.* London, Chapman and Hall, 1987, pp 17–31.

2. Soulier JP: Diseases transmissible by blood transfusion. *Vox Sang* 47:1–6, 1984.

3. Prince AM, Horowitz B, Horowitz MS, Zang E: The development of virus-free labile blood derivatives: A review. *Eur J Epidemiol* 3:103–118, 1987.

4. Gomperts ED: Procedures for the inactivation of viruses in clotting factor concentrates. *Am J Hematol* 23:295–305, 1986.

5. Beeson PB: Jaundice occurring one to four months after transfusion of blood or plasma: Report of seven cases. *JAMA* 121:1332–1334, 1943.

6. Seeler RA, Mufson MA: Development and persistence of antibody to hepatitis-associated (Australian) antigen in patients with hemophilia. *J Infect Dis* 123:279–283, 1971.

7. Essien EM, Smith JA, Francis TI: The prevalence of Australian antigen and antibody in haemophilia. *Acta Haematol* 50:293–298, 1973.

8. Burrell CJ, Parker AC, Ramsay DM, Proudfoot E: Antibody to hepatitis B antigen in haemophiliacs and their household contacts. *J Clin Pathol* 27:323–325, 1974.

9. Peterson MR, Barker LF, Schade DS: Detection of antibody to hepatitis-associated antigen in hemophilia patients and voluntary blood donors. *Vox Sang* 24:66–75, 1973.

10. Morfini M, Rafanelli D, Longo G, et al: Hepatitis-free interval after clotting factor therapy in first infused haemophiliacs. *Thromb Haemost* 56:268–270, 1986.

11. Hilgartner MW, Giardina P: Liver dysfunction in patients with hemophilia A, B, and von Willebrand's disease. *Transfusion* 17:495–499, 1977.

12. Enck RE, Betts RF, Brown MR, Miller G: Viral serology (hepatitis B virus, cytomegalovirus, Epstein-Barr virus) and abnormal liver function tests in transfused patients with hereditary hemorrhagic diseases. *Transfusion* 19:32–38, 1979.

13. Rizzetto M, Purcell RH, Gerin JL: Epidemiology of HBV-associated delta agent: Geographical distribution of anti-delta and prevalence in polytransfused HBsAg carriers. *Lancet* 1:1215–1218, 1980.

14. Lewis JH: Hemophilia, hepatitis and HAA. *Vox Sang* 19:406–409, 1970.

15. Lewis JH, Maxwell NG, Brandon JM: Jaundice and hepatitis B antigen/antibody in hemophilia. *Transfusion* 14:203–211, 1974.

16. Mannucci PM, Capitanio A, del Ninno E, et al: Asymptomatic liver disease in hemophiliacs. *J Clin Pathol* 28:620–624, 1975.

17. Colombo M, Mannucci PM, Carnelli V, et al: Transmission of non-A, non-B hepatitis by heat-treated factor VIII concentrate. *Lancet* 2:1–4, 1985.

18. Kernoff PBA, Miller EJ, Savidge GF, et al: Reduced risk of non-A, non-B hepatitis after a first exposure to 'wet heated' factor VIII concentrate. *Br J Haematol* 67:207–211, 1987.

19. Schimpf K, Mannucci PM, Kreutz W, et al: Absence of hepatitis after treatment with a pasteurized factor VIII concentrate in patients with hemophilia and no previous transfusions. *N Engl J Med* 316:918–922, 1987.

20. Mannucci PM, Zanetti AR, Colombo M, et al: Prospective study of hepatitis after factor VIII concentrate exposed to hot vapor. *Br J Haematol* 68:427–430, 1988.

21. Hay CRM, Preston FE, Triger DR, Underwood JCE: Progressive liver disease in haemophilia: An understated problem? *Lancet* 1:1495–1498, 1985.

22. Schimpf K: Liver disease in haemophilia. *Lancet* 1:323, 1986.

23. Aledort LM, Levine PH, Hilgartner M, et al: A study of liver biopsies and liver disease among hemophiliacs. *Blood* 66:367–372, 1985.

24. Bianchi L, Desmet VJ, Popper H, et al: Histologic patterns of liver disease in hemophiliacs with special reference to morphologic characteristics of non-A, non-B hepatitis. *Semin Liver Dis* 7:203–209, 1987.

25. Drake JH, Parmley RT, Britton HA: Loss of hepatitis B antibody in human immunodeficiency virus–positive hemophilia patients. *Pediatr Infect Dis* 6:1051–1054, 1987.

26. Buchanan GR, Richards N, Holtkamp CA, Rutledge J: Hepatitis in household contacts of patients with hemophilia who have received multiple transfusions. *J Pediatr* 108:937–939, 1986.

27. Kahn RA, Staggs SD, Oskins PD, Miller WV: Household contacts of hemophiliacs: Risk of developing hepatitis in the household contacts of hemophiliacs. *Blood* 54 (suppl 1):124a, 1979.

28. Johnson CA: Prevalence of hepatitis B core antibody in family members treating patients with hemophilia. *Pediatr Infect Dis* 3:593–594, 1984.

29. Search for elusive NANB hepatitis virus may be over. *Council Comm Blood Centers Newslett* May 13, 1988, pp 1–2.

30. Alter HJ, Jett DW, Polito AJ, et al: Overview of hepatitis C virus disease and its detection: Analysis of the role of HCV in transfusion-associated hepatitis. *Proceedings of the 1990 International Symposium on Viral Hepatitis and Liver Disease.* In Press.

31. Fletcher ML, Trowel JM, Craske J, et al: Non-A, non-B hepatitis after transfusion of factor VIII in infrequently treated patients. *Br Med J* 287:1754–1757, 1983.

32. Kernoff PBA, Lee CA, Karayiannis P, Thomas HC: High risk of non-A, non-B hepatitis after first exposure to volunteer or commercial clotting factor concentrates: Effects of prophylactic immune serum globulin. *Br J Haematol* 60:469–479, 1985.

33. Carnelli V, Gomperts KD, Friedman A, et al: Assessment for evidence of non A-non B hepatitis in patients given *N*-heptane suspended heat-treated clotting factor concentrates. *Thromb Res* 46:827–834, 1987.

34. Horowitz MS, Rooks C, Horowitz B, Hilgartner MW: Virus safety of solvent/detergent-treated antihaemophilic factor concentrate. *Lancet* 2:186–188, 1988.

35. Rizzetto M, Canese MG, Arico S, et al: Immunofluorescence detection of new antigen-antibody system (delta/anti-delta) associated to hepatitis B virus in liver and in serum of HBsAg carriers. *Gut* 18:997–1003, 1977.

36. Rizzetto M, Morello C, Mannucci PM, et al: Delta infection and liver disease in hemophilic carriers of hepatitis B surface antigen. *J Infect Dis* 145:18–21, 1982.

37. Rosina F, Saracco G, Rizzetto M: Risk of post-transfusion infection with hepatitis delta virus: A multicenter study. *N Engl J Med* 312:1488–1491, 1985.

38. Centers for Disease Control: Surveillance of hemophilia-associated acquired immunodeficiency syndrome. *MMWR* 35:669–671, 1986.

39. Goerdert JJ, Sarngadharan MG, Eyster ME, et al: Antibodies reactive with human T cell leukemia viruses in the serum of hemophiliacs receiving factor VIII concentrate. *Blood* 65:492–495, 1985.

40. Gjerset GF, McGrady G, Counts RB, et al: Lymphadenopathy-associated virus antibodies and T cells in hemophiliacs treated with cryoprecipitate or concentrate. *Blood* 66:718–720, 1985.

41. Ragni MV, Tegtmeier GE, Levy JA, et al: AIDS retrovirus antibodies in hemophiliacs treated with factor VIII or factor IX concentrates, cryoprecipitate, or fresh frozen plasma: Prevalence, seroconversion rate, and clinical correlations. *Blood* 67:592–595, 1986.

42. Waskin H, Smith KJ, Simon TL, et al: Prevalence of HTLV-III antibody among New Mexico residents with hemophilia. *West J Med* 145:477–480, 1986.

43. Kreiss JK, Kitchen LW, Prince HE, et al: Human T cell leukemia virus type III antibody, lymphadenopathy, and acquired immune deficiency syndrome in hemophiliac subjects: Results of a prospective study. *Am J Med* 80:345–350, 1986.

44. Koerper MA, Kaminsky LS, Levy JA: Differential prevalence of antibody to AIDS-associated retrovirus in haemophiliacs treated with factor VIII concentrate versus cryoprecipitate: Recovery of infectious virus. *Lancet* 1:275, 1985.

45. Jason JM, Holman RC, Kennedy MS, Evatt BL: Longitudinal assessment of persons with hemophilia exposed to HTLV-VIII/LAV, in *Program and Abstracts of the 26th Interscience Conference on Antimicrobial Agents and Chemotherapy*. New Orleans, 1986, p. 97.

46. Mosseler J, Schimpf K, Auerswald G, et al: Inability of pasteurized factor VIII preparations to induce antibodies to HTLV-III after long-term treatment. *Lancet* 1:1111, 1985.

47. Sullivan JL, Brewster FE, Brettler DB, et al: Hemophiliac immunodeficiency influence of exposure to factor VIII concentrate, LAV/HTLV-III, and herpesviruses. *J Pediatr* 108:504–510, 1986.

48. McDougal JS, Martin LS, Cort SP, et al: Thermal inactivation of the acquired immunodeficiency syndrome virus, human T lymphotropic virus-III/lymphadenopathy-associated virus, with special reference to antihemophilic factor. *J Clin Invest* 76:875–877, 1985.

49. Centers for Disease Control. Update: Acquired immunodeficiency syndrome in person with hemophilia. *MMWR* 33:589–592, 1984.

50. Felding P, Nilsson IM, Hansson BG, Biberfeld G: Absence of antibodies to LAV/HTLV-III in haemophiliacs treated with heat-treated factor VIII concentrate of American origin. *Lancet* 2:832–833, 1985.

51. Rouzioux C, Chamaret S, Montagnier L, et al: Absence of antibodies to AIDS virus in haemophiliacs treated with heat-treated factor VIII concentrate. *Lancet* 1:271–272, 1985.

52. Berntorp E: No evidence of HIV transmission after long-term follow-up of haemophiliacs treated with heat-treated factor VIII concentrate of American origin. *Lancet* 2:283, 1987.

53. Van den Berg W, ten Cate JW, Breederveld C, Goudsmit J: Seroconversion to HTLV-III in haemophiliac given heat-treated factor VIII concentrate. *Lancet* 1:803–804, 1986.

54. Mariani G, Ghirardini A, Mandelli F, et al: Heated clotting factors and seroconversion for human immunodeficiency virus in three hemophilic patients. *Ann Intern Med* 107:113, 1987.

55. White GC, Mathews TJ, Weinhold KJ, et al: HTLV-III seroconversion associated with heat-treated factor VIII concentrate. *Lancet* 1:611–612, 1986.

56. Centers for Disease Control: Survey of non-U.S. hemophilia treatment centers for HIV seroconversions following therapy with heat-treated factor concentrates. *MMWR* 36:121–124, 1987.

57. Centers for Disease Control: Safety of therapeutic products used for hemophilic patients. *MMWR* 37:441–450, 1988.

58. Transfusion Safety Study Group: HIV transmission by anti-HIV donor screened, heat-treated clotting factor concentrates. In: Abstracts of the fourth international conference on acquired immunodeficiency syndrome. Stockholm, Sweden, June 1988.

59. Remis RS, Tsoukas C, Schechter MT, et al: Case-control study of a cluster of HIV seroconversions among hemophilia patients implicating heat-treated donor-screened factor concentrates. In: Abstracts of the fourth international conference on acquired immunodeficiency syndrome. Stockholm, Sweden, June 1988.

60. Centers for Disease Control: Revision of the CDC surveillance case definition for acquired immunodeficiency syndrome. *MMWR* 36:1S, 1987.

61. Stehr-Green JK, Jason JM, Evatt BL: Geographic variability of hemophilia-associated AIDS in the United States. *Am J Hematol* 32:178–183, 1989.

62. Centers for Disease Control. Update: Serologic testing for antibody to human immunodeficiency virus. *MMWR* 37:833–845, 1988.

63. Mortimer PP, Luban NLC, Kelleher JF, Cohen BJ: Transmission of serum parvovirus-like virus by clotting-factor concentrates. *Lancet* 2:482–484, 1983.

64. Crocchiolo PR, Lizioli A, Leopardi O: HIV and aplastic anemia. *Lancet* 2:109, 1988.

65. Akizuki S, Nakazato O, Higuchi Y, et al: Necropsy findings in HTLV-I associated myelopathy. *Lancet* 1:156–157, 1987.

66. Okochi K, Sato H, Hinuma Y: A retrospective study on transmission of adult T cell leukemia virus by blood transfusion: Seroconversion in recipients. *Vox Sang* 46:245–253, 1984.

67. Chorba TL, Jason JM, Ramsey RB, et al: HTLV-I antibody status in hemophilia patients treated with factor concentrates prepared from U.S. plasma sources and in hemophilia patients with AIDS. *Thromb Haemost* 53:180–182, 1985.

68. Rodeghiero F, Castaman GC, Chisesi T, et al: One year follow-up study of T-cell subsets and incidence of seropositivity for HTLV-I and HTLV-III antibodies in

patients treated "on demand" or sporadically with clotting concentrates. *Thromb Haemost* 54:665–668, 1985.

69. Schochetman G, Schable CA, Goldstein LC, Epstein J: Screening of U.S. populations for HIV-2. In: Abstracts of the fourth international conference on acquired immunodeficiency syndrome. Stockholm, Sweden, June 1988.

70. Hilfenhaus J, Gregersen JP: Inactivation of HIV-1 and HIV-2 by various manufacturing procedures for human plasma proteins. In: Abstracts of the fourth international conference on acquired immunodeficiency syndrome. Stockholm, Sweden, June 1988.

16
Decreasing the Incidence of Transfusion-Transmitted Infection: Avoiding Unnecessary Transfusions

Gary Stack, MD, PhD
Edward L. Snyder, MD

The best way to decrease the incidence of transfusion-transmitted disease is to decrease the frequency of transfusion. More stringent indications for the transfusion of blood and components benefit patients since infusion of unnecessary and potentially infectious units of blood is avoided. Although the principal risk associated with the transfusion of blood components is the transmission of hepatitis, other diseases, including AIDS and CMV infection, are also of concern.

Although we are unlikely to ever achieve an ideal "zero-risk" blood supply,[1] efforts toward that end mandate the screening of donor blood for the infectious agents of greatest concern as well as exclusion of donors at high risk of being infected with those or other agents. At best, however, this approach only can provide a "minimal risk" blood supply. The reasons for this are varied and include the following: (1) no test is 100% sensitive, (2) economic considerations prevent testing for many other low-incidence infectious agents; (3) new infectious agents are continually being identified, such as the prion of Creutzfeldt-Jakob disease[2]; (4) the occurrence of a "window period" early in hepatitis B and HIV-1 infection before antibodies are produced hampers identification of infected units of blood[3]; and (5) a small percentage of HIV antibody–positive patients can serorevert, ie, stop making antibodies to HIV-1.[4,5]

In this regard a new sensitive assay to detect "silent sequences" of viral DNA integrated into the genome of infected cells has been developed.[6] It is based on an in vitro DNA amplification technique using the PCR. Although it is a most sensitive assay, the technology is still too cumbersome and costly to be applied to donor blood screening.[7]

Given that donor history and donor blood screening cannot provide a zero-risk blood supply, other methods of decreasing the incidence of transfusion-transmitted disease need to be considered. Alternative approaches to be discussed in this chapter include: (1) a reevaluation of the "transfusion triggers" to effect a more judicious use of blood products, (2) selection of the appropriate blood component to ensure more efficient use of transfusion therapy, (3) use of autologous as opposed to homologous transfusion whenever possible, (4) use of pharmacologic agents to decrease or circumvent the need for blood transfusion, and (5) development of mechanical or chemical means to inactivate or eliminate infectious agents from blood products.

The Transfusion Trigger: Avoiding Unnecessary Transfusions

The risk of disease transmission increases with the number of donor exposures. The "transfusion trigger," a term coined by Friedman et al,[8] refers to "the clinical events and laboratory data which cause physicians to transfuse blood to patients." An understanding of transfusion triggers and a determination of whether they are valid is important in eliminating unnecessary transfusions. One 1985 survey concluded that 11% of red blood cell transfusions were of doubtful benefit to the patient.[9] The most abused blood component, however, is probably fresh-frozen plasma.[10] A 1986 survey indicated that as many as 73% of fresh-frozen plasma transfusions were unjustified.[11]

The standard approach to a transfusion trigger has been to use a cut-off value for a single laboratory measure, such as hematocrit or platelet count. This is appealing because it allows for rapid and uncomplicated decision making, but is often not justifiable. It is difficult to determine precisely the minimum requirement for red blood cells, platelets, and other blood components in humans because the necessary studies cannot be justified on ethical grounds. Furthermore, each patient's ability to tolerate deficiencies in various blood components depends on the patient's current clinical status, medical history, and numerous other variables. Thus, clinical judgment based on an evaluation of relevant clinical events and laboratory values remains the ultimate criterion for blood transfusion. Nevertheless, some guidelines are necessary.

It is the responsibility of the prescribing physician to evaluate the specific need of the patient and to transfuse only the appropriate blood component. This requires a scientific approach based on documentation of a deficiency with appropriate laboratory tests. The need for such documentation is becoming greater in our increasingly litigious society. A responsive clinical laboratory is needed to provide timely measurements of hematologic criteria such as hematocrit, platelet count, prothrombin time, partial thromboplastin time, and fibrinogen. In the absence of laboratory results clinicians may "blindly" transfuse numerous and often unnecessary blood components.

Red Blood Cell Products

Whole Blood

A unit of whole blood contains 450 ± 45 mL of blood collected into an anticoagulant-preservative solution such as CPDA-1. It initially contains all the cellular and plasma constituents of blood. Platelets and granulocytes in whole blood, however, lose their activity within 24 to 48 hours of storage at 4 °C. Factor VIII is also labile in vitro at 4°C and its coagulant activity falls to less than 50% of initial levels after 24 hours of storage.[12]

Whole blood is indicated when a patient needs red blood cell mass and volume expansion. The transfusion of whole blood, per se, however, is rarely required. Most patients can be treated as effectively with red blood cells diluted with a suitable crystalloid solution rather than with whole blood. For restoring the oxygen-carrying capacity of blood in euvolemic anemic patients, the component of choice is red blood cells rather than whole blood. Whole blood raises the red blood cell mass the same amount as a unit of red blood cells; however, whole blood also provides twice the volume of the red blood cell unit. In fact, where volume overload is a concern, as in congestive heart failure or renal failure, whole blood is contraindicated. For multiple clotting factor deficiencies, fresh-frozen plasma, not whole blood, is the component of choice. In the frozen state (≤ -18 °C) the lability of factors V and VIII is much lower than that at 4 °C in stored whole blood. Similarly, for thrombocytopenia, platelet concentrates should be transfused since the platelets in stored whole blood are not functional.

For the replacement of blood volume alone, crystalloid or nonplasma colloid solutions are indicated. In acute hemorrhage loss of up to 15% of total blood volume often can be tolerated without treatment[13] and losses of up to 20% to 25% can be corrected by crystalloid[14] or nonplasma colloid solutions alone. Whole blood is indicated, however, for actively bleeding patients who have lost over 25% of their blood volume.[15] Whole blood in this situation simultaneously replenishes oxygen-carrying capacity and blood volume. If whole blood is not available, then packed red blood cells plus 0.9% sodium chloride or a suitable colloid solution should be used. Use of whole blood or human plasma solely as a volume expander is contraindicated because of the risk of transfusion-transmitted diseases.

Another valid indication for use of whole blood is for neonatal exchange transfusion to simultaneously reduce hyperbilirubinemia and correct the anemia associated with hemolytic disease of the newborn. The units of whole blood chosen should be as fresh as possible, usually less than 7 days old. Use of fresher blood ensures that electrolyte concentrations are at levels better tolerated by infants, and that red blood cell levels of 2,3-diphosphoglycerate (2,3-DPG), which decreases on storage, will be high enough to assure desirable posttransfusion hemoglobin-oxygen exchange characteristics. As an alternative to whole blood in this situation, red blood cells can be reconstituted with fresh-frozen plasma. The major disadvantage with the use of fresh-frozen plasma, however, is that the patient will receive components from two donors instead of one, thereby doubling the risk of transfusion-transmitted disease. Many physicians would use a 5% albumin solution in place of fresh-frozen plasma in such cases.

Red Blood Cells and Additive Solution Red Blood Cells

Red blood cells are obtained from whole blood by removing 200 to 250 mL of plasma after centrifugation or sedimentation. Additive solution red blood cells contain an additional 100 mL of adenine and saline solution.[16] Although the shelf-life of additive solution red blood cells is longer (42 days), the risks of transfusion-transmitted disease are the same as those of red blood cell units. Additive solution red blood cell units and red blood cell units can be considered interchangeably in the discussion that follows.

Red blood cells are the component of choice to enhance oxygen-carrying capacity in the treatment of anemia by increasing the circulating red blood cell mass. The transfusion trigger for red blood cells has generally been a hematocrit of less than 0.3 or a hemoglobin concentration of less than 6.2 mmol/L. However, the best available evidence indicates that the appropriate transfusion trigger below which most patients are justifiably transfused is a hemoglobin concentration of 4.3 mmol/L (hematocrit of 0.21). This hemoglobin level in an otherwise healthy individual with normal intravascular volume and tissue perfusion is sufficient to adequately meet tissue oxygen requirements.[17] A hemoglobin value of 4.4 mmol/L is gaining wider acceptance as a more appropriate value for the red blood cell transfusion trigger.

With appropriate compensatory mechanisms, such as increased cardiac output and an elevated oxygen extraction ratio, even lower hemoglobin levels can be tolerated without adverse effect. Some patients, however, may not tolerate this level because of inadequate cardiac output, ischemic heart disease, pulmonary disease, cerebrovascular disease, or peripheral vascular disease. These patients may require a transfusion when the hemoglobin level is higher. In general, however, few patients require transfusion when their hemoglobin level is above 6.2 mmol/L or the hematocrit is 0.3. For hemoglobin levels ranging from 4.3 to 6.2 mmol/L, clinical judgment must come into play and the complete clinical picture must be evaluated.[18] Symptoms such as tachycardia, tachypnea, and vertigo must be considered, as well as abnormal laboratory values for oxygen delivery such as PaO_2, mixed venous oxygen content, and the tissue oxygen extraction ratio.

Whether the anemia is acute or chronic is also important. Because of compensatory increases in plasma volume as well as red blood cell 2,3-DPG levels, chronically anemic patients can tolerate lower hemoglobin levels than can patients who have become acutely anemic. The increase in red blood cell 2,3-DPG in chronic anemia causes a right shift in the oxyhemoglobin dissociation curve, which results in an increased release of oxygen to the tissues.

Washed Red Blood Cells

Washed red blood cells are obtained from whole blood from which most of the plasma and at least 70% of the leukocytes have been removed, while leaving at least 70% of the red blood cell mass. When washed red blood cells are prepared with automated or semiautomated machines, it is possible to remove an average of 85% of the starting leukocytes, over 90% of the platelets, and as much as 90% of the plasma. The average red blood cell loss is approximately 15%.[19] Additional washing cycles remove even more white blood cells, but at the cost of further red blood cell loss. Patients who have had two documented febrile or allergic transfusion reactions or an anaphylactic reaction are candidates for washed red blood cells.[20,21]

Frozen Deglycerolized Red Blood Cells

Red blood cells can be stored frozen in glycerol at < -70 °C for up to 10 years. Frozen deglycerolized red blood cells are usually reserved for patients who have multiple red blood cell alloantibodies and for whom compatible blood is not otherwise available. It also permits storage of multiple units of autologous blood for future transfusions.

Frozen deglycerolized red blood cells have lower levels of residual leukocytes, platelets, and plasma than do liquid washed red blood cell preparations. For reasons of cost and convenience, however, washed red blood cells are the component of choice for patients requiring plasma- or leukocyte-poor red blood cells. Patients who continue to have severe allergic or febrile reactions despite use of washed red blood cells may benefit from frozen-deglycerolized red blood cells.

CMV infections are a significant cause of morbidity and mortality in low birth weight (<1200 g) infants. For this reason blood components having a reduced risk of CMV transmission currently are recommended for seronegative infants weighing less than 1200 g or for infants whose CMV antibody status is unknown. CMV transmission by blood can be reduced by transfusing red blood cells that have been screened and shown to be CMV-seronegative. Since CMV is a leukocyte-associated virus, and because frozen deglycerolized red blood cells are leukocyte-depleted, this blood component also has a reduced risk of CMV transmission.[22] New-generation leukocyte-depletion blood filters have recently been developed.[23-25] They are efficient at removing leukocytes from units of red blood cells as well as platelet concentrates and accordingly are indicated to prevent febrile transfusion reactions. From early data, their ability to decrease CMV transmission from blood transfusion appears promising.[26,27] The actual incidence of transmission of CMV infection in low birth weight seronegative infants transfused with CMV-seropositive or unscreened blood has varied widely in different studies, with results ranging from 0.8 to 30%.[28] For this reason there is still some controversy regarding the cost-effectiveness of providing special seronegative or leukocyte-depleted blood products to all neonates. AABB standards suggest that CMV-negative blood should be provided if transfusion-transmitted CMV infection is a problem in the local hospital community.[29] The need for CMV-negative blood likely will increase. The trend in modern transfusion practice is to provide CMV-negative blood for various types of transplant recipients as concern over the mortality and morbidity of CMV infection grows.[30]

Alternatives to Homologous Red Blood Cell Transfusion

In the treatment of any chronic anemia a transfusion should always be the last resort. Initially, the need for iron, vitamin B_{12}, or folate should be thoroughly evaluated. If blood is needed, however, alternatives to standard homologous transfusion are available. For anticipated transfusion in the perioperative period, predeposit autologous blood donations can often be utilized. Indeed, most elective surgical patients are eligible for autologous blood collection. While this practice is rapidly increasing, it is still underutilized.[31,32] Autologous transfusions have been shown to significantly decrease the need for homologous transfusions in patients undergoing elective surgery.[33,34] Donations can be made at 4- to 7-day intervals, particularly when iron supplementation is given. Other forms of conservation such as perioperative autologous blood salvage and intraoperative hemodilution have been used to decrease the need for homologous red blood cell transfusions in major surgical procedures in which substantial blood loss is expected.[35,36] In one pediatric study the combination of preoperatively collected autologous blood and intraoperatively salvaged blood was successful in supplying all blood needs for 77% of the patients.[37]

Alternatives to transfusion are also being evaluated. Recombinant human erythropoietin (r-HuEPO) is a growth factor that stimulates erythropoiesis. In the appropriate setting r-HuEPO may decrease the need for homologous red blood cell transfusions. Clinical studies have shown intravenous r-HuEPO to be effective in correcting the anemia of chronic renal failure in which endogenous erythropoietin levels ar deficient.[38,39] In one nonhuman primate study the blood collected in an aggressive autologous donation program was increased 35% by use of r-HuEPO.[40] Moreover, r-HuEPO has been reported to increase autologous blood donation yields in humans.[41]

Desmopressin (1-desamino-8-D-arginine vasopressin [DDAVP]) is a synthetic analogue of the antidiuretic hormone L-arginine vasopressin.[42] Compared with natural antidiuretic hormone, DDAVP has increased antidiuretic activity, a longer half-life, and minimal vasoconstrictive activity. DDAVP has been shown to induce short-term increases in levels of circulating endogenous von Willebrand's factor and factor VIII. DDAVP when given preoperatively has been shown to be effective in decreasing blood loss in cardiac and orthopedic surgery.[43,44] It is unclear whether this effect is specifically mediated by the release of factor VIII and von Willebrand's factor or some other mechanism.[45] Other studies, however, showed that desmopressin had no appreciable effect on total blood loss or transfusion requirements.[45] The most promising synthetic red blood cell substitute being tested at this time is a polymerized, pyridoxylated, stroma-free hemoglobin solution (poly-SFH-P).[46,47] Hemoglobin prepared from outdated blood is polymerized to decrease its colloid osmotic pressure to physiologic levels (20 to 25 mm Hg) at a hemoglobin concentration of 8.8 to 10 mmol/L. It is further modified by the addition of pyridoxal 5-phosphate, which causes a right shift in the oxyhemoglobin dissociation curve. This mimics the effect of 2,3-DPG, which is lost during hemoglobin preparation. Poly SFH-P (T 1/2 = 38 hours) has been shown to support life in baboons at a hematocrit of <0.1 with no significant change in heart rate, cardiac output, oxygen consumption, or mean arterial pressure.[46,48] A clinical trial completed in 1988 on six male volunteers given 0.25 g/kg of poly-SFH-P disclosed no adverse effects after 6 weeks of followup. Renal function was unaffected and, surprisingly, there was no gross hemoglobinuria.[49] Should it prove safe and effective in the treatment of anemia, poly-SFH-P would have the advantage over red blood cells of being universally compatible, having a long shelf life, and being free of infectious agents. The potential antigenicity of poly-SFH-P has yet to be determined, as has any possible adverse effect on immune or phagocytic reticuloendothelial cell function.

The perfluorochemical emulsion Fluosol-DA, 20%, has also been evaluated as a potential synthetic oxygen carrier,[47,50] since oxygen is highly soluble in perfluorocarbon compounds. Fluosol-DA is composed primarily of two compounds, perfluorodecalin and perfluorotripropylamine, emulsified with a surfactant. A high partial pressure is required for these compounds to carry needed amounts of oxygen. As a consequence, patients often need intubation and supplemental oxygen. Fluosol-DA has a short in vivo half-life of approximately 24 hours. Results of clinical studies have not been promising and Fluosol-DA has not been shown to be an effective red blood cell substitute.[51] Fluosol-DA is being evaluated for use in cardiac catheterization and in the treatment of stroke and sickle cell anemia patients.

Attempts have also been made to produce artificial red blood cells by encapsulating purified human hemoglobin and 2,3-DPG in synthetic liposomes.[52,53] These artificial red blood cells have shown some limited success in studies with rats, but require much further development.

Platelets

Random-Donor Platelets

One unit of random-donor platelet concentrate is prepared from 1 unit of whole blood. Platelets are suspended in approximately 50 mL of plasma and stored at room temperature with gentle agitation for up to 5 days. Typically, 6 to 8 units of platelets are pooled into one component bag to provide an adult dose of approximately 1 unit of platelet concentrate per 10 kg of body weight. Accordingly, one transfusion of pooled random donor platelets exposes the adult recipient to risks of infection from six to eight donors. Platelets are indicated to prevent bleeding or to control active bleeding when there is a deficiency in either platelet number or function. As in the case of red blood cells, it has been difficult to arrive at an appropriate transfusion trigger based on a threshold level of platelets. If there is platelet dysfunction, as in Bernard-Soulier syndrome, Glanzmann's thrombasthenia, postcardiopulmonary bypass, or drug-induced platelet dysfunction, bleeding or the risk of bleeding is often unrelated to the patient's platelet count. In these cases a prolonged bleeding time can be used as part of the transfusion trigger.

Many physicians prophylactically transfuse to maintain a platelet count of at least 20×10^9/L.[54] However, there are few studies to support a platelet level of $\leq 20 \times 10^9$/L as an appropriate transfusion trigger. This figure is based on studies from the late 1950s to mid 1960s, which now are seen to have had confounding variables.[55] Many physicians feel that stable patients with an intact vascular system without any coagulopathy do not require a transfusion when platelet levels are above 10×10^9/L. However, nonbleeding patients who have other risk factors for bleeding, such as those within the perioperative period or with an associated coagulopathy or thrombocytopathy, may benefit from platelet levels maintained above 50 × 10⁹/L. In patients who are actively bleeding, particularly when there are extensive vascular injuries, a platelet level approaching 100 × 10⁹/L may be necessary for adequate hemostasis. The decision to transfuse platelets must take into account the cause of the thrombocytopenia or platelet dysfunction, not just the absolute platelet count.

In patients with idiopathic thrombocytopenic purpura, circulating platelet levels are low because of immune-mediated peripheral destruction while platelet production in the bone marrow is actually increased. The result is an increase in the percentage of young platelets, which often function more effectively. Accordingly, in idiopathic thrombocytopenic purpura the bleeding time is not prolonged to the extent predicted by the platelet count and these patients are less likely to bleed than are other patients with similar platelet counts.[56]

Thus, platelet transfusions in acute or chronic idiopathic thrombocytopenic purpura are often unnecessary even at low platelet counts unless the patient is actively bleeding. Specifically, most surgeons feel that platelet transfusions are not indicated for patients with idiopathic thrombocytopenic purpura who are undergoing splenectomy. Moreover, the posttransfusion platelet count increments in patients with this disorder are generally poor. When various treatment modalities fail, however, and when faced with life-threatening hemorrhage, platelet transfusions are indicated and, indeed, may be effective. Carr et al[57] showed that 42% of platelet transfusions in 11 of 13 patients with idiopathic thrombocytopenic purpura yielded clinically significant posttransfusion platelet level increases.

Primary therapies for idiopathic thrombocytopenic purpura involve immunosuppression with corticosteroids, other chemotherapeutic agents, and splenectomy. High-dose, intravenous immune globulin therapy also has been shown to be effective in increasing platelet counts.[58,59] The exogenous immunoglobulin apparently blocks Fc receptors on phagocytic macrophages, thereby preventing the binding and removal of antibody-coated platelets. Unfortunately, response to this therapy has a lag time of several days and is often transient. Moreover, some patients become refractory to this treatment. Bussel et al have shown that concurrent plasmapheresis may be useful in augmenting the effectiveness of intravenous immune globulin in patients with refractory idiopathic thrombocytopenic purpura.[60]

Baumann et al[61] have shown that the posttransfusion platelet increment in idiopathic thrombocytopenic purpura can be substantially augmented if a single dose of intravenous immune globulin is administered just before transfusion. Patients with refractory idiopathic thrombocytopenic purpura have also been successfully treated with danazol, a synthetic, attenuated androgen. Danazol treatment is associated with a decrease in the number of Fc receptors on monocytes.[62] It is hypothesized that this allows reduced clearance of IgG-coated platelets and a concomitant increase in platelet levels.

Even if the various therapeutic interventions fail, platelet transfusions should not be routinely provided to patients with idiopathic thrombocytopenic purpura; one cannot predict a priori the likelihood of a successful response. If truly indicated for active bleeding, platelet transfusions in ITP may be effective. Knowing the risks of transfusion-transmitted diseases, however, physicians should review the indications for platelet transfusion carefully before each infusion.

Patients with uremia have an extended bleeding time and are at risk of hemorrhage because of platelet dysfunction. Thrombocytopenia is not usually a problem in these patients. It is believed that some metabolite accumulates in the plasma of uremic patients, which can inhibit platelet function. Guanidinosuccinic acid and phenolic acids are among the substances that have been implicated.[63,64] Because transfused platelets are also inhibited after transfusion into uremic patients, they offer limited benefit. Dialysis, however, is often able to reverse the thrombocytopathy transiently. DDAVP and cryoprecipitate have both been shown to produce a transient correction of the bleeding tendency in uremia.[65,66] These agents should be considered for control of acute bleeding or prophylaxis before invasive procedures. The effect of DDAVP is manifest within 1 to 2 hours. The lag time before the onset of the effect of cryoprecipitate is longer, but so is cryoprecipitate's duration of action. DDAVP has the added advantage of not transmitting infectious disease.

Conjugated estrogens administered daily for 5 days have been shown to shorten the bleeding time in patients with uremia.[67,68] The duration of estrogen effect (14 days) is much longer than that of cryoprecipitate or DDAVP. The mechanism by which estrogen corrects the bleeding time is not known and seems to be unrelated to von Willebrand's factor levels or multimer formation.

In patients with uremia an inverse relationship has been observed between the hematocrit and the bleeding time. Red blood cell transfusion to a hematocrit of approximately 0.3 has been shown to normalize the bleeding time and decrease bleeding tendencies.[69] The mechanism of this effect is not known, but red blood cells seem to play a role in facilitating the adherence of platelets to the subendothelium.[70] More recently, several studies showed that infusion of recombinant human erythropoietin in uremic patients with severe anemia both raised the hematocrit and decreased the bleeding time to a significant degree.[71,72] Thus, in many uremic patients recombinant human erythropoietin may both replace the need for transfusion of red blood cells and simultaneously correct platelet dysfunction.

Aspirin inhibits platelet function by blocking the enzyme cyclo-oxygenase. Aspirin may prolong the bleeding time and predispose patients with other hemostatic abnormalities such as a coagulopathy or vascular defect to bleeding. Platelet transfusion may be indicated occasionally in such patients to prevent abnormal bleeding during surgery or during invasive procedures. The patient should not be taking aspirin since exogenous platelets will be equally inhibited. It may be prudent to discontinue administration of the aspirin and wait 2 or 3 days, if possible, before surgery to allow for correction of the bleeding time toward normal. In most patients without other hemostatic abnormalities, however, aspirin ingestion will only minimally elevate the bleeding time (2 or 3 minutes) and should not bring about a substantial risk of hemorrhage; surgery need not be postponed. To routinely transfuse platelets into such patients may needlessly place them at serious risk of disease transmission without justifiable benefit being derived from the platelet infusion.

Patients undergoing cardiopulmonary bypass as a part of open-heart surgery often acquire a transient defect in platelet function (prolonged bleeding time) as well as thrombocytopenia. This may be due in part to a partial depletion of platelet alpha granules that contain platelet factor IV and β-thromboglobulin.[73] The transient platelet dysfunction leads to excessive postoperative bleeding in some patients. Curiously, a randomized trial in which patients undergoing cardiopulmonary bypass surgery were given prophylactic platelet transfusions showed that correction of the bleeding time did not correlate with decreased blood loss.[74] Another study, however, did show a correlation between total platelet mass and risk of postoperative hemorrhage.[75] Thus, platelet transfusion in the post–cardiopulmonary bypass setting is controversial. At present they should be reserved for patients in whom there is excessive bleeding.

DDAVP, which presents no risk of transmission of infectious disease, has been shown to be effective for some patients. A controlled, randomized trial of prophylactic DDAVP showed that it decreased blood loss and transfusion requirements in patients undergoing cardiac surgery with cardiopulmonary bypass.[76] Another agent, aprotinin, is a serine protease inhibitor that has been shown by some researchers, but not by all, to decrease blood loss and transfusion requirements by fivefold to eightfold, respectively, during cardiac surgery.[77,78] How aprotinin decreases hemorrhage after cardiopulmonary bypass is unclear. Prostacyclin has also been used to protect platelets during cardiac bypass surgery.[79]

Single-Donor Platelets

Single-donor platelets are collected from a single donor by apheresis on a cell separator for 2 to 3 hours. The number of platelets in 1 unit of single-donor platelets ($>3 \times 10^{11}$) is equivalent to that in 5 to 8 units of random-donor platelets. Single-donor platelets that have been HLA-matched to the recipient are indicated for patients who are refractory to random-donor platelets because of alloimmunization to class I HLA antigens. Non-HLA–matched "random" single-donor platelets offer some advantages to non-alloimmunized patients who require a platelet transfusion. One advantage is a decreased risk of transfusion-transmitted infection because the recipient is exposed to one, as opposed to many (five to eight), donors.

In determining the eligibility of a patient for HLA-matched single-donor platelets, the response to random-donor platelets should be monitored with the determination of a corrected count increment (CCI).

$$CCI = \frac{(\text{posttransfusion platelet count} - \text{pretransfusion platelet count}) \times (\text{body surface area/m}^2)}{(\text{No. of platelets transfused}) \times 10^{-11}}$$

A reasonable posttransfusion CCI is >7500.

The criteria for collecting and transfusing HLA-matched single-donor platelets are as follows: (1) the recipient should have had a poor response (CCI <7500) to two consecutive transfusions of random donor platelet concentrates; (2) the refractoriness to random donor platelets likely should be the consequence of HLA alloimmunization, as shown by evidence of HLA alloantibody; (3) other causes of platelet refractoriness should be ruled out.

The platelet count should be determined before transfusion and at 10 minutes to 2 hours after transfusion.[80,81] Low CCIs calculated at later times are less specific for alloimmunization as the cause of platelet destruction. The likelihood of HLA alloimmunization as the cause of a low 1-hour CCI is determined by excluding other possible causes. Bishop et al[82] have shown that major factors other than HLA alloantibody correlating with a low 1-hour posttransfusion CCI were bone marrow transplantation, disseminated intravascular coagulation, amphotericin B treatment, splenomegaly, concurrent administration of antibiotics, and fever. Should the cause of platelet refractoriness not be HLA alloimmunization, then the patient is not a good candidate for HLA-matched-single-donor platelets. Once the decision is made to proceed with a transfusion of HLA-matched single-donor platelets, it is the responsibility of the ordering physician to determine whether the patient is responding better to them than to random-donor platelets; again, the 1 hour CCI should be monitored. If there is no significant improvement in the CCI after HLA-matched single-donor platelet transfusions using the best matches available, then there is not sufficient justification for continuing to use HLA-matched single-donor platelets.

A number of additional strategies have been proposed to improve responses of patients who have become refractory to platelet transfusions. Platelets express ABO antigens, and while ABO-incompatible platelet transfusions are effective, there are reports that ABO-compatible platelets can give a somewhat better recovery.[83] Thus, refractory patients, as well as others, might benefit from receiving ABO-compatible platelets. In addition, just as in idiopathic thrombocytopenic purpura, some selected refractory patients have obtained better responses to platelet transfusions when administered intravenous immunoglobulin; this treatment, however, has had variable results.[58,84] Such variability could be due to the unsuspected simultaneous occurrence of platelet alloantibody and autoantibody in the same patient.[85] Plasmapheresis that transiently decreases the HLA antibody level has also produced modest improvement in some alloimmunized patients.[86] Again, however, the results have been variable. Platelet cross-matching has been applied with some success in refractory alloimmunized patients.[87] However, the patient's serum needs to be tested against numerous pheresis donors and not all hospitals or blood centers have access to a sufficiently large pool of such donors. Accordingly, platelet cross-matching is not widely available.

New techniques currently under investigation to prevent or delay HLA alloimmunization include (1) transfusion of HLA-matched single-donor platelets to all patients, (2) the use of new-generation leukocyte-depleting blood filters[88,89] for red blood cell and platelet transfusions, and (3) the irradiation of platelet concentrates with ultraviolet light (UV-B, 290 to 320 nm) to decrease the immunogenicity of the carrier lymphocytes.[90-92]

Granulocytes

Granulocyte concentrates prepared via leukapheresis contain $>1.0 \times 10^{10}$ granulocytes in 200 to 300 mL of plasma along with variable amounts of lymphocytes, red blood cells, and platelets. Although the shelf-life of granulocyte concentrates is 24 hours, they are best used as soon as possible. Daily granulocyte transfusions for a minimum of 4 days is the usual treatment plan; one or two transfusions are unlikely to be of benefit and are not indicated.

Candidates for granulocyte transfusions should satisfy the following criteria: (1) an absolute granulocyte count of $<500/\mu L$, (2) a documented or suspected infection that has been unresponsive to 24 to 48 hours of appropriate antibiotic therapy, and (3) a reasonable chance of recovery from the underlying disease.

The number of granulocyte transfusions prescribed nationally has decreased progressively in recent years because of improvements in antibiotic therapy.[15] While some studies have shown that granulocyte transfusions may be beneficial for neutropenic patients with gram-negative septicemia[93,94] and newborns with sepsis,[95] early antibiotic therapy is the most effective treatment. Unfortunately, as many as 26% of full-term infants and a higher percentage of preterm infants with neonatal sepsis die despite prompt initiation of broad-spectrum antibiotic therapy.[96] Granulocyte transfusions for neonatal sepsis have been shown to be efficacious in decreasing mortality in some studies,[95,97] but not in a more recent report[98]; controlled randomized multicenter studies are needed. At present, most physicians reserve granulocyte transfusions for critically ill patients who show no improvement despite maximal antibiotic therapy. Some researchers feel that granulocyte transfusions would be more effective if enough granulocytes could be given, and that the current dose of 1 or 2×10^{10} granulocytes per transfusion is likely too small to be of clinical benefit.

Granulocyte transfusions are often associated with serious side effects. These must be weighed against their questionable efficacy when making a decision to transfuse or not. Many patients receiving granulocyte transfusions develop fever and chills, while some become severely hypotensive, or develop pulmonary infiltrates.[99] With a significant risk of adverse reactions and a lack of evidence of additional benefit when appropriate antibiotic therapy is used, granulocyte transfusions are no longer considered a primary therapeutic option for adults.[100]

As an alternative to homologous granulocyte transfusions, endogenous granulocyte production can be stimulated using recombinant human granulocyte and granulocyte-macrophage colony-stimulating factors (rhG-CSF, rhGM-CSF). These are growth factors that stimulate the proliferation of hematopoietic cells. The DNA coding sequences for G-CSF and GM-CSF have been cloned and used to synthesize large amounts of recombinant gene products. Recombinant rhG-CSF has been shown to stimulate a sustained rise in neutrophil counts in cancer patients and to reduce the period of neutropenia after administration of cytotoxic chemotherapy and after bone marrow transplantation.[101-103] Recombinant hGM-CSF has dramatically stimulated circulating granulocyte levels in patients with malignancy or bone marrow failure.[104-107] Not only does GM-CSF stimulate the proliferation of myeloid progenitor cells, but it also stimulates certain functions of mature granulocytes, such as their ability to phagocytize bacteria.[108] Both rhG-CSF and rhGM-CSF appear promising as an alternative therapy for granulocytopenia.

Plasma Products and Derivatives

Fresh-Frozen Plasma

One unit of fresh-frozen plasma is separated from 1 unit of whole blood and rapidly frozen within 8 hours of donation. It is stored at ≤ -18 °C or colder for up to 12 months. One unit of FFP contains all of the coagulation factors ordinarily present in approximately 200 mL of plasma, including both the stable and labile factors.[15]

Transfusion of FFP is indicated for replacing clotting factors in patients with multiple factor deficiencies who are bleeding or about to undergo surgery, or for similar patients with isolated factor deficiencies when a specific factor concentrate is not available.[109] As with other blood components, fresh-frozen plasma should not be transfused empirically.[110] A clotting factor deficiency should be documented in the laboratory with an increase in the prothrombin time or a partial thromboplastin time in the range of >1.5 times the normal value or with an abnormal result from the specific factor assay.

One mL of fresh-frozen plasma is defined as containing 1 unit of a coagulation factor; 200 mL of fresh-frozen plasma contains 200 units each of factors V, VIII, X, etc. Thus, 1 unit (bag) of fresh-frozen plasma contains a theoretical maximum of 6% to 7% of the clotting factors circulating in a 70-kg person, based on a total plasma volume of 2800 mL (40 mL/kg). In practice, however, the clotting factor increment from transfusion of 1 unit of FFP is less than 6% to 7%. Assuming a patient is completely deficient in one or more factors, 4 or more units of fresh-frozen plasma are usually needed to restore factor levels to 30% of normal, which has been shown to provide an adequate level of hemostasis. The therapeutic effect of fresh-frozen plasma is transient with a duration dependent on the half-life of the deficient factor.

The specific indications for transfusion of fresh-frozen plasma are as follows:

1. Replacement of documented deficiencies in multiple coagulation factors in patients who are bleeding or about to undergo surgery. Such multifactor deficiencies occur in the setting of disseminated intravascular coagulation or liver failure, or after massive transfusion.
2. Reversal of the anticoagulant effect of warfarin in patients who are bleeding or are in preparation for emergency surgery. The use of fresh-frozen

plasma should be reserved for times when waiting hours for the reversal effect of administered vitamin K would be life-threatening. In this situation a transfusion of 1 to 2 units of fresh-frozen plasma may be sufficient.[111]

3. Replacement of documented isolated deficiencies of factors for which no concentrate exists, eg, factors V or XI, in patients who are bleeding or are in preparation for surgery. Specific concentrates are the treatment of choice for factor VIII and IX deficiencies, although fresh-frozen plasma may be used in mild to moderate forms of hemophilia B; cryoprecipitate is also available for treatment of factor VIII deficiency.

4. Treatment of thrombotic thrombocytopenic purpura, usually in conjunction with plasmapheresis.

5. Reconstitution with red blood cells if whole blood is not available for transfusion in neonates. To decrease the risk of disease transmission many physicians will substitute 5% albumin for fresh-frozen plasma in such patients.

6. Treatment of thrombotic episodes due to congenital deficiencies of antithrombin III or protein C, as well as treatment of C1-esterase inhibitor deficiency and of protein-losing enteropathy in infants.[112]

Fresh-frozen plasma is considered one of the most abused blood components in terms of unnecessary transfusion.[10] It is not indicated for volume expansion; crystalloid and colloid solutions are as effective and are safer for this purpose. In addition, there is no evidence to support the use of prophylactic fresh-frozen plasma transfusions without at least laboratory evidence of a coagulation factor deficiency.

Cryoprecipitated Antihemophilic Factor

Cryoprecipitated antihemophilic factor (cryoprecipitate) is the cold-insoluble precipitate obtained when 1 unit of fresh-frozen plasma is thawed in the cold. The cold-thawed plasma is spun on the centrifuge, and the cryoprecipitate along with 10 to 15 mL of plasma is immediately refrozen. It can be stored at $-18\,°C$ or lower for up to 12 months.

One bag of cryoprecipitate contains at least 80 IU of factor VIII,[29] representing approximately 40% to 50% of the amount present in the starting unit of fresh-frozen plasma, but which is concentrated about tenfold per unit volume. One bag of cryoprecipitate also contains approximately 150 to 250 mg of fibrinogen plus von Willebrand's factor and fibronectin. Cryoprecipitate also contains some factor XIII. Transfusion of cryoprecipitate typically requires the pooling of as many as ten or more units (bags) of cryoprecipitate, depending on the particular patient's needs. Cryoprecipitate is currently the only available source of concentrated fibrinogen. Cryoprecipitate transfusions are indicated in the following cases:

1. Patients with von Willebrand's disease who are bleeding or being prepared for invasive procedures.

2. Patients with laboratory-confirmed hypofibrinogenemia or dysfibrinogenemia who are bleeding or are being prepared for surgery. Note that fresh-

frozen plasma is often the component of choice for fibrinogen replacement when there are multiple factor deficiencies. Cryoprecipitate should not be used as sole therapy for disseminated intravascular coagulation, since it does not contain factor V; fresh-frozen plasma is indicated in such clinical situations.

3. Patients with documented factor XIII deficiency who are bleeding or being prepared for an invasive procedure.
4. Patients with uremic bleeding.[66]
5. Patients with factor VIII deficiency (hemophilia A) when purified factor VIII concentrates are not available.

Cryoprecipitate, like fresh-frozen plasma, is not routinely treated to remove or inactivate viruses and can transmit hepatitis and HIV. Before the institution of donor screening to eliminate individuals at high risk of HIV infection, 17% of hemophiliacs who received only cryoprecipitate were reported to have become HIV-seropositive.[113] One way to decrease the risk of viral infection from cryoprecipitate is to decrease the number of donor exposures per transfusion episode. To that end, McLeod et al[114] have demonstrated the feasibility of using plasmapheresis as a source of cryoprecipitate to supply regional and individual needs. In addition, efforts are continually being made to enhance the yields of factor VIII and von Willebrand's factor in cryoprecipitate.

Pharmacologic alternatives to cryoprecipitate transfusions can be used in some clinical settings. DDAVP, which stimulates the release of high molecular weight multimers of von Willebrand's factor, can be used in place of cryoprecipitate in some patients with mild to moderate forms of type I von Willebrand's disease.[115] Type IIb von Willebrand's disease cannot be treated with DDAVP because of the risk of platelet aggregation.[116] Other types of von Willebrand's disease show variable responses to DDAVP.[42] A dose of 0.3 μg/ kg given intravenously can correct the bleeding time in some patients in as few as 30 minutes; the effect persists for several hours. Patients should be pretested to determine if, in fact, they will respond to DDAVP. DDAVP treatment may be sufficient to allow patients to undergo minor procedures such as dental extractions without the need for transfusion, but DDAVP alone is not likely to be effective for major surgical procedures. Some commercial preparations of factor VIII contain sufficient levels of biologically active von Willebrand's factor for use in treatment of von Willebrand's disease. These heat-treated factor VIII concentrates have a lower risk of transmission of HIV and hepatitis B and C.[117-119] Virally attenuated forms of fresh-frozen plasma and cryoprecipitate are under development.

Albumin

Albumin is prepared by fractionation of large pools of human plasma, most of which are obtained by plasmapheresis. Different plasma proteins are selectively and sequentially precipitated from the plasma by the Cohn-Oncley cold-ethanol fractionation technique.[120,121] Because of the large donor pool size, and despite the screening of all donors for hepatitis and HIV markers, the source plasma starting material is still assumed to be contaminated with hepatitis and AIDS viruses. Accordingly, albumin is heat-treated in the presence of stabilizing agent at 60 °C for 10 hours in the liquid state to inactivate any residual viruses. As a result, albumin administration presents no known risk of transmission of hepatitis B or HIV infection.[122,123] Albumin contains 96% albumin and 4% globulins. It is useful for volume expansion in a variety of situations when use of fresh-frozen plasma is unwarranted. Five percent and 25% products are available. Indications for albumin replacement include plasmapheresis, burns, acute nephrotic syndrome, and acute liver failure.[124]

Heat-Treated Factor VIII

Factor VIII, or anti-hemophilic factor, concentrate is prepared from pooled units of human plasma. All units of plasma used are screened and found nonreactive for markers of HIV and hepatitis infection. However, because this testing does not eliminate all units of infectious plasma, the starting plasma pool is assumed to be contaminated with HIV and hepatitis viruses.

Factor VIII concentrates are available in two grades of purity, intermediate and monoclonal purified. Intermediate purity concentrates also contain varying amounts of von Willebrand's factor, fibrinogen, anti-A and anti-B blood group antibodies, and traces of other plasma proteins. Since the factor isolation process does not itself eliminate or inactivate viral contaminants, additional viral inactivation measures are taken. In most cases various heat treatments are used. Depending on the supplier, heating is done in the dry state at 68 °C for 72 hours, in a solvent suspension at 60 °C for 20 hours, or in an aqueous state at 60 °C for 10 hours.[125] Heat treatment is less effective when the material is dry.[126] The risk of hepatitis or HIV infection from the newer heat-treated factor VIII concentrates is lower.[127,128]

Another fractionation process uses a solvent-detergent treatment consisting of tri(*N*-butyl)phosphate with sodium cholate, which inactivates hepatitis B virus, non-A, non-B hepatitis virus, and HIV while maintaining high recovery of factor VIII activity.[129] Data show that the risk of HIV and hepatitis transmission is lower with this product.[130,131]

Monoclonal purified factor VIII concentrates are also available. The specific activity of factor VIII in these preparations is several thousand-fold higher than in the intermediate-purity products, based on estimates from the package insert for the product. One product is purified with an immunoaffinity chromatography step using a mouse monoclonal antibody to factor VIII. The preparation includes a viral inactivation step using organic solvent-detergent (tri[*N*-butyl]-phosphate plus Triton X-100). Another product is purified from plasma proteins by affinity chromatography using a mouse monoclonal antibody to von Willebrand's factor, which is used first to isolate the factor VIII–von Willebrand's factor complex. Factor VIII is then dissociated from von Willebrand's factor and recovered. For viral inactivation the product is heated at 60 °C for 30 hours in the dry state. Early results with the monoclonal purified preparations in a limited number of patients indicate no transmission of hepatitis or HIV.[125] More data are required to assess the risk of transfusion-transmitted viruses with these products.

Replacement therapy with factor VIII concentrates is indicated for the treatment or prophylaxis of bleeding in patients with documented hemophilia A. As an alternative, in some patients with mild or moderate hemophilia A DDAVP can increase circulating levels of factor VIII several-fold.[132] DDAVP should be used in preference to factor VIII concentrates in these patients whenever possible. Cryoprecipitates obtained from a small number of screened donors, when feasible, can be considered as an alternative for reducing the risk of hepatitis. In addition, hemophilia patients not already infected by hepatitis B should receive hepatitis B vaccination. Recombinant human factor VIII is currently being tested and will be free of transfusion-transmitted diseases.

Heat-Treated Factor IX Complex

Like factor VIII concentrate, factor IX complex is prepared from source plasma pooled from large numbers of screened donors. Factors IX concentrate is heat-treated in an attempt to inactivate viruses. Nevertheless, HIV and hepatitis transmission have been reported to occur. While monoclonal purified factor IX has been prepared for research purposes, it is not commercially available at this time.[133]

Factor IX complex consists of clotting factors II, IX, X, low levels of factor VII, and trace amounts of other plasma proteins. It is indicated for the treatment of severe hemophilia B.

Factor IX complex has been associated with the development of postoperative thrombosis and disseminated intravascular coagulation, apparently because of the presence of activated clotting factors in the preparation.[134] Patients who have liver disease may be at particular risk of contracting this occasionally fatal complication. Factor IX complex has been used to treat bleeding in patients with hemophilia A who are refractory to factor VIII because of factor VIII antibodies.[135] In patients who have such an inhibitor, porcine factor VIII and anti-inhibitor coagulation complex concentrates may also be of value.

Anti-Inhibitor Coagulant Complex

The anti-inhibitor coagulant complex concentrates contain variable amounts of vitamin K–dependent clotting factors II, IX, and X (mainly nonactivated), and factor VII (mainly activated). A small amount of factor VIII as well as other plasma proteins are present. Just as with factor VIII and factor IX complex concentrates, the anti-inhibitor coagulant complex is prepared from plasma from many screened donors. The risk of viral infection and the viral inactivation methods used are similar to those used for factor IX complex concentrates. Anti-inhibitor coagulant complex may be indicated for use in hemophilia A or B patients with high levels (>10 Bethesda units) of inhibitors to factor VIII or IX, and who are bleeding or being prepared for surgery.[136] The exact mechanism by which anti-inhibitor coagulant complex bypasses the need for factor VIII (or factor IX) in the clotting cascade is unknown, but is thought to be due to the presence of activated factors VII and X.

When the factor VIII inhibitor level is <10 Bethesda units, human factor VIII concentrate is the treatment of choice. Alternative techniques for treatment of factor VIII inhibitors include porcine factor VIII concentrate and plasmapheresis.[136-138] Porcine factor VIII has been effectively used when the inhibitor antibody is not highly cross-reactive. Porcine factor VIII may be limited in usefulness because it can be immunogenic in humans. Plasmapheresis may be effective in some patients by transiently lowering inhibitor levels.[138] The reported effectiveness of anti-inhibitor coagulant complex is variable.[135]

Immune Globulin

Immune globulin is also prepared from screened plasma by the Cohn-Oncley cold ethanol fractionation process. Two different preparations are available, one for intramuscular use, the other modified for intravenous use.[139-141] In the United States immune globulin preparations containing specific antibodies, such as Rh immune globulin, are available only for intramuscular use. The intramuscular preparations should not be given intravenously because of the possibility of anaphylactic reactions. They contain immunoglobulin aggregates that have strong complement-fixing activity. The intravenous preparations are modified to prevent in vitro aggregation. The indications for immune globulins have been reviewed.[58,84,139-141] As with albumin, which is also prepared by cold ethanol fractionation, there are no confirmed cases of HIV transmission by either intravenous or intramuscular immune globulin.[142] Immune globulin preparations for intramuscular use are also considered to be free of hepatitis infectivity. This may be partly because of the efficacy of the Cohn-Oncley fractionation process for separating and inactivating viruses, and the large amounts of neutralizing antiviral antibody present in the immunoglobulin. Intravenous immune globulin, however, has been reported to transmit non-A, non-B hepatitis.[139,140]

Viral Inactivation: Future Prospects

A long-term goal of transfusion medicine is to provide blood products which are free of infectious risk. Significant progress toward this end has been made in just a few years. The spread of AIDS provided the needed impetus. Blood collection centers screen out donors at high risk of being infected with HIV and other transfusion-transmitted pathogens. Indeed, the virus which causes hepatitis C was identified and testing began within a very short period of time.[143-146] Methods have been developed for obtaining safer, more highly purified plasma protein derivatives, in particular for factor concentrates. New viral inactivation or attenuation steps have been developed and implemented. While these can be viewed as initial stop-gap measures, they have rather quickly minimized viral contamination of the blood supply. In the meantime more effective solutions can be developed.

It seems likely that disease transmission by coagulation factor concentrates and other plasma protein derivatives will be eliminated through the production and use of synthetic recombinant coagulation factor proteins.

Technical difficulties, such as those related to obtaining nonimmunogenic and biologically active conformations of these proteins, do not seem insurmountable. Indeed, recombinant human factor VIII is at this writing being tested. The genes for factor IX, von Willebrand's factor, albumin, antithrombin III and others have already been isolated.[147]

Virus-free cellular blood components represent unique challenges. Thermal or chemical techniques currently employed for sterilizing plasma protein fractions are not suitable for cellular components. Some progress has been made toward developing synthetic substitutes for cellular components, in particular for red blood cells, and cell culture technology holds the potential for in vitro blood cell production. However, elimination of the need for all donated human cellular blood components is not likely to occur in the foreseeable future. Expanded use of recombinant hematopoietic growth factors, other pharmacologic agents, autologous transfusions, and perioperative blood salvage can reduce transfusion requirements in some settings, but will not likely eliminate them.

What is needed is a technique to inactivate all viruses present in donated blood that at the same time will not harm cellular components. Photoinactivation and irradiation techniques have shown promise in some preliminary studies.[148] Pulsed laser–ultraviolet radiation, which delivers rapid nanosecond pulses of ultraviolet radiation at 308 nm, has been shown to inactivate poliovirus test viruses without significantly inhibiting platelet function.[149] In another approach, herpes simplex virus type I and HIV-1 have been photoinactivated with visible light (630 nm) in flowing blood to which a hematoporphyrin-derived photosensitizing agent has been added. There was no apparent deleterious effect on the blood components.[150] Ultraviolet light treatment of psoralen-containing platelet concentrates has been reported to inactivate a variety of viruses.[151] These results are preliminary and whether these treatments will inactivate intracellular viruses is under investigation. This type of approach does offer numerous important advantages that will likely enhance and improve upon, but again are unlikely to eliminate the need for, donor blood donations and screening.

References

1. Zuck TF: Greetings: A final look back with comments about a policy of a zero-risk blood supply. *Transfusion* 27:447–448, 1987.

2. Holland PV: Why a new standard to prevent Creutzfeldt-Jakob disease. *Transfusion* 28:293, 1988.

3. Ward JW, Holmberg SD, Allen JR, et al: Transmission of human immunodeficiency virus (HIV) by blood transfusions screened as negative for HIV antibody. *N Engl J Med* 318:473–478, 1988.

4. Farzadegan H, Polis MA, Wolinsky SM, et al: Loss of human immunodeficiency virus type 1 (HIV-1) antibodies with evidence of viral infection in asymptomatic homosexual men. *Ann Intern Med* 108:785–790, 1988.

5. Zuck TF: Silent sequences and the safety of blood transfusions. *Ann Intern Med* 198:895–897, 1988.

6. Ou CY, Kwok S, Mitchell SW, et al: DNA amplification for direct detection of HIV-1 in DNA of peripheral blood mononuclear cells. *Science* 239:295–297, 1988.

7. Stanier P, Taylor DL, Kitchen AD, et al: Persistence of cytomegalovirus in mononuclear cells in peripheral blood from blood donors. *Br Med J* 299:897–898, 1989.

8. Friedman BA, Burns TL, Schork MA: An analysis of blood transfusion of surgical patients by sex: A quest for the transfusion trigger. *Transfusion* 20:179–188, 1980.

9. Ali A: Evaluation of current use of red cell transfusion in the perioperative period, in *Perioperative Red Cell Transfusion, Program and Abstracts, NIH Consensus Development Conference, June 27–29.* 1988, pp 25–27.

10. Jones J: Abuse of fresh-frozen plasma. *Br Med J* 295:287, 1987.

11. Blumberg N, Laczin J, McMican A, et al: A critical survey of fresh-frozen plasma use. *Transfusion* 26:511–513, 1986.

12. Nilsson L, Hedner U, Nilsson IM, Robertson B: Shelf-life of bank blood and stored plasma with special reference to coagulation factors. *Transfusion* 23:377–381, 1983.

13. Moore FD: The effects of hemorrhage on body composition. *N Engl J Med* 273:567–577, 1965.

14. Gollub S, Svigals R, Bailey CP, et al: Electrolyte solutions in surgical patients refusing transfusion. *JAMA* 215:2077–2083, 1971.

15. Widmann FK (ed): *Technical Manual,* ed 9. Arlington, VA, American Association of Blood Banks, 1985.

16. Heaton A, Miripol J, Aster R, et al: Use of Adsol preservative solution for prolonged storage of low viscosity AS-1 red blood cells. *Br J Haematol* 57:467–478, 1984.

17. Consensus Conference: Perioperative red blood cell transfusion. *JAMA* 260:2700–2703, 1988.

18. Spence RK, Carson JA, Poses R, et al: Elective surgery without transfusion: Influence of preoperative hemoglobin level and blood loss on mortality. *Am J Surg* 159:320–324, 1990.

19. Hughes A, Mijovic V, Brozovic B, et al: Leukocyte-depleted blood: A comparison of cell-washing techniques. *Vox Sang* 42:145–150, 1982.

20. Kevy SV, Schmidt PJ, McGinniss MH, et al: Febrile, nonhemolytic transfusion reactions and the limited role of leukoagglutinins in their etiology. *Transfusion* 2:7–16, 1962.

21. Menitove JE, McElligott MC, Aster RH: Febrile transfusion reaction: What blood component should be given next? *Vox Sang* 42:318–321, 1982.

22. Taylor BJ, Jacobs RF, Baker RL, et al: Frozen deglycerolyzed blood prevents transfusion-acquired cytomegalovirus infections in neonates. *Pediatr Infect Dis* 5:188–191, 1986.

23. Sirchia G, Wenz B, Rebulla PO, et al: Removal of white cells from red cells by transfusion through a new filter. *Transfusion* 30:30–33, 1990.

24. Kickler TS, Bell W, Ness PM, et al: Depletion of white cells from platelet concentrates with a new adsorption filter. *Transfusion* 29:411–414, 1989.

25. Snyder EL: Clinical use of white cell–poor blood components. *Transfusion* 29:568–571, 1989.

26. Adler SP: Cytomegalovirus and transfusions. *Trans Med Rev* 2:235–244, 1988.

27. Bowden RA, Sayers MH, Cays M, Slichter SJ: The role of blood product filtration in the prevention of transfusion associated cytomegalovirus (CMV) infection after marrow transplant (abstract). *Transfusion* 29(suppl):57S, 1989.

28. Tegtmeier GE: The use of cytomegalovirus-screened blood in neonates. *Transfusion* 28:201–203, 1988.

29. Holland PV (ed): *Standards for Blood Banks and Transfusion Services*, ed 13. Arlington, VA, American Association of Blood Banks, 1989.

30. Tegtmeier GE: Posttransfusion cytomegalovirus infections. *Arch Pathol Lab Med* 113:236–245, 1989.

31. Toy PT, Strauss RG, Stehling LC, et al: Predeposited autologous blood for elective surgery: A national multicenter study. *N Engl J Med* 316:517–520, 1987.

32. Anderson BV, Tomasulo PA: Current autologous transfusion practices. *Transfusion* 28:394–396, 1988.

33. Love TR, Hendren WG, O'Keefe DD, Daggett WM: Transfusion of predonated autologous blood in elective cardiac surgery. *Ann Thorac Surg* 43:508–512, 1987.

34. Bailey TE Jr, Mahoney OM: The use of banked autologous blood in patients undergoing surgery for spinal deformity. *J Bone Joint Surg* 69:329–332, 1987.

35. Giordano GF, Goldman DS, Mammana RB, et al: Intraoperative autotransfusion in cardiac operations. *J Thorac Cardiovasc Surg* 96:382–386, 1988.

36. Kafer ER, Isley MR, Hansen T, et al: Automated acute normovolemic hemodilution reduces homologous blood transfusion requirements for spinal fusion. *Anesth Analg* 65:S76, 1986.

37. Novak RW: Autologous blood transfusion in a pediatric population: Safety and efficacy. *Clin Pediatr* 27:184–187, 1988.

38. Eschbach JW, Egrie J-C, Downing MR, et al: Correction of anemia of end-stage renal disease with recombinant human erythropoietin: Result of a phase I and II clinical trial. *N Engl J Med* 319:73–78, 1987.

39. Winearls CG, Oliver DO, Pippard MJ, et al: Effect of human erythropoietin from recombinant DNA on the anemia of patients maintained by chronic hemodialysis. *Lancet* 2:1175–1178, 1986.

40. Levine EA, Rosen AL, Gould SA, et al: Recombinant human erythropoietin and autologous blood donation. *Surgery* 104:365–369, 1988.

41. Goodnough LT, Rudnick S, Price TH, et al: Increased preoperative collection of autologous blood with recombinant human erythropoietin therapy. *N Engl J Med* 321:1163–1168, 1989.

42. Mannucci PM: Desmopressin: A nontransfusional form of treatment for congenital and acquired bleeding disorders. *Blood* 72:1449–1455, 1988.

43. Salzman EW, Weinstein MJ, Weintraub RM, et al: Treatment with desmopressin acetate to reduce blood loss after cardiac surgery: A double-blind randomized trial. *N Engl J Med* 314:1402–1406, 1986.

44. Kobrinsky NL, Letts RM, Patel LR, et al: 1-Desamino-8-D-arginine vasopressin (Desmopressin) decreases operative blood loss in patients having Harrington rod spinal fusion surgery. *Ann Intern Med* 107:446–450, 1987.

45. Hackman T, Gascoyne RD, Naiman SC, et al: A trial of desmospressin (1-deamino-8-D-arginine vasopressin) to reduce blood loss in uncomplicated cardiac surgery. *N Engl J Med* 321:1437–1443, 1989.

46. Gould SA, Sehgal LR, Rosen AL, et al: The development of polymerized pyridoxylated hemoglobin solution as a red cell substitute. *Ann Emerg Med* 15:1416–1419, 1986.

47. Kahn RA, Allen RW, Baldassare J: Alternate sources and substitutes for therapeutic blood components. *Blood* 66:1–12, 1985.

48. Gould SA, Sehgal LR, Rosen AL, et al: The efficacy of polymerized pyridoxylated hemoglobin solution as an O_2 carrier. *Ann Surg* 211:394–398, 1990.

49. Moss G: Synthetic blood substitutes, presented at *Update in Transfusion Medicine*. Boston, Sept 9–10, 1988.

50. Waxman K: Perfluorocarbons as blood substitutes. *Ann Emerg Med* 15:1423–1424, 1986.

51. Gould SA, Rosen AL, Sehgal LR, et al: Fluosol-DA as a red-cell substitute in acute anemia. *N Engl J Med* 314:1653–1656, 1986.

52. Djordjevich L, Miller IF: Synthetic erythrocytes from lipid encapsulated hemoglobin. *Exp Hematol* 8:584–592, 1980.

53. Hunt CA, Burnette RR, MacGregor RD, et al: Synthesis and evaluation of a prototypal artificial red cell. *Science* 230:1165–1168, 1985.

54. Consensus conference: Platelet transfusion therapy. *JAMA* 257:1777–1780, 1987.

55. Anderson KC: Platelet transfusion therapy, in Churchill WH, Kurtz SR (eds): *Transfusion Medicine*. Boston, Blackwell Scientific Publications, 1988, pp 145–167.

56. Harker LA, Slichter SJ: The bleeding time as a screening test for evaluation of platelet function. *N Engl J Med* 287:155–159, 1972.

57. Carr JM, Kruskall MS, Kaye JA, Robinson SH: Efficacy of platelet transfusions in immune thrombocytopenia. *Am J Med* 80:1051–1054, 1986.

58. Nelson JM: Intravenous immunoglobulin: Silver bullet of the 80s. *Lab Med* 19:799–805, 1988.

59. Bussel JB, Pham LC: Intravenous treatment with gammaglobulin in adults with immune thrombocytopenic purpura: Review of the literature. *Vox Sang* 52:206–211, 1987.

60. Bussell JB, Saal S, Gordon B: Combined plasma exchange and intravenous gammaglobulin in the treatment of patients with refractory immune thrombocytopenic purpura. *Transfusion* 28:38–41, 1988.

61. Baumann MA, Menitove JE, Aster RH, Anderson T: Urgent treatment of idiopathic thrombocytopenic purpura with single-dose gammaglobulin infusion followed by platelet transfusion. *Ann Intern Med* 104:808–809, 1986.

62. Schreiber AD, Chien P, Tomaski A, Cines DB: Effect of danazol in immune thrombocytopenia purpura. *N Engl J Med* 316:503–508, 1987.

63. Horowitz HI, Stein M, Cohen BD, White JG: Further studies on the platelet inhibitor effect of guanidinosuccinic acid and its role in uremic bleeding. *Am J Med* 49:336–345, 1970.

64. Rabiner SF, Molinas F: The role of phenol and phenolic acids on the thrombocytopathy and defective platelet aggregation of patients with renal failure. *Am J Med* 49:346–351, 1970.

65. Mannucci PM, Remuzzi G, Pusineri F, et al: Deamino-8-D-arginine vasopressin shortens the bleeding time in uremia. *N Engl J Med* 308:8–12, 1983.

66. Janson PA, Jubelirer SJ, Weinstein MJ, Deykin D: Treatment of the bleeding tendency in uremia with cryoprecipitate. *N Engl J Med* 303:1318–1322, 1980.

67. Liu YK, Kosfeld RE, Marcum SG: Treatment of uraemic bleeding with conjugated oestrogen. *Lancet* 2:887–890, 1984.

68. Livio M, Mannucci PM, Vigano G, et al: Conjugated estrogens for the management of bleeding associated with renal failure. *N Engl J Med* 315:731–735, 1986.

69. Livio M, Gotti E, Marchesi D, et al: Uraemic bleeding: Role of anaemia and beneficial effect of red cell transfusions. *Lancet* 2:1013–1015, 1982.

70. Castillo R, Lozano T, Escolar G, et al: Defective platelet adhesion on vessel subendothelium in uremic patients. *Blood* 68:337–342, 1986.

71. Eschbach JW, Egrie J-C, Downing MR, et al: Correction of anemia of end-stage renal disease with recombinant human erythropoietin: Result of a phase I and II clinical trial. *N Engl J Med* 310:73–78, 1987.

72. Moia M, Mannucci PM, Vizzotto L, et al: Improvement in the haemostatic defect of uraemia after treatment with recombinant human erythropoietin. *Lancet* 2:1227–1229, 1987.

73. Harker LA, Malpass TW, Branson HE, et al: Mechanism of abnormal bleeding in patients undergoing cardiopulmonary bypass: Acquired transient platelet dysfunction associated with selective alpha granule release. *Blood* 56:824–834, 1980.

74. Simon TL, Akl BF, Murphy W: Controlled trial of routine administration of platelet concentrates in cardiopulmonary bypass surgery. *Ann Thorac Surg* 37:359–364, 1984.

75. Mohr R, Martionwitz U, Golan M, et al: Platelet size and mass as an indicator for platelet transfusion after cardiopulmonary bypass. *Circulation* 74:153–158, 1986.

76. Salzman EW, Weinstein MJ, Weintraub RM, et al: Treatment with desmopressin acetate to reduce blood loss after cardiac surgery: A double-blind randomized trial. *N Engl J Med* 314:1402–1406, 1986.

77. Royston D, Bidstrup BP, Taylor KM, Sapsford RN: Effect of aprotinin on need for blood transfusion after repeat open-heart surgery. *Lancet* 2:1289–1291, 1987.

78. Bidstrup BP, Royston D, Sapsford RN, Taylor KM: Reduction in blood loss and blood use after cardiopulmonary bypass with high dose aprotinin (Trasylol). *J Thorac Cardiovasc Surg* 97:364–372, 1989.

79. Longmore DB, Bennett JG, Hoyle PM, et al: Prostacyclin administration during cardiopulmonary bypass in man. *Lancet* 1:800–804, 1981.

80. Daly PA, Schiffer CA, Aisner, et al: Platelet transfusion therapy: One-hour posttransfusion increments are valuable in predicting the need for HLA-matched preparations. *JAMA* 243:435–438, 1980.

81. O'Connell B, Lee EJ, Schiffer CA: The value of 10-minute posttransfusion platelet counts. *Transfusion* 28:66–67, 1988.

82. Bishop JF, McGrath K, Wolf MM, et al: Clinical factors influencing the efficacy of pooled platelet transfusions. *Blood* 71:383–387, 1988.

83. Murphy S: ABO blood groups and platelet transfusion. *Transfusion* 28:401–402. 1988.

84. Berkman SA, Lee ML, Gale RP: Clinical uses of intravenous immunoglobulins. *Ann Intern Med* 112:278–292, 1990.

85. Thompson BY, Snyder EL, Beardsley DS: Autoantibodies against platelet GPIb/IX and GPIIb/IIIa associated with refractoriness to platelet transfusions (abstract). *Transfusion* 29(suppl):46S, 1989.

86. Bensinger WI, Buckner CD, Clift RA, et al: Plasma exchange for platelet alloimmunization. *Transplantation* 41:602–605, 1986.

87. Kickler TS, Ness PM, Braine HG: Platelet crossmatching. *Am J Clin Pathol* 90:69–72, 1988.

88. Sniecinski I, O'Donnell MR, Nowicki B, Hill LR: Prevention of refractoriness and HLA-alloimmunization using filtered blood products. *Blood* 71:1402–1407, 1988.

89. Saarinen UM, Kekomaki R, Siimes MA, Myllyla G: Effective prophylaxis against platelet refractoriness in multitransfused patients by use of leukocyte-free blood components. *Blood* 75:512–517, 1990.

90. Deeg HJ, Aprile J, Graham TC, et al: Ultraviolet irradiation of blood prevents transfusion-induced sensitization and marrow graft rejection in dogs. *Blood* 67:537–539, 1986.

91. Buchholz DH, Miripol J, Aster RH, et al: Ultraviolet irradiation of platelets to prevent recipient alloimmunization. *Transfusion* 28(suppl):26S, 1988.

92. Murphy MF, Waters AH: Platelet transfusions: The problem of refractoriness. *Blood Rev* 4:16–24, 1990.

93. Alavi JB, Root RK, Djerassi I, et al: A randomized clinical trial of granulocyte transfusions for infection in acute leukemia. *N Engl J Med* 296:706–711, 1977.

94. Herzig RH, Herzig GP, Graw RG Jr, et al: Successful granulocyte transfusion therapy for gram-negative septicemia. *N Engl J Med* 296:701–705, 1977.

95. Cairo MS: Granulocyte transfusions in neonates with presumed sepsis. *Pediatrics* 80:738–740, 1987.

96. Freedman RM, Ingram DL, Cross I, et al: A half century of neonatal sepsis at Yale. *AJDC* 135:140–144, 1981.

97. Christensen RD, Rothstein G, Anstall HB, et al: Granulocyte transfusions in neonates with bacterial infection, neutropenia, and depletion of mature marrow neutrophils. *Pediatrics* 70:1–6, 1982.

98. Baley JE, Stork EK, Warkentin PI, et al: Buffy coat transfusions in neutropenic neonates with presumed sepsis: A prospective randomized trial. *Pediatrics* 80:712–720, 1987.

99. Higby DJ, Burnett D: Granulocyte transfusions: Current status. *Blood* 55:2–8, 1980.

100. Winston DJ, Ho WG, Gale RP: Therapeutic granulocyte transfusions for documented infections *Ann Intern Med* 97:509–515, 1982.

101. Morstyn G, Campbell L, Souza LM, et al: Effect of granulocyte colony stimulating factor on neutropenia induced by cytotoxic chemotherapy. *Lancet* 1:667–672, 1988.

102. Kodo H, Tajika K, Takahashi S, et al: Acceleration of neutrophilic granulocyte recovery after bone-marrow transplantation by administration of recombinant human granulocyte colony-stimulating factor. *Lancet* 2:38–39, 1988.

103. Glaspy JA, Baldwin GC, Robertson PA, et al: Therapy for neutropenia in hairy cell leukemia with recombinant human granulocyte colony-stimulating factor. *Ann Intern Med* 109:789–795, 1988.

104. Vadhan-Raj S, Buescher S, LeMaistre A, et al: Stimulation of hematopoiesis in patients with bone marrow failure and in patients with malignancy by recombinant human granulocyte-macrophage colony stimulating factor. *Blood* 72:134–141, 1988.

105. Groopman JE, Mitsuyasu RT, DeLeo MJ, et al: Effected of recombinant human granulocyte-macrophage colony-stimulating factor on myelopoiesis in the acquired immunodeficiency syndrome. *N Engl J Med* 317:593–598, 1987.

106. Antin JH, Smith BR, Holmes W, et al: Phase I/II study of recombinant human granulocyte-macrophage colony-stimulating factor in aplastic anemia and myelodysplastic syndrome. *Blood* 72:705–713, 1988.

107. Nemunaitis J, Binger JW, Buckner CD, et al: Use of recombinant human granulocyte-macrophage colony-stimulating factor in autologous marrow transplantation for lymphoid malignancies. *Blood* 72:834–836, 1988.

108. Fleischmann J, Golde DW, Weisbart RH, Gasson JC: Granulocyte-macrophage colony-stimulating factor enhance phagocytosis of bacteria by human neutrophils. *Blood* 68:708–711, 1986.

109. Consensus Conference: Fresh-frozen Plasma: Indications and risks. *JAMA* 253:551–553, 1985.

110. Braunstein AH, Oberman HA: Transfusion of plasma components. *Transfusion* 24:281–286, 1984.

111. Mollison PL, Engelfriet CP, Contreras M: *Blood Transfusion in Clinical Medicine.* London, Blackwell Scientific Publishers, 1988.

112. Huestis DW, Bove JR, Case J: *Practical Blood Transfusion.* Boston, Little, Brown & Co, 1988.

113. Ragni MV, Tegtmeier GE, Levy J, et al: AIDS retrovirus antibodies in hemophiliacs treated with factor VIII or factor IX concentrates, cryoprecipitate, or fresh frozen plasma: Prevalence, seroconversion rate, and clinical correlations. *Blood* 67:592–595, 1986.

114. McLeod BC, Sassetti RJ, Cole ER, Scott JP: A high-potency, single donor cryoprecipitate of known factor VIII content dispensed in vials. *Ann Intern Med* 106:35–40, 1987.

115. Ruggeri ZM, Mannucci MP, Lombardi R, et al: Multimeric composition of factor VIII/von Willebrand factor following administration of DDAVP: Implications for

pathophysiology and therapy of von Willebrand's disease subtypes. *Blood* 59:1272–1278, 1982.

116. Holmberg L, Nilsson IM, Borge L, et al: Platelet aggregation induced by 1-deamino-8-D-arginine vasopressin (DDAVP) in type IIB von Willebrand's disease. *N Engl J Med* 309:816–821, 1983.

117. Frick WA, Yu MY: Characterization of von Willebrand factor in factor VIII concentrates. *Am J Hematol* 31:41–45, 1989.

118. Berntorp E, Nilsson IM: Biochemical and in vivo properties of commercial virus-inactivated factor VIII concentrates. *Eur J Haematol* 40:205–214, 1988.

119. Berntorp E, Nilsson IM: Use of a high-purity factor VIII concentrate (Humate P) in von Willebrand's disease. *Vox Sang* 56:212–217, 1989.

120. Cohn EF, Strong LE, Hughes WL Jr, et al: Preparation and properties of serum and plasma proteins IV: A system for the separation into fractions of protein and lipoprotein components of biological tissues and fluids. *J Am Chem Soc* 68:459–475, 1946.

121. Oncley JL, Melin M, Fichert DA, et al: The separation of the antibodies, isoagglutinins, prothrombin, plasminogen and beta-1-lipoprotein into subfractions of human plasma. *J Am Chem Soc* 71:541–550, 1949.

122. Trepo C, Hantz O, Jacquier MF, et al: Different fates of hepatitis B virus markers during plasma fractionation: A clue to the infectivity of blood derivatives. *Vox Sang* 35:143–148, 1978.

123. Wells MA, Wittek AE, Epstein JS, et al: Inactivation and partition of human T-cell lymphotrophic virus, type III, during ethanol fractionation of plasma. *Transfusion* 26:210–213, 1986.

124. Tullis JL: Albumin: I. Background and use; II: Guidelines for clinical use. *JAMA* 237:355–360, 460–463, 1977.

125. Safety of therapeutic products used for hemophilia patients. *MMWR* 37:441–450, 1988.

126. Horowitz B, Prince AM: Laboratory and preclinical evaluation of the virus safety of coagulation factor concentrates. *Dev Biol Stand* 67:291–302, 1987.

127. Schimpf K, Mannucci PM, Kreutz W, et al: Absence of hepatitis after treatment with a pasteurized factor VIII concentrate in patients with hemophilia and no previous transfusions. *N Engl J Med* 316:918–922, 1987.

128. Schimpf K, Brackmann HH, Kreuz W, et al: Absence of anti-human immunodeficiency virus types 1 and 2 seroconversion after the treatment of hemophilia A or von Willebrand's disease with pasteurized factor VIII concentrate. *N Engl J Med* 321:1148–1152, 1989.

129. Prince AM, Horowitz B, Brotman B: Sterilization of hepatitis and HTLV-III viruses by exposure to tri(n-butyl) phosphate and sodium cholate. *Lancet* 1:706–710, 1986.

130. Horowitz MS, Rooks C, Horowitz B, Hilgartner MW: Virus safety of solvent/detergent-treated antihaemophilic factor concentrate. *Lancet* 2:186–189, 1988.

131. Piszkiewicz D, Sun CS, Tondreau SC: Inactivation and removal of human immunodeficiency virus in monoclonal purified antihemophilic factor (human) (Hemofil M). *Thromb Res* 55:627–634, 1989.

132. Mannucci PM, Ruggeri ZM, Paretti FI, Capitanio A: 1-deamino-8-D-arginine vasopressin: A new pharmacological approach to the management of hemophilia and von Willebrand's disease. *Lancet* 1:869–872, 1977.

133. Bessos H, Prowse CV: Immunopurification of human coagulation factor IX using monoclonal antibodies. *Thromb Haemost* 56:86–89, 1986.

134. Kasper CK: Postoperative thrombosis in hemophilia. *N Engl J Med* 289:160, 1973.

135. Lusher JM, Shapiro SS, Palascak JE, et al: Efficacy of prothrombin-complex concentrates in hemophiliacs with antibodies to factor VIII: A multicenter therapeutic trial. *N Engl J Med* 303:421–425, 1980.

136. Lusher JM: Factor VIII inhibitors: Etiology, characterization, natural history, and management. *Ann NY Acad Sci* 509:89–102, 1987.

137. Gatti L, Mannucci PM: Use of porcine factor VIII in the management of seventeen patients with factor VIII antibodies. *Thromb Haemost* 51:379–384, 1984.

138. Wensly RT, Stevens RF, Burn AM, et al: Plasma exchange and human factor VIII concentrate in managing hemophilia A with factor VIII inhibitors. *Br J Med* 281:1388–1389, 1980.

139. Stiehm ER, Ashida E, Kim KS, et al: Intravenous immunoglobulins as therapeutic agents. *Ann Intern Med* 107:367–382, 1987.

140. Steele RW, Burks AW Jr, Williams LW: Intravenous immunoglobulin: New clinical applications. *Ann Allergy* 60:89–94, 1988.

141. Consensus Conference: Intravenous immunoglobulin. *JAMA* 264:3189–3193, 1990.

142. Safety of therapeutic immune globulin preparations with respect to transmission of human T-lymphotropic virus type III lymphadenopathy associated virus infection. *MMWR* 35:231–232, 1986.

143. Rumi MG, Colombo M, Gringeri A, Mannucci PM: High prevalence of antibody to hepatitis C virus in multitransfused hemophiliacs with normal transaminase levels. *Ann Intern Med* 112:379–380, 1990.

144. Kuo G, Choo Q-L, Alter HJ, et al: An assay for circulating antibodies to a major etiologic virus of human non-A, non-B hepatitis. *Science* 244:362–364, 1989.

145. Alter MJ, Purcell RH, Shih JW, et al: Detection of antibody to hepatitis C virus in prospectively followed transfusion recipients with acute and chronic non-A, non-B hepatitis. *N Engl J Med* 321:494–500, 1989.

146. Choo Q-L, Kuo G, Weiner AJ, et al: Isolation of a cDNA clone derived from a blood-borne non-A, non-B viral hepatitis genome. *Science* 244:359–362, 1989.

147. Furie B, Furie BC: The molecular basis of blood coagulation. *Cell* 53:505–518, 1988.

148. Prodouz KN, Fratantoni JC: Inactivation of virus in blood products. *Transfusion* 28:2–3, 1988.

149. Prodouz KN, Fratantoni JC, Boone EJ, Bonner RF: Use of laser-UV for inactivation of virus in blood products. *Blood* 70:589–592, 1987.

150. Matthews JL, Newman JT, Sogandares-Bernal F, et al: Photodynamic therapy of viral contaminants with potential for blood banking applications. *Transfusion* 28:81–83, 1988.

151. Lin L, Wiesehahn GP, Morel PA, Corash L: Use of 8-methoxypsoralen and long-wavelength ultraviolet radiation for decontamination of platelet concentrates. *Blood* 74:517–525, 1989.

Index

Numbers in **boldface** refer to pages on which figures appear; numbers followed by a *t* indicate tabular material.

Amyloid, 149–150
Amyotrophic lateral sclerosis, 150
Anaphylactic transfusion reaction,
    11
Anemia, 7, 14, 290–292
Anti-HBc test, 120–121, 257
    cost of, 263t
    in delta agent infection, 127
    in non-A, non-B hepatitis, 124–
        126
Antihemophilic factor, cryoprecipi-
    tated. *See* Cryoprecipitate
Anti-HIV tests, 244–247
Anti-inhibitor coagulant complex
    concentrate, 303–304
Antireceptor, 35
Antithrombin III deficiency, 300
Aplastic crisis, 157, 264, 279–280
Aprotinin, 14–15, 296
Apthovirus, 32
Arbovirus, 27–28t, 150–154
ARC. *See* AIDS-related complex
Arenaviridae, 27t, 33, 36
Argentine hemorrhagic fever virus,
    154
Arrhythmia, transfusion-associated,
    11
Artervirus, 32
Arthropod vector, 47, 151
    of babesiosis, 188
    of Chagas' disease, 182
    of filariasis, 185–186
    of Lyme disease, 191–192
    of malaria, 168–169
Aspartate aminotransferase (AST),
    in hepatitis, 120
Aspirin, 295
AST. *See* Aspartate aminotrans-
    ferase
Atherosclerosis, CMV infection and,
    138
Autologous donation, 3, 15, 77–78,
    128, 210, 292
Azidothymidine. *See* Zidovudine
AZT. *See* Zidovudine

B
Babesia divergens, 188
Babesia microti, 188–189

Babesiosis, 176, 188–190
Bacterial contamination
    detection of, 197
    mechanisms for, 195–196
    of platelets, 198–201
    of red blood cells, 196–198, 200–
        201
    of whole blood, 196–198, 200–
        201
Bacterial sepsis. *See* Sepsis
Bedbug vector, in Chagas' disease,
    182
Benzonidazol, 183
Bernard-Soulier syndrome, 293
Birnaviridae, 34
BK virus, 26t, 31
Blackwater fever, 167, 170, 172
Bleeding time, 293–295
Blood collection, bacterial contami-
    nation during, 195–197, 202–
        203
Blood culture, 201
Blood donation. *See* Donation
Blood donor. *See* Donor
Blood processing, bacterial contam-
    ination during, 195–196
Blood products
    production per year, 4–5, 4t
    radiation treatment of, 142
    transfusions per year, 4–5, 4t
Blood shortages, 251–252, 259
Blood storage
    bacterial contamination during,
        196–198, 202–203
    outdating, 203
Bolivian hemorrhagic fever virus,
    154
Bone-break fever. *See* Dengue fe-
    ver virus
Bone marrow transplantation, 7, 13,
    137, 140–142, 262, 297
Borrelia burgdorferi, 191–192
Borreliosis, 191–192
B19 parvovirus, 157–158, 264
Bronchiolitis, 28t
Brugia malayi, 185
Brugia timori, 185

Cost, of laboratory testing, 262–
263, 263t
Cotrimoxazole, 190
Counterelectrophoresis assay, for
HBV, 253
Country of origin, 211, 226–227
Cowpox virus, 26t, 30
Coxsackievirus, 27t, 32
Creutzfeldt-Jakob disease, 29t, 35,
48, 147–150, 157
  donor screening for, 233
  epidemiology of, 148–149
  infectious agent in, 149
  prevention of, 150
Crimean-Congo hemorrhagic fever
virus, 156
Crossover donation, 210
Croup, 28t
Cryoprecipitate
  bacterial contamination of, 196,
198
  delta agent in, 276–277
  HBV in, 272–274
  HCV in, 274–275
  HIV in, 277–279, 278t
  indications for, 300–301, 303
  production per year, 5
  transfusions per year, 4t, 5
  transmission of malaria in, 175
  units per transfusion, 4t
  usage pattern, **2**, 9, 15
Crystalloid solution, 289
Cutaneous T-cell lymphoma, 81, 87
Cyst, *Toxoplasma*, 187
Cystitis, hemorrhagic, 26t
Cytomegalovirus (CMV), 26t, 30–
31, 41, 48–49, 133–134
  characteristics of, 135–137
  cytopathic effect of, **38**, 135,
139–140
  in frozen deglycerolized red
blood cells, 291
  genome of, 136
  inactivation in blood products,
141–142
  infection with

diseases associated with, 137–
138
  epidemiology of, 134–135
  latent, 139
  prevention of, 140–142
laboratory testing for, 39, **39–40**,
138–140, 243, 280–282
oncogenic potential of, 138
serologic response to, **44**
Cytomegalovirus (CMV) immune
globulin, 50
Cytopathic effect, 38
  of CMV, **38**, 135, 139–140

D
Danazol, 294
Dane particle, 119
DDAVP. *See* Desmopressin
1-Deamino-8D-arginine vasopressin. *See* Desmopressin
Deferral, 116
  after blood transfusion, 213–215,
220–221
  Chagas' disease-related, 184
  by country of origin, 211, 226–
227
  deferral registry, 208, 209t, 212–
213
  after dental surgery, 202–203,
234
  of health care worker, 220
  hemodialysis patient-related,
219–220
  hepatitis-related, 213–222
  HIV-related, 76, 222–230
  HTLV-related, 234
  malaria-related, 175, 179
  pituitary-derived growth hormone
and, 150, 233
  rate of, 2
  travel history-based, 150, 175,
226–227, 230–233
Delta agent, 29t, 35
  characteristics of, 126
  in hemophiliacs, 276–277
  infection with
    diagnosis of, 126–127

of delta agent infection, 126
of filariasis, 185
of hepatitis A, 117
of hepatitis B, 119, 258
of HIV infection, 102–103
of HTLV infection, 82–85
of Lyme disease, 191
of malaria, 167–170
of non-A, non-B hepatitis, 121–122
of syphilis, 161–162
of viral infections, 47–48
Epstein-Barr virus (EBV), 26t, 30–31, 133–134
Equine encephalitis virus, 27t, 32
Erythema infectiosum, 157
Erythema migrans, 191
Erythropoietin, recombinant human, 14–15, 292, 295
Escherichia coli, 200
Exanthem subitum, 134
Extravascular hemolysis, 10–11

F
Fansidar, 176
Febrile nonhemolytic transfusion reaction, 10t, 11
Fibrinogen replacement, 300–302
Fibrin sealant, 9
Fibronectin, 300
Fifth disease. *See* Erythema infectiosum
Filariasis, 185–186
Filoviridae, 28t, 33
Financial aspects, of laboratory testing, 262–263, 263t
Flaviviridae, 27t, 32–33
Fluorescent treponemal antibody absorption (FTA-ABS) test, 164, 260
Fluosol-DA, 293
Foamy virus. *See* Spumavirinae
Fracture, transfusion in, 7
Fresh-frozen plasma
  HAV in, 117
  indications for, 289, 299–300
  production per year, 5

transfusions per year, 4t, 5
units per transfusion, 4t
usage pattern, **2**, 8–9, 15, 77
Frozen deglycerolized red blood cells, 291
FTA-ABS. *See* Fluorescent treponemal antibody absorption test

G
gag gene, retroviral, 58–59, **59**, 82, 88t, 103, 248–249, 252
Gametocyte, *Plasmodium*, 169
Gancyclovir (DHPG), 49–50
Gastroenteritis, viral, 27t, 32
Gastrointestinal disorder, transfusion in, 7
G-CSF. *See* Granulocyte colony-stimulating factor
Gene amplification. *See* Polymerase chain reaction assay
Genital herpes, 26t, 30
Geographic distribution. *See* Epidemiology
German measles, 27t, 32
Gerstmann-Straussler syndrome, 147–150
Glanzmann's thrombasthenia, 293
GM-CSF. *See* Granulocyte-macrophage colony-stimulating factor
Graft-*v*-host disease, 10t, 13
Granulocyte colony-stimulating factor (G-CSF), 14–15, 298–299
Granulocyte concentrate, 298–299
Granulocyte-macrophage colony-stimulating factor (GM-CSF), 14–15, 298–299
Growth factors, human recombinant, 14–15
Growth hormone. *See* Pituitary-derived human growth hormone

H
Hairy cell leukemia, 29t, 34, 81, 91, 252
Haitian entrant, 226–227
Hantann virus, 28t
HAV. *See* Hepatitis A virus

Hepatocellular carcinoma, 119, 123
Herpangina, 32
Herpes simplex virus type 1 (HSV-1, HHV-1), 26t, 30, 133–134
Herpes simplex virus type 2 (HSV-2, HHV-2), 26t, 30, 133–134
Herpesviridae, 24, 26t, 30, 37
Herpes virus, 48–49, 133
  latent infection with, 133–134
Heterophile-negative mononucleosis, 26t
Heterosexual, risk of HIV exposure, 227
HHV. *See* Herpes simplex virus; Human herpes virus
Hip replacement surgery, 6
HIV. *See* Human immunodeficiency virus
Homologous donation, 1–2
Homosexual, male, 209, 211, 223–230
HSV. *See* Herpes simplex virus
HTLV. *See* Human T-cell leukemia virus
Human B-cell lymphotrophic virus (HBLV), 26t, 30
Human B-lymphotrophic virus. *See* Human herpes virus type 6
Human herpes virus type 6 (HHV-6), 133–134
Human herpes virus type 7 (HHV-7), 133–134
Human immunodeficiency virus (HIV), 48–49
  infection with, CMV infection and, 137
  receptor for, 54, 60
Human immunodeficiency virus type 1 (HIV-1), 29t, 34, 82
  alternative sites for testing donors, 225
  characteristics of, 103–104
  donor screening for, 211–212, 222–230, 250
  genome of, 58, **59**, 63–65
  infection with
    epidemiology of, 74, 102

in hemophiliacs, 274, 277–280, 278t
  natural history of, 74–75
  prevention of, 76–78, 279
  risk of, 75–76
  serologic characteristics of, 41–44, **42–43**
  syphilis and, 165
laboratory testing for, 75–77, 103–105, 244–252, 263t
  donor notification of results, 247–249
  false-positive, 246–247
  impact on blood safety, 249–251, 250t
  impact on blood supply, 251–252
  seronegative but infectious blood, 251
receptor for, 35–36
surrogate test for, 165
Human immunodeficiency virus type 2 (HIV-2), 29t, 82, 101–102, 226
characteristics of, 103–104
genome of, **59**, 63–65
infection with
  diseases associated with, 104
  epidemiology of, 102–103
  in hemophiliacs, 280
  seroprevalence of, 102–103
laboratory testing for, 104–105, 249, 263
Human pituitary-derived growth hormone, 150, 157, 233
Human T-cell leukemia virus types I and II (HTLV-I/II), 29t, 34, 48, 81
characteristics of, 87–89
donor screening for, 234
genome of, 58, **59**, 62, 87–89, 88t
infection with
  diseases associated with, 89–91
  epidemiology of, 82–85
  in hemophiliacs, 280
  in United States, 84–85

Perfluorochemical emulsion, 14,
293
Pestivirus, 32
Photoinactivation of viruses, 305
Picornaviridae, 27t, 32, 36, 117
Pituitary-derived human growth
hormone, 150, 157, 233
Placental blood, 197
Plantar warts, 26t, 31
Plasma, fresh-frozen. *See* Fresh-frozen plasma
Plasmapheresis, 302
Plasmodium falciparum, 168–173,
175t, 176–178, 230–232
Plasmodium knowlesi, 168
Plasmodium malariae, 168–171,
173–174, 175t, 231–232
Plasmodium ovale, 168–169, 173,
175t, 231–232
Plasmodium vivax, 168, 172–173,
175t, 231–232
Platelet concentrate
ABO-compatible, 297
bacterial contamination of, 195–
196, 198–201
indications for, 289, 293–298
irradiated, 297–298
outdating of, 199
preparation of, 3–4
production per year, 4–5
random-donor, 293–296
single-donor, 3–4, 296–298
transfusions per year, 4–5, 4t
units per transfusion, 4t
usage pattern, **2**, 7–8, 77
Platelet count, 293–294, 297
Platelet dysfunction, 15, 293–294
Pleurodynia, 32
Pneumonia, viral, 28t
Pneumovirus, 28t, 33
pol gene, retroviral, 59, **59**, 82, 88t,
103, 248
Poliovirus, 27t, 32
Polymerase chain reaction (PCR)
assay, 40, 46–47, **46**, 287
for HCV, 122
for HIV, 105, 249

for HTLV, 92t, 98–101, **99–100**
Polymerized, pyridoxylated, stroma-
free hemoglobin solution
(poly-SFH-P), 292–293
Polyomavirus, 26t, 31
Poly-SFH-P. *See* Polymerized, pyri-
doxylated, stroma-free hemo-
globin solution
Posttransfusion case follow-up, 209t
hepatitis, 221–222
Poxviridae, 24, 26t, 30, 37
PPA. *See* Passive particle agglutina-
tion assay
Pregnant women, CMV-seronega-
tive units for, 262
Preselection of donors, 209, 209t
CMV-seronegative, 260–261
Prion, 35, 149, 233
Prison inmate, 209, 214, 219
Probe. *See* Nucleic acid probe
Proficiency testing, in laboratory,
263
pro gene, retroviral, 88t
Progressive multifocal leukoence-
phalopathy, 26t, 31, 148, 150
Promoter insertion, 61
Prophylaxis, malaria, 175–176
Prostatic cancer, 138
Prostitute contact, 223, 227
Protease, viral, 59
Protein immunoblot assay
for HIV, 103, 105
for HTLV, 92t, 93–94, **95**
Protein-losing enteropathy, 300
Prothrombin time, 299
Proto-oncogene, 60
Provirus, 54, 56
Pseudomonads, 198
Pseudomonas aeruginosa, 199
Pseudomonas cepacia, 196
Psychrophilic bacteria, 197–198,
200
Public education, 116, 209t, 211,
224–225
Pulmonary edema, transfusion-as-
sociated, 10t, 11–12

Pulsed laser-ultraviolet radiation, 305
Purpura, posttransfusion, 10t, 13
Pyrimethamine, 188

Q
Qinghaosu, 176
Quality control, in laboratory testing, 263
Quartan malaria, 171, 173–175
Quinine, 176

R
Rabies virus, 28t, 34
Radiation treatment, of blood products, 142
Radioimmunoassay, 41
  for HBV, 253–254
  for HIV, 105
  for HTLV, 92t, 93–98, **96–97**
Random-donor platelet concentrate, 293–296
Rapid plasma reagin test, for syphilis, 164, 259
Rapid tests
  for CMV, 261
  for HIV, 245
Red blood cells, 77
  additive solution, 289–290
  alternatives to, 291–293
  artificial, 293
  bacterial contamination of, 196–198, 200–201
  frozen deglycerolized, 291
  indications for, 289–291
  pediatric units, 4
  production per year, 4
  transfusion rate, 5
  transfusions per year, 4, 4t
  units per transfusion, 4t
  usage patterns, 1, **2**, 6–7
  washed, 290–291
Redwater, 190
Relapsing malaria, 172
Reoviridae, 27t, 34
Replacement donor, 210
Respiratory disorder, 7, 27t

Respiratory syncytial virus, 28t, 33–34, 49
Restriction endonuclease, 45
Retroviridae, 29t, 34, 37, 53
Retrovirus, 48
  characteristics of, 34
  culture of, 39–40
  genome of, 57–65, **59**
  integration into host genome, 56
  life cycle of, 54–57, **55**
  oncogenes in, 60–62
  structure of, 53–54
  taxonomy of, 53
  transformation by, 60–62
Reverse transcriptase, 34, 37–38, 45, 49, 54–56, **55**, 59
  assay of, 40, 101
rev gene, retroviral, 63
rex gene, retroviral, 62, 88t, 89
Rhabdoviridae, 28t, 34, 36
Rhinovirus, 27t, 32
Ribavirin, 49, 156
Ridoviridae, 24
Rift Valley fever virus, 28t, 151
Rimantadine, 49
RNase H, 56, 59
RNA virus, 24, 27–29t, 32–35
  (−)-stranded, 36
  (+)-stranded, 36
Romana sign, 183
Roseola infantum. *See* Exanthem subitum
Ross River virus, 27t, 32
Rotavirus, 27t, 34
R region, of retroviral genome, 58
Rubella virus, 27t
Rubeola virus. *See* Measles virus
Rubivirus, 27t

S
Saddleback fever. *See* Dengue fever virus
St. Louis encephalitis virus, 27t, 33
Salmonella, 195, 199–200
Salmonella typhi, 199
Schizogony, 168
Schizont, 173

Scrapie, 149
Self-deferral, 209t, 211
Sepsis, 10t, 12
  clinical manifestations of, 200
  diagnosis of, 201
  donor screening for, 233–234
  neonatal, 298
  after platelet transfusion, 198–
    201
  prevention of, 202–203
  after red blood cell transfusion,
    196–198, 200–201
  transfusion-associated, 195
  treatment of, 202
  after whole blood transfusion,
    196–198, 200–201
Seroconversion, in HIV infection,
    41–43, **42–43**
Serologic diagnosis. *See* Laboratory
    test
Serologic test for syphilis (STS),
    161–165
Serratia marcescens, 196
Shell vial centrifugation culture, of
    CMV, 140
Shingles, 26t, 30, 133
Sindbis virus, 27t, 32
Single-donor platelet concentrate,
    3–4, 296–298
Slow virus, 35, 48, 147–150. *See
    also* Creutzfeldt-Jakob disease
Smallpox virus, 26t, 30
Southern blotting, 46
Sperm donor, 150
Sporozoite, 168–169
Spumavirinae, 34, 53, 82
Staphylococci, 197, 199–200
Staphylococcus aureus, 199
Staphylococcus epidermidis, 198–
    200
Stevens-Johnson syndrome, 176
STS. *See* Serologic test for syphilis
Subacute sclerosing panencephalitis,
    28t, 33, 150
Subacute spongiform encephalop-
    athy, 35

Sub-Saharan Africans, 226
Sulfadiazine, 188
Surgical patient, 6
Surrogate test, 165, 243, 256–259
Syphilis, 161–165
  clinical manifestations of, 163
  epidemiology of, 161–162
  HIV infection and, 165
  laboratory testing for, 163–164,
    243, 259–260
  latent, 163

T
Tacaribe virus, 27t, 33
Tachyzoite, 187
tat gene, retroviral, 63
Tattoo, 116, 214–215, 219
tax gene, retroviral, 58, 61–62, 88t,
    90
T cells, transformation of, 61
Telephone call-back, 209t, 212, 228
Thalassemia, 117
Thrombocytopenia, 15, 289, 294
Thrombotic thrombocytopenic pur-
    pura, 8, 300
Tick vector
  of babesiosis, 188
  of Lyme disease, 191–192
Togaviridae, 27t, 151
Toxoplasma gondii, 186–188
Toxoplasmosis, 186–188
Transfer RNA, 57
Transformation
  by CMV, 138
  by HTLV, 91
  by retroviruses, 60–62
Transfusion
  pharmacologic agents to reduce,
    14–15
  reducing number of, 8t, 14–15,
    77, 287–305
  usage patterns, 1, **2**, 5–9, 15
Transfusion history, deferral and,
    213–215, 220–221
Transfusion reaction
  acute, 9–12, 10t, 291

delayed, 10t, 12–13
frequency of, 10t
Transfusion trigger, 7, 8t, 9, 288
Trauma patient, 7
Travel history, deferral due to, 175,
    211, 226–227, 230–233
Treponemal test, for syphilis, 164,
    260
Treponema pallidum, 161–163
Treponema peretenue, 164
Trophozoite, 169, 173, 187
Tropical pulmonary eosinophilia,
    186
Tropical spastic paraparesis (TSP),
    29t, 34, 90–91, 234, 252, 280
Tropical splenomegaly syndrome,
    177–178
Tropical virus, 150–154
Trypanosoma cruzi, 181–185, 182t,
    264
Trypanosomiasis, 181–185, 182t
TSP. *See* Tropical spastic parapa-
    resis

U

U3 region, of retroviral genome,
    57–58
U5 region, of retroviral genome, 58
Uremia, 15, 295, 301
Urine test, for CMV, 261
Urticaria, transfusion-associated, 11

V

Vaccine, 50
  hepatitis A, 119
  hepatitis B, 50, 121, 127, 219,
      273–274
  malaria, 176–179
  yellow fever, 152
Vaccinia virus, 26t, 30
Varicella-zoster immune globulin,
    50
Varicella-zoster virus, 26t, 30, 133–
    134

Variola virus. *See* Smallpox virus
VDRL test, for syphilis, 164, 259
Venipuncture site, 196, 234
Vidarabine, 49
vif gene, retroviral, 63–64
Virus
  classification of, 24–35, 25–29t
  definition of, 23–24
  gene sequence detection in, 44–
      47
  inactivation in blood products,
      127, 141–142, 272, 304–305
  infection with
    epidemiology of, 47–48
    laboratory diagnosis of, 37–47
    pathogenesis of, 48–49
    prevention of, 49–50
    treatment of, 49–50
  isolation of, 37–41
  receptor, 35
  replication of, 24, **25**, 35–37
  serology of, 41–44
  transmission of, 47–48
Visna virus, 34, 149
Volume expansion, 8, 289, 302
Volume overload, 289
v-*onc* sequences, 60–62
von Willebrand's disease, 9, 15,
    300–301
von Willebrand's factor, 292, 300–
    302
vpr gene, retroviral, 64
vpu gene, retroviral, 64, 103
vpx gene, retroviral, 64–65, 103

W

Warfarin reversal, 299–300, 303
Washed red blood cells, 290–291
Western blot assay, 42, **43**
  for HIV, 247–249, 279–280
  for HTLV, 93–94, **95**, 252
Whole blood
  bacterial contamination of, 196–
      198, 200–201

indications for, 288–289
production per year, 4
transfusion rate, 5
transfusions per year, 4
usage patterns, **2**, 6–7, 77
Wilms' tumor, 138
Wuchereria bancrofti, 185–186

Y
Yaws, 164
Yellow fever virus, 27t, 33, 151–
153
Yersinia enterocolitica, 197

Z
Zidovudine, 49